Recent Results in Cancer Research

163

W0050515

Managing Editors
P.M. Schlag, Berlin · H.-J. Senn, St. Gallen

Associate Editors
P. Kleihues, Lyon · F. Stiefel, Lausanne
B. Groner, Frankfurt · A. Wallgren, Göteborg

Founding Editors
P. Rentchnik, Geneva

Springer-Verlag Berlin Heidelberg GmbH

H.-J. Senn · R. Morant (Eds.)

Tumor Prevention and Genetics

With 26 Figures and 32 Tables

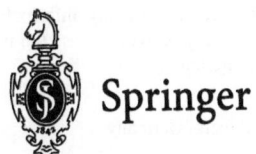 Springer

Prof. Dr. Hans-Jörg Senn
Dr. Rudolf Morant

Zentrum für Tumordiagnostik und Prävention
Rorschacherstr. 150
9006 St. Gallen, Switzerland

Indexed in Current Contents and Index Medicus

ISBN 978-3-642-62892-4   ISBN 978-3-642-55647-0 (eBook)
DOI 10.1007/978-3-642-55647-0

ISSN 0080-0015

Library of Congress Cataloging-in-Publication Data

International Conference on Tumor Prevention + Genetics (2nd: 2002: Saint Gall,
Switzerland). Tumor prevention and genetics / H.-J. Senn, R. Morant (eds.).   p.;   cm.
– (Recent results in cancer research, ISSN 0080-0015; 163). Includes bibliographical
references and index. ISBN 978-3-642-62892-4   1. Cancer – Genetic aspects.
2. Cancer – Prevention. 3. Cancer – Chemoprevention. I. Senn, Hansjörg. II. Morant,
R. (Rudolf), 1951–   III. International Society of Cancer Chemoprevention. Conference (7th: 2002: Saint Gall, Switzerland) IV. Title. V. Series. [DNLM: 1. Neoplasms –
prevention & control – Congresses. 2. Chemoprevention – Congresses. 3. Neoplasms –
genetics – Congresses. QZ 267 I457:2003] RC268.4 .I585 2002   616.99'4042–dc21
2002030613

Cataloging-in-Publication Data applied for
Bibliographic information published by Die Deutsche Bibliothek
Die Deutsche Bibliothek lists this publication in the Deutsche Nationalbibliografie;
detailed bibliographic data is available in the Internet at <http://dnb.ddb.de>.

http://www.springer.de

© Springer-Verlag Berlin Heidelberg 2003
Originally published by Springer-Verlag Berlin Heidelberg New York in 2003
Softcover reprint of the hardcover 1st edition 2003

Typesetting: Stürtz AG, 97080 Würzburg, Germany
Cover design: design & production GmbH, 69121 Heidelberg, Germany

Printed on acid-free paper   21/3150/ag – 5 4 3 2 1 0

Contents

4 Secondary Prevention of Breast Cancer: The Mammography Controversy

5 Chemoprevention of Skin and Lung Cancer

6 Prevention and Screening of Prostate Cancer

7 Prevention and Screening of Colorectal Cancer

Summary and Conclusions............................. 264

Introduction

Hans-Jörg Senn

H.-J. Senn (✉)
Center for Tumor Detection and Prevention, Rorschacherstr. 150,
CH-9006 St. Gallen, Switzerland

Clinical oncology has centered mainly on developing new strategies and a multitude of new drugs for fighting relapsing and progressive cancer during the last two decades. Furthermore, it has done this with respectable success in quite a number of neoplastic diseases such as acute leukemias and sarcomas in pediatric patients and certain types of aggressive lymphomas, as well as selected solid tumors such as testicular cancer and choriocarcinoma in adult age. Curatively intended adjuvant chemo- and endocrine-therapies of several "main killers" among prevalent cancer types, especially breast and colon cancer, have also become successful and health-politically meaningful therapeutic targets [1, 2].

However, the net gain in "cure" of these (mostly pharmacologic) therapeutic approaches has to be realistically judged as having a moderate impact on the cancer problem as a whole, and the mortality rate of the most frequent tumor types, which are prevalent in adult life, has with very few exceptions not been substantially decreased over the past two to three decades. Increasingly, health politicians, epidemiologists, and medical journal editors are asking for alternative strategies of lowering cancer incidence and increasing survival, ventilating new and hitherto mostly neglected areas of research such as primary and secondary cancer prevention.

This "new dimension" in oncology of favoring tumor prevention has been greatly fertilized by dramatic evolutions in molecular biology and cancer genetics, providing new and unprecedented insight into the development of neoplastic transformation and fostering new ways of cancer risk assessment by uncoding an increasing number of disease-associated mutations. Cancer as a familial and even genetic disease has entered modern oncologic research and the thinking of open-minded clinical oncologists. Yet, the communication between laboratory researchers and developments in molecular genetics and the patient- or population-based efforts of (mostly epidemiologically oriented) preventionalists and clinicians has hindered the rapid evolution of intelligent common strategies for more successful clinical tumor prevention at the practical and society level.

Recent Results in Cancer Research, Vol. 163
© Springer-Verlag Berlin Heidelberg 2003

It is the declared aim of a new conference line of St. Gallen Oncology Conferences, located in the historic, cultural and medical capital city of eastern Switzerland and in the very center of old Continental Europe, to overcome this communication gap between cancer genetics and tumor prevention by creating a repetitive conference platform, whereby laboratory scientists, epidemiologists, and prevention-minded clinical oncologists from surgery, radiology, and internal medicine can meet and join forces. After launching an exploratory pilot conference in 1997, a first official "International Conference on Tumor Prevention and Genetics" (TUP-2000) was held at St. Gallen University in February 2000, introducing these topics as a new dimension in oncology at the brink of the new millennium.

The success of this first TUP-2000 conference and its successful and immediate publication in a special issue of the prestigious *European Journal of Cancer* [3] prompted the organizers of St. Gallen Oncology Conferences to convoke another (second) Conference on Tumor Prevention and Genetics at the same academic venue on 14–16 February 2002. The goal of this second event was clearly set to intensify the scientific liaison between molecular genetics and epidemiologic as well as clinical tumor prevention. Some 260 delegates from more than 50 countries attended the conference, which in its second edition prompted considerably more pharmaceutical company support, with AstraZeneca, Macclesfield/UK, becoming its main sponsor. The TUP-2002 conference induced a variety of highly interesting interactions between laboratory researchers and clinical oncologists, hitherto used to "cure" neoplastic diseases rather than "care" about how to intelligently prevent the sad and potentially lethal diseases from happening.

This new volume in the well-recognized Springer series *Recent Results in Cancer Research* contains most of the invited guest presentations of the TUP-2002 conference in St. Gallen. It leads from evolutions in basic research in molecular genetics through the role of preclinical models in cancer prevention to the application of gained knowledge – not at the "bedside" (which is to be prevented), but rather at the "street level"; that is, to people with increased cancer risk within normal, "healthy" society, gathering in tumor prevention centers and primary care medical facilities, where cancer prevention has to finally prove its ultimate value.

St. Gallen Oncology Conferences are committed to supporting the evolution of primary and secondary tumor prevention with the same enthusiasm as they have promoted the successful development of tertiary cancer prevention (which is adjuvant systemic therapy) of breast cancer during the last 24 years in eight consecutive international consensus conferences, thus greatly influencing the standardized therapeutic approach to this frequent neoplastic disease at a worldwide level.

References

1. Senn HJ, Gelber RD, Goldhirsch A, Thürlimann B (1998) Adjuvant therapy of primary breast cancer, vi. Recent results in cancer research. Springer, Berlin Heidelberg New York
2. Goldhirsch A, Glick JH, Gelber RD, Coates AS, Senn HJ (2001) Meeting highlights: international consensus panel on the treatment of primary breast cancer. J Clin Oncol 19:3917–3827
3. Senn HJ, Canellos GP (2000) Tumor prevention and genetics: introduction. Eur J Cancer 36:1187–1188

Latest News in Cancer Genetics 1

Genetic Susceptibility, Predicting Risk and Preventing Cancer

Paul D. P. Pharoah

P.D.P. Pharoah (✉)
Strangeways Research Laboratories, Department of Oncology,
University of Cambridge, Worts Causeway, Cambridge CB1 8RN, UK

Abstract

A polygenic approach to disease prevention has become a realistic goal that has arisen from the sequencing of the human genome. Some believe it will be possible to identify individuals as susceptible by their genotype and to prevent disease by targeting interventions to those at risk. However, doubts have been expressed about the magnitude of these genetic effects, and hence the potential to apply them either to individuals or to populations. Published data suggest that the familial aggregation of breast cancer not due to the known high penetrance genes is polygenic, which implies that the distribution of risk in the population is continuous. This model is likely to apply to other common cancers. The utility of a continuous distribution for identifying a high-risk group of the population for targeted preventive intervention depends on the spread of that risk distribution. For breast cancer, the data are compatible with a log-normal distribution of genetic risk in the population which is sufficiently wide to provide useful discrimination of high- and low-risk groups. Assuming all the susceptibility genes could be identified, the half of the population at highest risk would account for 88% of all cases. In contrast, if currently identified risk factors for breast cancer were used to stratify the population, the half of the population at highest risk would account for only 62% of all cases. These results suggest that in the future the construction and use of genetic risk profiles may provide significant improvements in the efficacy of population-based programmes of intervention for cancers and other diseases.

Introduction

Until recently, the main focus of the research effort into the inherited basis of cancer has been based on the Mendelian inheritance of single, strong, but uncommon predisposing genes. The completion of the human genome sequence has provided the opportunity to obtain detailed information about the range of genetic differences between individuals. Knowledge of the genetic variation across many loci in the population will then allow a "polygenic" approach, in which risks will be estimated from the combined effect of this variation. The promise of a polygenic approach to the prevention and treatment of common diseases has generated much excitement. Some have claimed (Beaudet 1999; Bell 1998) that the greater understanding of genetic risk factors and their interactions with the environment will allow diseases to be predicted and to be prevented at both individual and population levels, by directing interventions at individuals shown to be at high risk. Others are less sure (Friend 1999; Holtzman and Marteau 2000; Vineis et al. 2001): in particular, they question whether molecular testing for common genetic variants can have sufficient predictive power to be of practical use either for the individual or for defining risk groups in the population at large. In this chapter, I will use data derived from a large population-based study of breast cancer to explore the potential for disease prevention using multiple genetic markers of risk.

Disease Prevention in Individuals at High Risk

The concept of sick individuals and sick populations in the context of disease prevention was first proposed by Geoffrey Rose. He described two alternative approaches to preventive medicine. The first seeks to identify high-risk individuals and to offer them individual protection. In contrast, the population strategy seeks to control the determinants of disease incidence in the population as a whole. The high-risk approach has several advantages. In particular it is likely to maximize the benefit:harm ratio of a preventive intervention and so the intervention can be restricted to those in whom benefit outweighs harm. The high-risk approach also maximizes the cost-effectiveness of an intervention, which is critically dependent on its absolute (rather than relative) benefit – even where there is a net benefit to individuals at low risk, the cost effectiveness of the intervention may be prohibitive in low-risk groups. For example, many published clinical guidelines recommend that the use of cholesterol-lowering drugs should be restricted to those at highest risk of coronary heart disease, even though there is ample evidence of benefit even for those at low risk. Other advantages of the high-risk approach include improved compliance because of subject motivation and physician motivation.

The main disadvantages of the high-risk approach were said to be: difficulties in identifying the at risk group; limited potential for the population; limited potential for the individual; and behaviourally inappropriate. Perhaps the major concern is that the high-risk approach has limited potential for the population. The range of risk associated with single risk factors tends to be relatively small, even for well-established risk factors like serum cholesterol and coronary heart disease. Because of this, single risk factors are, in themselves, weak predictors of future disease. It then follows that the majority of disease occurs in individuals who are not at high risk, and consequently, the reduction of risk in high-risk individuals has a limited impact on disease incidence in the population as a whole.

However, these concepts were based on classic lifestyle and environmental determinants of disease incidence, and some of the principles may not apply to genes as determinants of disease.

Prevention in Those at High Genetic Risk

What then, might be the impact of the identification of genetic risk factors for disease, in terms of disease prevention at the level of the population? Several authors have pointed out that individual susceptibility genes are unlikely to contribute much to disease prevention (Vineis et al. 2001). For example, consider a highly penetrant gene mutation that is rare in the population (0.2%). Suppose that the mutation confers a tenfold increase in risk in carriers and the lifetime risk of disease in a carrier is 50%. The mutation would be present in 2% of all cases. If we have an intervention that reduces risk by 40% the absolute risk reduction in carriers is 20% (40% of 50%). Thus for every five (100/20) carriers treated, we would prevent one case. This is the numbers needed to treat (NNT). However, if we identified carriers by testing (or "screening") the population, we would need to screen 2,500 individuals (5/ 0.002) to prevent one case. This is the number needed to screen (NNS). A population screening programme to detect and treat carriers would reduce total disease burden by 0.8% if uptake of testing and treatment were complete.

Let us now consider a more common, low-penetrance genetic variant, which carries a twofold increase in disease risk and a lifetime risk of disease of 10%, and is present in 5% of the population. The variant would be present in 9.5% of all cases. An intervention that reduces risk by 40% (absolute risk reduction 4%) will have an NNS of 500, and, at best, could reduce total disease burden by 3.8%.

However, the potential impact of identifying multiple susceptibility genes is less clear. To examine the potential for prediction of risk based on common genetic variation three questions have to be addressed: (1) What is the likely distribution of genetically determined risk in the population? (2) What are the implications of these risk distributions for the effective targeting of interventions to individuals, and within the population? It is also of interest to compare the discriminatory power of genetic risk prediction with that using established lifestyle and environmental risk factors, and so a third question can be posed: (3) What is the distribution of risk described by established risk factors?

These questions have been explored for breast cancer, using data collected from a large population-based study of breast cancer carried out in East Anglia, UK (Pharoah et al. 2002).

Distribution of Genetic Risk in Population

Breast cancer, like other common cancers, shows familial clustering. Depending on age, the risk is typically two- to threefold increased in first-degree relatives of a case. Such familial clustering may either be the result of inheritance or due to lifestyle and environmental factors that are shared within families. Twin studies suggest that most of the familial aggregation of cancer results from inherited susceptibility (Lichtenstein et al. 2000; Peto and Mack 2000). However, the known predisposing genes for breast cancer, including *BRCA1* and *BRCA2*, account for only 20%–25% of this effect (Easton 1999), suggesting that there are other susceptibility genes yet to be identified. The number and properties of these genes are unknown.

Mathematical modelling of the familial aggregation of breast cancer in the population can provide important clues about the range of genetic models that best account for the familial aggregation of breast cancer not due to the high-penetrance BRCA genes. Two such studies have been published. The first study used data from a series of 856 breast cancer cases from Australia that were diagnosed under the age of 40 years and had been tested for mutations in *BRCA1* and *BRCA2* (Cui et al. 2001). The model that fit these data the best was that of a single recessive allele that conferred a high disease risk. Another study analysed the occurrence of breast cancer in the relatives of patients in the Anglian Breast Cancer Study, a population-based series of approximately 1,500 cases, all of whom were screened for mutations in *BRCA1* and *BRCA2* (Antoniou et al. 2001). Two models were found to fit the data well. The model best describing these data was a polygenic model, in which susceptibility to breast cancer is conferred by a large number of alleles. The risk associated with any individual allele is small; but the effects are multiplicative so that a woman with several susceptibility alleles is at high risk. The second model was that of a single common recessive allele (frequency 0.24). The risk allele was estimated to confer a relative risk of 21 for rare homozygotes compared common homozygotes and heterozygotes, corresponding to a moderately high penetrance of 42%. The polygenic and recessive models were also applied to a series of multiple case families not due to *BRCA* mutations (Antoniou et al. 2001). The polygenic model fitted these data well, but the fit of the recessive model was not so good. Furthermore, a recent large meta-analysis found that the familial breast cancer risk to siblings is similar to that of mothers, suggesting that any recessive component for the excess familial risk is at best small (Collaborative Group on Hormonal Factors in Breast Cancer 2001). The polygenic model is likely to be an appropriate model for many common cancers and other diseases.

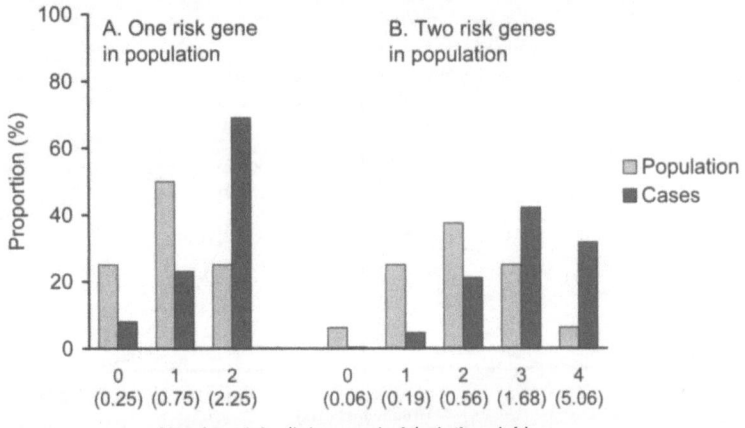

Fig. 1. Proportion of population and cases by number of risk alleles carried for (*A*) a single codominant gene (*B*) two codominant genes. Each additional risk allele carried results in a threefold increase in risk

Implications of the Polygenic Model for Risk Distribution in the Population

The implications of the polygenic model for the distribution of breast cancer risk in the population are illustrated in the following paragraphs and in Fig. 1.

Let us assume that one dominant susceptibility allele has been identified, and half the population carry the high-risk allele (risk allele frequency of 0.29). If "high-risk" individuals have a breast cancer relative risk (RR) of three compared to "low-risk" individuals, the high-risk group will have a RR of 1.5 and the low-risk group will have a RR of 0.5 (1.5=3×0.5), giving a population average RR of one. Absolute risks of breast cancer will depend on underlying incidence rates. Using rates typical of northern Europe and the United States, the absolute risk of breast cancer by age 70 years in the two risk groups will be 2.9% and 8.4%, corresponding to an average population risk of 5.7% (Pharoah and Mackay 1998). It then follows that 75% of all breast cancer cases will occur in high-risk women and 25% in low-risk women. An intervention targeted to "high-risk" women thus has the potential to reduce breast cancer morbidity by a maximum of 75%. Now assume that the risk allele of the gene acts in a codominant manner and the allele frequency is 0.5. There will now be three risk groups in the population (Fig. 1): one quarter of the population will have no high-risk alleles and a RR of 0.25 (0.5×0.5); half the population will have one high-risk allele (RR of 0.75); and one quarter of the population will have two high-risk alleles (RR of 2.25). The breast cancer risks by age 70 years in these three groups are 1.5%, 4.3%, and 12.3%, and they account for 8%, 23%, and 69% of all breast cancer cases, respectively. Figure 1 also shows the effect of two codominant genes with five risk groups. As the num-

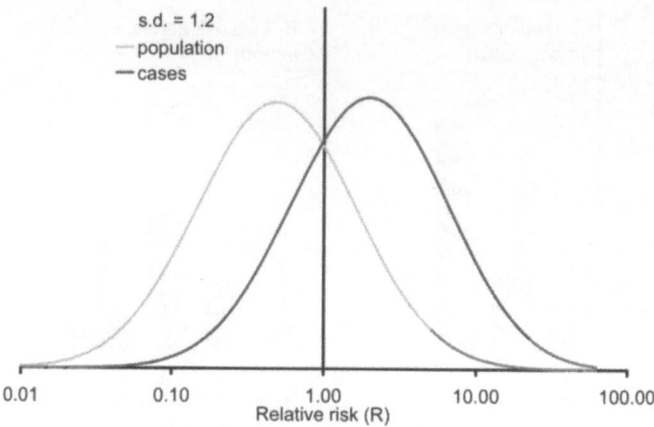

Fig. 2. Log-normal distribution of genetic risk in population. Relative risks are shown on a log scale, while the arithmetical average risk for the entire population has been set at 1.0. The risk distribution in individuals who will develop breast cancer (cases) is shifted to the right. The standard deviation describes the spread of risk between high and low values within the population, and thus the potential to discriminate different levels in different individuals

ber of susceptibility genes increases, the number of risk groups will increase and risk in the population tends towards a continuous distribution.

Under the polygenic model, the (continuous) distribution of RR in the population is predicted to be log-normal; that is, the logarithm of RR for all individuals in the population will follow a normal distribution (Fig. 2).

A normal distribution is defined by its mean value and its standard deviation. The standard deviation of the log-normal distribution of genetic risk was estimated to be 1.2 (Antoniou et al. 2001). Once the standard deviation is defined, the mean of the distribution can be set so that the arithmetical average risk (RR) is equal to 1. The standard deviation describes the variation in risks that can be defined within the population, and thus is the key indicator of the power to discriminate individuals in groups at low or high risk.

It can be shown that the distribution of (initial) risk among cases of the disease is also log-normal and has a simple relationship to the distribution of risk in the population. The standard deviation of the log-normal distribution in cases is the same as in the population, but the average risk is higher (Fig. 2). (A complication occurs because at older ages the distribution of risk in both the general population and among cases changes as higher risk individuals are more likely to have been "eliminated".)

Figure 2 shows the distribution of genetic risk in the population for a standard deviation of 1.2. The area under the curve gives the proportion of the population in any risk group. The risk to the highest quintile of the distribution is 40-fold higher than that of the lowest quintile. The figure also shows the risk distribution in cases according to their initial level of risk; that is, the risk distribution of women in the population who will subsequently develop breast cancer.

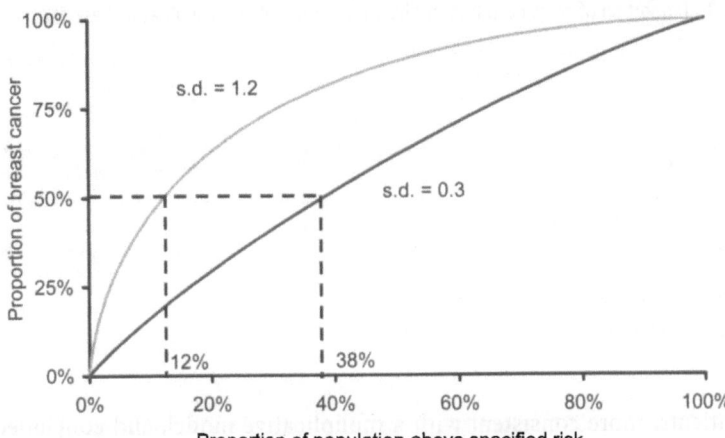

Fig. 3. The proportion of cases accounted for by a given proportion of population above a specified risk according to the standard deviation (SD) of underlying risk distribution. Thus the 12% of the population with the highest risk account for half of all cases if SD=1.2, whereas for SD=0.3, 38% of population account for half the cases

The proportion of the population that have a risk greater than a given level, and the proportion of cases that will occur within this high-risk subgroup, provides more useful information. These figures are obtained from the area under the population and case curves in Fig. 1 to the right of any given risk cut-off. Thus, for a standard deviation of 1.2, half the population have a RR of 0.46 or higher and this half of the population accounts for 88% of all breast cancer cases.

It can also be shown that the 12% of the population at highest risk account for 50% of cases. Another way of depicting these data is to plot the proportion of cases that occur in women above a given level of risk against the proportion of the population above that level of risk as shown in Fig. 3.

In practice, the estimated power of the genetic risk distribution is an upper limit, because some disease-associated genes may prove difficult to detect, and this will reduce the width of the distribution and hence the predictive value. We therefore recalculated the model assuming that genes responsible for half the variation in genetic risk could be identified. The risk to the highest quintile of the distribution is now 12-fold higher than that of the lowest quintile. The results are shown in Table 1.

The assumption that the putative polygenes act in a multiplicative manner may not be correct. Risch has argued, on the basis of the ratio of risks to monozygotic and dizygotic twins of cancer cases, that an additive model provides the best fit for most common cancers including breast cancer (Risch 2001). The effect of an additive model would be to reduce the standard deviation of the risk distribution from 1.2 to 1.05, and hence slightly reduce the predictive power of genetic testing. In contrast, a recent analysis of twin data reported by Peto and Mack found a very high incidence in monozygotic twins

Table 1. Proportion of cases occurring in given proportion of population at highest risk

	Standard deviation	Relative risk[a]	Cumulative risk[b]	Percentage of population at highest risk		
				50%	20%	10%
Classic risk factors	0.30	0.91	7.3%	62%	28%	15%
Genetic factors						
50% genes	0.84	0.67	3.8%	80%	50%	32%
100% genes	1.20	0.46	2.7%	88%	63%	44%

[a] Modal value for relative risk distribution.
[b] Modal value for cumulative risk by age 70 years.

of patients, more consistent with a muliplicative model, and concluded that a high proportion, and perhaps the majority, of breast cancers arise in a susceptible minority of women (Peto and Mack 2000). If this were true, the discriminatory power could be substantially improved.

Implications of the Recessive Model for Risk Distribution in the Population

Under the recessive model there would be a single risk allele with frequency 0.24. Thus, women with the at risk genotype (RR=9.8) would comprise 6% of the population and account for 56% of cases. The remaining 94% of the population (RR=0.46) would account for 44% of cases. However, in view of the failure of genetic linkage studies to identify further breast cancer susceptibility genes, such a model seems less plausible than a polygenic model of inheritance (Risch 2001; Vaittinen and Hemminki 2000).

Distribution of Risk Due to Established Risk Factors

Several risk factors which do not require molecular genotyping (although they may in part have a genetic basis) are already used to stratify individuals into high- and low-risk groups for breast cancer. We have used data on 3,209 breast cancer cases from the same population-based study as we used for the genetic risk estimates, to estimate the risk distribution for breast cancer in the premenopausal women that is provided by these "established" risk factors (Kelsey et al. 1993). We included age at menarche (under 13 versus 13 and over), number of full-term pregnancies, age at first full-term pregnancy, oral contraception use (current, past, never) and family history. The RR associated with each factor was assumed to act independently, with multiple risk factors combining multiplicativity. The distribution of RR in the cases was found to be approximately log normally distributed with a standard deviation of 0.3. It follows that the distribution of risk in the population determined by these risk factors should also be log normal, with the same standard deviation. The width of this distribution corresponds to a 3.5-fold difference in risk between the highest quintile to the lowest; but it is considerably narrower than the distribution with SD 1.2 predicted for genetic risk factors. However, the addition of other risk factors, such as mammographic patterns or serum markers such as sex steroid hormone or cytokine levels, may enhance the discriminatory power considerably.

Discussion

The possibility that genetic susceptibility to breast cancer is due to several loci, each conferring a modest independent risk, seems reasonable. In practice, the number of loci involved will be finite, but once there are more than 4–5 loci the distribution of risk will be similar to the polygenic model except at the extreme tails.

A key aspect of the model is the standard deviation, because this determines the power of the risk distribution to discriminate high- and low-risk individuals. The estimate of the standard deviation is tightly specified by the segregation analysis and is also close to that predicted by other studies of familial risk. The RR of disease in monozygotic twins ($\lambda_{\text{monozygotic}}$) and siblings ($\lambda_{\text{sibling}}$) are related to each other and to the predicted standard deviation of the polygenic log-normal risk distribution by the equation:

$$\lambda_{\text{monozygotic}} = \lambda^2_{\text{sibling}} = e^{\sigma^2}$$

Assuming λ_{sibling} to be equal to 2, as estimated by many observational epidemiologic studies (Pharoah et al. 1997), this equation solves to predict a standard deviation of 1.2. The familial RRs for many other common cancers are also around 2, which suggests that the distribution of risk for these cancers will be similar to that we have observed for breast cancer. Thus, the potential benefits of a targeted high-risk approach to disease prevention are also likely to be similar.

The practical use of risk information should be considered in two contexts: that of the individual, and that of the population as defined by Rose (Rose 1985). In both cases, our analysis suggests that a "risk profile" that is based on the combination of known genotype and other risk factors is likely to provide risk discrimination which will be of practical value in health care terms. Whether genetic testing in whole populations would be socially or economically acceptable remains unknown, and is likely to depend on whether useful action can be seen to result. But it does seem clear that the use of combinations of risk factors is potentially able to overcome many of the limitations of single risk factors, which have been the cause of scepticism about the practical utility of molecular genotyping for common, low-risk genes (Holtzman and Marteau 2000).

For example, in respect of individual risk, a single gene which conferred a RR of breast cancer of 1.5-fold – the size of effect that seems plausible from reported studies (Dunning et al. 1999) – would increase the risk of breast cancer to an individual from the UK population average of 5.7% by age 70 years to around 8.5%. On the other hand, inspection of Fig. 2 suggests that a genotypic risk profile might identify one woman in 30 who has a risk by age 70 of 20% or more. Little is known about how individuals will perceive and respond to such risks; but the discriminatory power of the polygenic risk profile is clear.

At the population level, the effects are even more striking. According to the genetic model, 12% of the population have a risk of breast cancer of 1 in 10 or more by age 70 years; and that half the total breast cancer incidence falls within that 12% of the population. Different cut-offs can be chosen to give the best combination of high risk and proportion of total breast cancer incidence that is included within the high-risk group, to suit the purpose in hand. A single genotypic marker would, by contrast, provide far weaker discrimination: for example, a dominant predisposing allele with frequency 10% and RR 1.5 would result in 26% of cancer incidence occurring in the 19% of the population who carried at least one allele – very poor enrichment in terms of targeting interventions. An important feature of the high-risk groups defined by the model is that most of the individuals within them will be at risk because of the combined effect of several predisposing alleles. This implies that interventions that are based on specific mechanisms of predisposition will individually deal with only a proportion of the excess cancer risk; and that except for predisposing genes with major effects, generic interventions are more likely to be appropriate.

Risk profiles may also be used to define low-risk groups. Thus, in Fig. 2, only 12% of breast cancer incidence falls within the 50% of women at lowest risk. Exclusion of the low-risk groups from interventions, if it were socially acceptable, might be very cost-effective. For example, screening of the whole population by mammography should reduce breast cancer mortality by approximately 30% (Kerlikowske et al. 1995). If mammography were offered only to the half of the population in the highest risk group by the genetic profile, total breast cancer mortality would still be reduced by 26%–a "loss" of only 4%. There would be additional benefits, since the benefit:harm ratio is likely to be improved by targeting to the high-risk group. (These arguments assume that the efficacy of any intervention is independent of genotype: if that is not the case, the dividend from genotyping may be greater or smaller depending on whether the cancers in high-risk individuals are more or less responsive to the intervention.)

These arguments and examples assume that all of the genetic factors that contribute to the estimated risk distribution can be identified and typed. In practice, this goal is some way off. Nevertheless, the figures in Table 1 suggest that even if only half the risk factors were typed, useful discrimination of risk might be possible. Our results also suggest that the power of risk profiles based solely on the currently available "classical" risk factors is quite weak, and that in the future genotypic data will potentially play a decisive role.

Acknowledgements. This work was supported by Cancer Research UK. The ideas on which this chapter is based were conceived after many lengthy discussions with Antonis Antoniou, Douglas Easton, Ron Zimmern, Martin Bobrow and Bruce Ponder.

References

Anglian Breast Cancer Study Group (2000) Prevalence and penetrance of BRCA1 and BRCA2 in a population based series of breast cancer cases. Br J Cancer 83:1301–1308

Antoniou AC, Pharoah PDP, McMullen G, Day NE, Ponder BAJ, Easton DF (2001) Evidence for further breast cancer susceptibility genes in addition to BRCA1 and BRCA2 in a population based study. Genet Epidemiol 21:1–18

Antoniou AC, Pharoah PDP, McMullen G, Day NE, Stratton MR, Peto J, Ponder BAJ, Easton DF (2001) A comprehensive model for familial breast cancer incorporating BRCA1, BRCA2 and other genes. Br J Cancer (in press)

Beaudet AL (1999) 1998 ASHG presidential address. Making genomic medicine a reality. Am J Hum Genet 64:1–13

Bell J (1998) The new genetics in clinical practice. Br Med J 316:618–620

Collaborative Group on Hormonal Factors in Breast Cancer (2001) Familial breast cancer: collaborative reanalysis of individual data from 52 epidemiological studies including 58,209 women with breast cancer and 101,986 women without the disease. Lancet 358:1389–1399

Cui J, Antoniou AC, Dite GS, Southey MC, Venter DJ, Easton DF, Giles GG, McCredie MR, Hopper JL (2001) After BRCA1 and BRCA2-what next? Multifactorial segregation analyses of three-generation, population-based Australian families affected by female breast cancer. Am J Hum Genet 68:420–431

Dunning AM, Healey CS, Pharoah PDP, Teare DM, Ponder BAJ, Easton DF (1999) A systematic review of genetic polymorphisms and breast cancer risk. Cancer Epidemiol Biomarkers Prev 8:843–854

Easton DF (1999) How many more breast cancer predisposition genes are there. Breast Cancer Res 1:14–17

Friend SH (1999) How DNA microarrays and expression profiling will affect clinical practice. Br Med J 319:1306–1307

Holtzman NA, Marteau TM (2000) Will genetics revolutionize medicine? N Engl J Med 343:141–144

Kelsey JL, Gammon MD, John EM (1993) Reproductive factors and breast cancer. Epidemiol Rev 15:36–47

Kerlikowske K, Grady D, Rubin SM, Sandrock C, Ernster VL (1995) Efficacy of screening mammography: a meta-analysis. JAMA 273:149–154

Lichtenstein P, Holm NV, Verkasalo PK, Iliadou A, Kaprio J, Koskenvuo M, Pukkala E, Skytthe A, Hemminki K (2000) Environmental and heritable factors in the causation of cancer- analyses of cohorts of twins from Sweden, Denmark, and Finland. N Engl J Med 343:78–85

Peto J, Mack TM (2000) High constant incidence in twins and other relatives of women with breast cancer. Nat Genet 26:411–414

Pharoah PDP, Antoniou A, Bobrow M, Zimmern RL, Ponder BAJ, Easton DF (2002) Polygenic susceptibility to breast cancer: implications for prevention. Nature Genet (in press)

Pharoah PDP, Day NE, Duffy S, Easton DF, Ponder BAJ (1997) Family history and the risk of breast cancer: a systematic review and meta-analysis. Int J Cancer 71:800–809

Pharoah PDP, Mackay J (1998) Absolute risk of breast cancer in women at increased risk: a more useful clinical measure than relative risk? Breast J 7:255–259

Risch N (2001) The genetic epidemiology of cancer: interpreting family and twin studies and
    their implications for molecular genetic approaches. Cancer Epidemiol Biomarkers Prev
    10:733–741
Rose G (1985) Sick individuals and sick populations. Int J Epidemiol 14:32–38
Vaittinen P, Hemminki K (2000) Risk factors and age-incidence relationships for contralater-
    al breast cancer. Int J Cancer 88:998–1002
Vineis P, Schulte P, McMichael AJ (2001) Misconceptions about the use of genetic tests in
    populations. Lancet 357:709–712

Novel Approaches to Identify Low-Penetrance Cancer Susceptibility Genes Using Mouse Models

John P. de Koning, Jian-Hua Mao, Allan Balmain

J.P. de Koning (✉)
UCSF Comprehensive Cancer Center and Cancer Research Institute,
Department of Biochemistry and Biophysics,
University of California San Francisco, 2340 Sutter Street,
San Francisco, CA 94115, USA

Present address: J.P. de Koning, Lab for Physiological Chemistry,
Center for Biomedical Genetics, University Medical Center Utrecht,
Universiteitsweg 100, 3584 CG Utrecht, The Netherlands

Abstract

Studies of cancer predisposition have largely concentrated on the role of high-penetrance susceptibility genes. Less than 10% of the total human tumor burden, however, is accounted for by mutations in these genes. More genetic variation in cancer risk is likely to be due to commoner but lower penetrance alleles. In man, such modifier genes will be difficult to find since they do not segregate as single Mendelian traits. The mouse offers a powerful system for studying polygenic traits such as cancer and has been widely used for this purpose. Novel approaches that might accelerate the identification of these low-penetrance cancer susceptibility genes by using mouse models will be discussed.

Epidemiological evidence has shown that the major causes of cancer include environmental agents such as radiation and chemicals. However, genetic background is also extremely important in determining cancer susceptibility. After all, although one individual in three develops sporadic cancer, two out of three do not, and it seems unlikely that this difference is accounted for only by variation in levels of exposure to dietary or environmental carcinogens. Certain individuals may therefore be predisposed to develop tumors, by virtue of their particular genetic background, while others appear to be more resistant.

Studies of germline genetic predisposition have so far mostly concentrated on high-penetrance susceptibility genes. If an individual is unlucky enough to inherit a mutation in one of these genes, the probability of developing a tumor in one of the affected tissues is extremely high. However, germline mutations in high-penetrance susceptibility genes occur infrequently and cancers arising in these high-risk families account therefore for only a very small proportion of total human cancers (Ponder 2001). Moreover, in families carrying particular mutant alleles of high-penetrance susceptibility genes with strong effects such as the neurofibromatosis type 1 (*NF1*) gene or breast cancer susceptibility genes *BRCA1* and *BRCA2*, phenotypes are dependent upon the genetic background, being most similar between monozygotic twins, but differing between distant relatives with the same mutation (Fodor et al. 1998; Nathanson et al. 2001). This indicates that genetic background in humans is able to control disease progression.

Sporadic cancers, constituting approximately 90%–95% of the total human tumor burden, probably also have a strong genetic component. This is supported by the observation that first-degree relatives of patients with most common cancers have a two- to threefold higher risk of developing cancer at the same site than the general population (Peto and Houlston 2001). Furthermore, studies involving monozygotic and dizygotic twins demonstrated that the risk of developing multiple cancer types has a strong genetic component (Lichtenstein et al. 2000). It is therefore likely that many, relatively common low-penetrance susceptibility, or modifier, genes segregate within the population that together make a strong contribution to individual probability of developing sporadic tumors (Balmain and Nagase 1998; Ponder 2001). The particular combination of resistance or susceptibility genes an individual inherits will thus be a major determinant of cancer risk. These low-penetrance susceptibility genes may control, for instance, intrinsic cellular growth functions, or may influence the ways in which environmental carcinogens interact with and cause mutations in target cells. The polygenic nature of the inheritance pattern and the variable penetrance of these modifier genes will mask any clear cut familial clustering and thereby complicate studies designed to find the loci involved.

The common way to find modifier genes that may contribute to sporadic cancer susceptibility in humans is to make an educated guess on the basis of possible involvement in cancer, find polymorphisms for the selected candidate gene in cancer patients and appropriate controls, and carry out an association study. In this design, frequencies of candidate genetic variants are compared between groups with different phenotypes, i.e., cancer cases and controls. The objective is to study polymorphisms that may either be causally related to disease risk or are in strong linkage disequilibrium with disease-causing variants. However, large studies are needed to provide adequate statistical power to detect small effects and these are thus expensive and time-consuming. In addition, the candidate gene approach requires prior knowledge of the gene for assignment of plausibility. Positional cloning, the standard strategy to identify novel genes, is not feasible in this setting because of the low-penetrance expected and the heterogeneity of cancer. Therefore, it is very difficult to identify novel genes using this strategy. The candidate modifiers studied so far include genes encoding steroid hormone receptors and paracrine growth factors, and genes involved in metabolism of carcinogens and in DNA repair (Dunning et al. 1999). Although the indications are that some of them are indeed involved in determination of risk, in general the numbers of cases and controls do not allow definitive conclusions to be reached, and some of the results are still controversial (Perera and Weinstein 2000). Studies involving large families that showed some initial effects have suffered from lack of confirmation in equally large studies of other populations. Naturally, this may be due to genetic heterogeneity, since the causal polymorphism responsible for the phenotype may differ between families. Alternatively, it may be that there are multiple weak interacting loci that only reach acceptable levels of significance in specific patient samples, dependent on the genetic background or environmental factors. In agreement with this, studies with mouse models of human cancer have revealed genetically interacting loci with major effects that are not detected as single loci (Fijneman et al. 1996; van Wezel et al. 1996; Nagase et al. 2001).

To circumvent the indicated limitations associated with human studies, the mouse is widely exploited as a model system for the identification of tumor modifier genes offering significant advantages (Balmain 2002). Many strains are available that either by chance or by selective breeding exhibit extreme sensitivity or resistance to tumor development in certain tissues. Crossing of resistant and sensitive strains can give valuable information about the dominant or recessive nature of resistance, as well as providing indications of the numbers of genes involved and their approximate locations in the genome. The ability to control the size of the population studied as well as the breeding enhances the statistical power to find loci of low penetrance linked to a particular trait. Furthermore, control of environmental factors allows a focus on genetic effects on tumorigenesis that is not possible with human populations. The development of novel techniques to manipulate the mouse germline has provided the opportunity to generate custom-made, more sophisticated models, e.g., transgenics, knockouts, knockins, and conditional gene expression systems (Macleod and Jacks 1999; Hann and Balmain 2001). Finally, mice exposed to environmental carcinogens develop tumors by a multistage process very similar to that seen in humans. The types of genetic alterations detected in mouse tumors involve genes encoding proteins such as Ras, cyclin D1, Rb, p53 and p16^{INK4a}, that are the most commonly altered genes in human tumors (Balmain and Harris 2000). This underlying similarity in the biology of carcinogenesis in mice and humans implies that the genes that control susceptibility to mouse tumor development may also be relevant to the human situation.

Another major advance was the development of statistical methods that take account of the effect that multiple genes make different quantitative contributions to the phenotype. Quantitative trait locus (QTL) analysis has accelerated the mapping of a large number of mouse tumor modifier loci that, e.g., control the size, growth rate, or number of lesions that develop (Fijneman et al. 1998; Nagase et al. 1999; van Wezel et al. 1999). A QTL typically spans an interval of 10–30 cM (Fig. 1A). The crucial, but difficult, next step in identification of the actual tumor modifier gene involves refinement of the initial region containing the QTL to an interval of 1–2 cM that is suitable for positional cloning and candidate gene approaches. Traditionally, this has been accomplished by generating multiple congenic lines, in which a small fragment of a chromosome from one parental strain has been bred onto the genetic background of the other strain (Fig. 1B). This requires repeated rounds of breeding resistant mice onto the sensitive background, i.e., backcrossing, to obtain

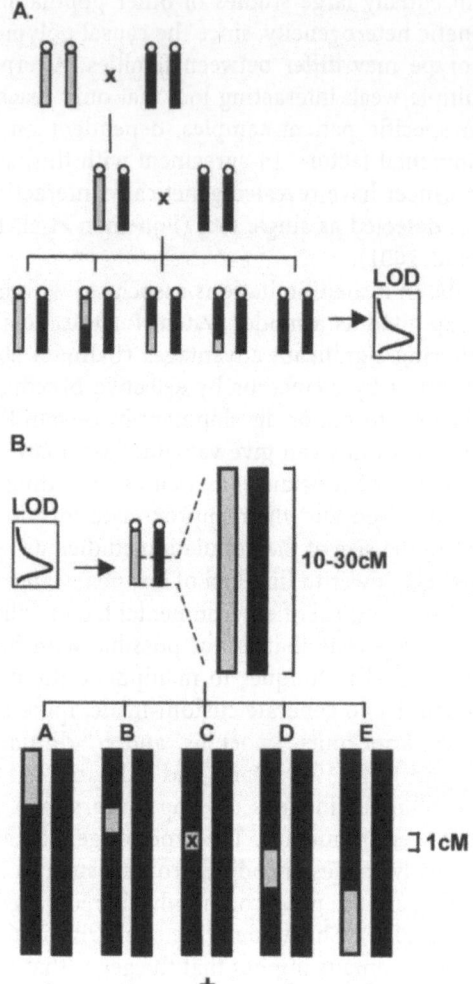

Fig. 1A,B. Classical approach to identify low-penetrance susceptibility genes. **A** Standard quantitative trait locus (QTL) analysis is carried out by genotyping and phenotyping backcross progeny from two different inbred *Mus musculus* strains based on a phenotypic difference between the two parental strains. Usually, this strategy identifies loci within regions spanning about 10–30 cM. **B** To refine the region of the identified QTL to an interval of 1 cM allowing candidate gene approaches, multiple congenic lines, e.g., A–E, need to be generated, each carrying different small regions of the QTL bred onto the genetic background of the other strain. Subsequently, progeny from each line is phenotyped to test for an effect of the isolated region on tumorigenesis, eventually leading to refinement of the locus based on the presence of a modifier gene (depicted by *X* in congenic line *C*)

multiple independent lines that carry different small regions of the QTL on a relatively pure, sensitive background. Subsequently, the effect of the isolated chromosomal region on tumorigenesis is determined by phenotyping large groups of mice generated from each congenic line. Obviously, this is an ex-

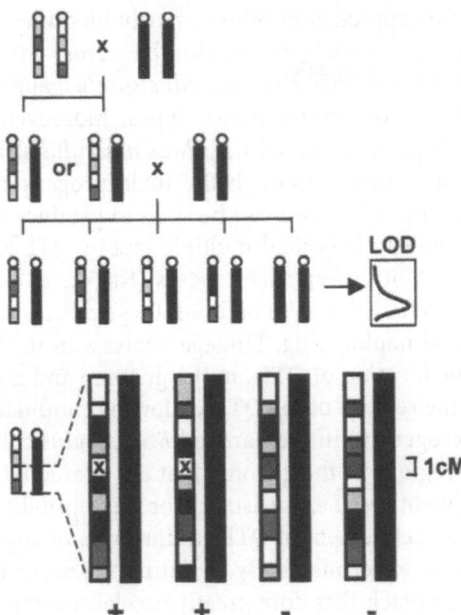

Fig. 2. Novel approach to rapidly identify low-penetrance susceptibility genes. To identify QTLs, the same backcross strategy is applied as in Fig. 1, except that outbred mice are used. In addition to linkage analysis, the genetic heterogeneity of the outbred colony is exploited to refine the identified region by constructing haplotypes using the same backcross data. By identifying shared regions between haplotypes with similar phenotypes, the QTL can be refined to an interval of, in this example, 1 cM containing the modifier (depicted by X)

pensive and time-consuming step. Moreover, it has been observed that in many cases the effect disappears as breeding progresses, either because of colocalization of multiple genes within the same QTL that contribute to the effect and which are successfully lost during breeding, or because of the presence of interacting genes on other chromosomal regions necessary for the phenotype (Legare et al. 2000). The final steps in identification of tumor modifiers involve screening of candidate genes within the refined region of the QTL. Functional or regulatory polymorphisms in the critical gene need to be identified, and their putative causal effect on the phenotype should ultimately be proven in vivo by transgenic or preferably knockin approaches. Pinpointing the causal polymorphism can be extremely complex because multiple genes in the immediate vicinity may exhibit sequence variants that correlate with the phenotype.

A novel strategy that resolves many of these problems is outlined in Fig. 2. By exploiting as much genetic information as possible in the initial screen, the requirement for generating congenic lines can be circumvented. This can be achieved by using an outbred stock of mice. The presence of recombinations and heterogeneity within outbred animals provides a resolution for QTL mapping that is not attainable by normal linkage analysis. Recently, we have successfully applied this approach to refine a newly identified susceptibility locus for skin carcinogenesis using interspecific backcross mice (Ewart-Toland et al., submitted). Wild mouse strains, i.e., *Mus spretus*, appear to carry numerous resistance alleles for several tumor types. Moreover, *Mus spretus* mice have retained the capacity to breed with *Mus musculus* strains, generating interspecific F1 hybrid mice. Although the male progeny of such crosses are sterile, the females are fertile and can be used to produce a backcross generation. We have previously identified multiple loci by QTL analysis that control skin tumor susceptibility using such crosses (Nagase et al. 1995, 1999). Since the original *Mus spretus* mice were outbred, these crosses can be used for both linkage analysis and haplotyping. Linkage analysis in the backcross provides information on the location of QTLs in the genome and haplotyping can then be used to refine the regions of the QTLs, allowing candidate gene approaches. Basically, the heterogeneity in the parental *Mus spretus* colony is exploited by identifying small regions of the genome that are shared by backcross progeny with the same phenotype, i.e., resistance or susceptibility to tumorigenesis (Fig. 2). This allows refinement of QTLs to intervals of approximately 1–2 cM, only using backcross experiments. By obviating the necessity to generate congenic lines, this approach therefore greatly accelerates the process of identification of tumor modifiers, potentially leading to enormous reductions in costs. Importantly, the strategy also applies to loci that cannot be refined by congenic lines due to epistatic interactions with other genes. A similar approach involving crosses between outbred heterogeneous stocks of *Mus musculus* with inbred *Mus musculus* mice was proposed as a theoretical solution to the time-consuming problem of refinement of a locus by classical techniques (Mott et al. 2000). However, this specific strategy may encounter practical difficulties because of the overall similarity between the genomes of the parental *Mus musculus* stocks, where allele sharing is common. Interspecific crosses involving *Mus spretus* do not suffer from this drawback, since in general both parental *Mus spretus* alleles can be distinguished from *Mus musculus* alleles in the backcross. Moreover, the phenotypic differences between different *Mus musculus* strains might be relatively small, whereas this is less likely if *Mus spretus* mice are used.

After localization of the QTL to a small interval, further problems exist in pinpointing the actual modifier gene within this region and in identifying the critical polymorphism. Although the availability of the complete mouse sequence from databases significantly simplifies sequence comparisons of all candidates between strains and individual mice, many potentially functional polymorphisms will have to be screened. Therefore, it is desirable to have several alleles, haplotypes, or strains of mice with the same phenotype for the locus studied, since this will help to narrow down the range of possible candidates. In a classical backcross strategy, a QTL is by definition the result of at least one difference between the two strains used. This means that any polymorphism of any candidate gene localized within the QTL will correlate with the phenotype and can thus be causal. The strategy as presented in Fig. 2 can also help to simplify this problem. Again, the heterogeneity in the outbred

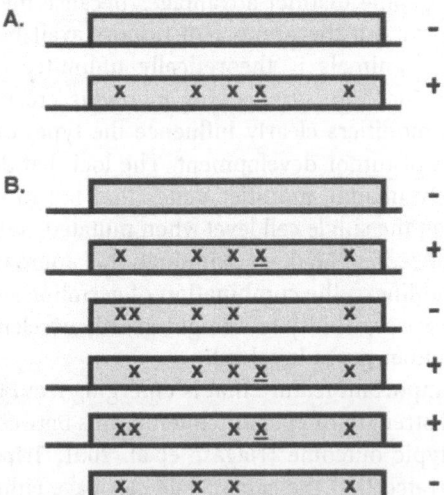

Fig. 3A,B. Rapid identification of the critical polymorphism in a candidate gene. **A** In a classical back-cross strategy as presented in Fig. 1, the phenotypic difference (either "-" or "+") between two inbred strains is exploited. Therefore, any polymorphism (indicated by *X*) of any candidate gene localized within the QTL can be the critical one and should therefore be tested for causality. **B** The novel strategy presented in Fig. 2 exploits the genetic heterogeneity in an outbred colony by comparing the phenotypes (either "-" or "+") of the various outbred alleles relative to the allele of the inbred strain. Polymorphisms that are not shared by alleles with similar phenotypes are discarded as being nonrelevant. If a polymorphism is shared by alleles with the same phenotype (underlined *X*), it is considered to be potentially critical requiring additional testing for causality

Mus spretus colony is exploited, now to filter out and discard nonrelevant polymorphisms. This additional screening method consists of comparing different alleles with similar phenotypes for the occurrence of shared polymorphisms in the candidate genes examined (Fig. 3). This criterion is rather stringent since it assumes that a single shared polymorphism causes the observed effect in the different alleles. Naturally, it should be taken into account that multiple different polymorphisms might be involved. Nevertheless, this approach may prevent costly functional screenings of polymorphisms and candidate genes that are not causally related to the QTL and may lead to rapid identification of potentially interesting polymorphisms for further testing.

Most of the high-penetrance genes responsible for familial cancer predisposition also act as classical tumor suppressor genes by showing loss-of-function mutations in sporadic human cancers. Subsequently, these mutations provide a strong driving force for loss of the remaining normal allele (Cavanee et al. 1983; Weinberg 1991). At this stage, it is unclear whether low-penetrance susceptibility genes can also act as oncogenes or tumor suppressor genes and acquire mutations leading to their activation or inactivation during carcinogenesis. The resolution of this question is important both conceptually and practically, since the observation of somatic genetic changes in tumors could enhance the process of refining the map location of the critical gene(s). The mouse again offers some distinct advantages because the parental origins of the alleles are known and the number of tumors available from informative, genetically uniform animals is theoretically unlimited. Preliminary results from our interspecific *Mus spretus/Mus musculus* cross demonstrated that some, but not all, modifiers clearly influence the types of genetic alterations during the process of tumor development. The loci that do not show somatic changes most likely include modifier genes that fail to confer any selective growth advantage at the single cell level when mutated and might encode non-cell autonomous or secreted factors. Although this approach is apparently not applicable to all modifiers, the combination of germline and somatic mapping of low-penetrance susceptibility loci might greatly accelerate identification of a subset of the modifier genes involved.

A particularly important feature that is emerging from the mouse studies is the frequency and strength of epistatic interactions between modifier loci that determine phenotypic outcome (Nagase et al. 2001; Tripodis et al. 2001). It has been demonstrated that the same allele can have either positive or negative effects depending on the genetic background of the host (Fijneman et al. 1996, 1998; van Wezel et al. 1996). Extrapolation to humans raises the possibility that a particular polymorphism may be detected as a tumor resistance modifier in one ethnic background but act in the opposite direction in another population. Furthermore, simple association studies designed to detect an effect of a specific polymorphism on cancer susceptibility may not show an effect if tested in isolation but could nevertheless be very important in combination with particular alleles of genes at other locations in the genome. A key goal of the Human Genome Project is to assemble a comprehensive map of single nucleotide polymorphisms (SNPs) that can be used for association studies (The International SNP Map Working Group 2001), but genome-wide scans for modifier genes are presently prohibitively expensive. At present, conventional approaches to identify human modifier genes mostly involve testing of known candidate genes, which means that the unknown and unexpected will be missed. The use of appropriate mouse models to guide the prioritizing of candidate genes, together with their interacting partners, for human association studies could have a major impact on the identification of modifier genes, ultimately leading to significant advances in understanding the polygenic basis of cancer.

Acknowledgments. This work was supported by NCI grants CA 84244 and CA 89520. John P. de Koning was supported by a grant from the Dutch Cancer Society "Koningin Wilhelmina Fonds".

References

Balmain A (2002) Cancer as a complex genetic trait: tumor susceptibility in humans and mouse models. Cell 108:145–152

Balmain A, Harris CC (2000) Carcinogenesis in mouse and human cells: parallels and paradoxes. Carcinogenesis 21:371–377

Balmain A, Nagase H (1998) Cancer resistance genes in mice: models for the study of tumour modifiers. Trends Genet 14:139–144

Cavanee WK, Dryja TP, Phillips RA, Benedict WF, Godbout R, Gallie BL, Murphree AL, Strong LC, White RL (1983) Expression of recessive alleles by chromosomal mechanisms in retinoblastoma. Nature 305:779–784

Dunning AM, Healey CS, Pharoah PDP, Teare MD, Ponder BAJ, Easton DF (1999) A systemic review of genetic polymorphisms and breast cancer risk. Cancer Epidemiol Biomarkers Prev 8:843–854

Ewart-Toland A, de Koning JP, Dunning AM, Mao JH, Pharoah PDP, Nagase H, Burns J, West S, Mannermaa A, Kataja V, Easton DF, Ponder BAJ, Balmain A (2002) Identification of STK6 (Aurora2) as a modifier of cancer risk in mouse and man (submitted)

Fijneman RJ, de Vries SS, Jansen RC, Demant P (1996) Complex interactions of new quantitative trait loci, Sluc1, Sluc2, Sluc3, and Sluc4, that influence the susceptibility to lung cancer in the mouse. Nat Genet 14:465–467

Fijneman RJ, Jansen R, van der Valk M, Demant P (1998) High frequency of interactions between lung cancer susceptibility genes in the mouse: mapping of Sluc5 to Sluc14. Cancer Res 58:4794–4798

Fodor FH, Weston A, Bleiweiss IJ, McCurdy LD, Walsh MM, Tartter PI, Brower ST, Eng CM (1998) Frequency and carrier risk associated with common BRCA1 and BRCA2 mutations in Ashkenazi Jewish breast cancer patients. Am J Hum Genet 63:45–54

Hann B, Balmain A (2001) Building "validated" mouse models of human cancer. Curr Opin Cell Biol 13:778–784

Legare ME, Bartlett FS, Frankel WN (2000) A major effect QTL determined by multiple genes in epileptic EL mice. Genome Res 10:42–48

Lichtenstein P, Holm NV, Verkasalo PK, Iliadou A, Kaprio J, Koskenvuo M, Pukkala E, Skytthe A, Hemminki K (2000) Environmental and heritable factors in the causation of cancer-analyses of cohorts of twins from Sweden, Denmark, and Finland. N Engl J Med 343:78–85

Macleod KF, Jacks T (1999) Insights into cancer from transgenic mouse models. J Pathol 187:43–60

Mott R, Talbot CJ, Turri MG, Collins AC, Flint J (2000) A method for fine mapping quantitative trait loci in outbred animal stocks. Proc Natl Acad Sci USA 97:12649–12654

Nagase H, Bryson S, Cordell H, Kemp CJ, Fee F, Balmain A (1995) Distinct genetic loci control development of benign and malignant skin tumours in mice. Nat Genet 10:424–429

Nagase H, Mao JH, Balmain A (1999) A subset of skin tumor modifier loci determines survival time of tumor-bearing mice. Proc Natl Acad Sci USA 96:15032–15037

Nagase H, Mao JH, de Koning JP, Minami T, Balmain A (2001) Epistatic interactions between skin tumor modifier loci in interspecific (spretus/musculus) backcross mice. Cancer Res 61:1305–1308

Nathanson KN, Wooster R, Weber BL (2001) Breast cancer genetics: what we know and what we need. Nat Med 7:552–556

Perera FP, Weinstein IB (2000) Molecular epidemiology: recent advances and future directions. Carcinogenesis 21:517–524

Peto J, Houlston RS (2001) Genetics and the common cancers. Eur J Cancer 37:S88–S96

Ponder BAJ (2001) Cancer genetics. Nature 411:336–341

The International SNP Map Working Group (2001) A map of human genome sequence variation containing 1.42 million single nucleotide polymorphisms. Nature 409:928–933

Tripodis N, Hart AAM, Fijneman RJA, Demant P (2001) Complexity of lung cancer modifiers: mapping of thirty genes and twenty-five interactions in half of the mouse genome. J Natl Cancer Inst 93:1484–1491

van Wezel T, Stassen AP, Moen CJ, Hart AA, van der Valk MA, Demant P (1996) Gene interaction and single gene effects in colon tumour susceptibility in mice. Nat Genet 14:468–470

van Wezel T, Ruivenkamp CA, Stassen AP, Moen CJ, Demant P (1999) Four new colon cancer susceptibility loci, Scc6 to Scc9 in the mouse. Cancer Res 59:4216–4218

Weinberg RA (1991) Tumor suppressor genes. Science 254:1138–1146

Assessing New Cancer Susceptibility Genes 2

Development of Novel Selective Cell Ablation in the Mammary Gland and Brain to Study Cell–Cell Interactions and Chemoprevention

Barry A. Gusterson, Wei Cui, A. John Clark

B.A. Gusterson (✉)
Department of Pathology, Western Infirmary, Glasgow G11 6NT, UK

Abstract

We have generated transgenic mice which express the gene encoding *Escherichia coli* nitroreductase (NTR) specifically in the luminal epithelial cells of the mammary gland and the glial cells of the brain. The enzyme activates an anti-tumour drug CB1954, to produce a cross-linking agent that kills all cells expressing the enzyme. We have shown that administration of the antitumour drug CB 1954 rapidly and selectively kills these cells. Original experiments demonstrated the ability to ablate the luminal cells in the mammary gland with no apparent bystander effect. Subsequently, astrocytes expressing nitroreductase under the targeting of the GFAP promoter were selectively ablated following administration of the prodrug CB 1954 produces a degeneration of granular neurones due to changes in glutamate levels. Recent experiments demonstrated inhibition of myc-dependent mammary tumours using the same enzyme (nitroreductase) – prodrug (CB 1954), combination. Owing to the ease of control of NTR-mediated cell ablation, we anticipate that this system will supersede herpes simplex virus type 1 thymidine kinase. There are widespread potential applications for this approach in the dissection of complex cellular interactions during development and in the adult organism. The present transgenic models also have important applications for the study in vivo of novel prodrugs that can be selected for variable degrees of bystander effects. Such studies will have particular significance for those groups advocating the use of NTR as an appropriate enzyme for gene-directed enzyme prodrug therapy by providing models of a wide range of human disease for mechanistic and therapeutic experimentation. The results clearly demonstrate that the model has potential to study chemoprevention and fundamental questions on cell–cell interactions in cell biology.

Methods of In Vivo Cell Ablation

Our primary interest is in the analysis of cell–cell interactions and lineage analysis in the intact mammary gland during development, but any system that develops a novel approach to cell ablation has potential advantages as a model system for gene therapy. The system to be described is cell-type specific, effective in nondividing cells, and cell killing is inducible. There is no apparent bystander effect in vivo, but some such effect can not be excluded.

Selective ablation of specific cell types enables the study of the developmental origin, fate, and physiological or developmental origin of particular cell types. There are two main approaches to selective cell ablation. Physical methods involve destruction of target cells by surgery (Smith 1989), current injection (Kuwada and Goodman 1985), UV laser ablation (Lohs-Schardin et al. 1979), and dye photoablation (Miller and Selverson 1979). Ablation methods (Bernstein and Breitman 1989) involve targeting expression of a potentially lethal toxin to a specific cell type using an appropriate gene promoter/enhancer in transgenic mice. Ablation methods provide a novel and powerful tool to study both the physiological importance and lineage of a target cell type in vivo. The genetic ablation approach is preferable when a tissue comprises various cell types which have different functions and are interspersed with each other, since physical means cannot be used to separate them.

Two strategies have been used in producing genetic ablation in transgenic mice. One involves targeting toxic genes to specific cell types of transgenic mice. Expression of the transgene provides high levels of the toxin and results in cell death in all toxin-expressing cells. The second strategy involves targeting expression of nontoxic genes to specific cell types of transgenic mice, and their products are not toxic unless they are in the presence of substances which are metabolized by these enzymes to cytotoxic compounds. Gene Directed Enzyme Prodrug Therapy (GDEPT) utilises this concept, but the major problem is delivery of the enzyme specifically to the target cell.

Toxins

Most work applying toxic genes in transgenic mice is based on two toxins, α-subunit of diphtheria toxin (DT) (Palmiter et al. 1987; Behringer et al. 1988, Burrows et al. 1996) and α-subunit of the lectin ricin (Landel et al. 1988). The DT is synthesized by the bacterium *Corynebacterium diphtheriae*, the causative agent in human diphtheria. In its native prototype form, DT consists of two subunits, a toxic α-subunit associated through disulphide bonds with a β-subunit to the cell-surface receptor initiates internalization of the associated α-subunit, which encodes an ADP-ribosyltransferase that catalyses the NA-dependent ADP ribosylation of elongation factor-2, resulting in the inhibition of protein synthesis and subsequent cell death (Collier 1975; Pappenheimer 1977). The lectin ricin is produced by castor bean (*Ricinus communis*). Similar to DT, ricin also consists of a toxic α-subunit and a cell-surface binding β-subunit. The α-subunit produces a ribonuclease which inactivates ribosomes by cleaving the adenosine from the A4365 of the 28S ribosomal RNA (Lamb et al. 1985). α-Subunits are unable to induce cell death without the cell-surface binding component of the β-subunit. Thus, when expressing α-subunit alone in transgenic mice, only host cells are killed and surrounding bystander cells are spared. This ablation strategy has been applied to several tissues, such as pancreas (Palmiter et al. 1987), and eye lens (Landel et al. 1988). The major disadvantage of this strategy is that the target cells are killed as soon as the toxin gene is expressed, which will result in early embryonic lethality and the investigators have no control over the timing of ablation.

Enzyme/Prodrug Methods

Herpes Simplex Virus Type 1 Thymidine Kinase (HSV-tk) Ablation

With the second strategy in which the products of the transgene are not toxic themselves, the investigators are able to control the timing of ablation by administering the downstream substances at appropriate times. The most widely used gene in this approach is HSV-tk (Borrelli et al. 1989; Al-Shaw et al. 1991; Canfield et al. 1996). HSV-tk is not, in itself, harmful to cells, but it is capable of selectively catalyzing the incorporation of certain nucleoside analogues, for example 1-(2-deoxy-2-fluoro-β-D-arabinofuranosil)-5-iodouracil, ganciclovir, and acyclovir, into host cell DNA, resulting in cell death. It was initially thought that the HSV-tk ablation system kills only proliferating cells, but not terminal differentiated cells. However, this view has been challenged by work which showed that HSV-tk with fluoro-idouracil or gancyclovir has effective inducible ablation in dividing cells (Archibald et al. 1990, Harris et al. 1991). In these cases the mode of action of the activated prodrug is unclear, although in nonproliferating thyrocytes it apparently occurs by p53-independent apoptosis (Wallace et al. 1996). A second problem with HSV-tk is that this gene is expressed ectopically in the testis from an internal cryptic promoter causing male sterility and results in considerable difficulties in the establishment of breeding lines (Al-Shaw et al. 1991). It has been shown recently that a truncated HSV-tk does not cause this problem although cells carrying this modified gene are considerably less sensitive to being killed by ganciclovir (Salomon et al. 1995).

Nitroreductase-CB 1954

We have described a new system for achieving the inducible ablation of specific cell types in transgenic mice that overcomes many of the problems associated with HSV-tk (Clark et al. 1997, Gusterson et al. 1997, Wei et al. 1999, Wei et al. 2001, Wei et al. 2002) The method is based on the *Escherichia coli* enzyme nitroreductase (NTR), which activates certain nitro compounds such as the antitumour drug 5-aziridin-1-yl-2-4-dinitrobenzamide (CB 1954). The compounds generated are secondarily activated in cells by thioesters (e.g., acetyl coenzyme A) to very reactive species that cross-link DNA (Knox et al. 1993). DNA cross-linking results in cell death that is independent of cell division. Moreover, its pharmacokinetics in mice and other animals is well characterized (Workman et al. 1986a, b). The human and mouse forms of DT diaphorase, the endogenous gene that can activate CB 1954, reduce CB 1954 very poorly (Chen et al. 1995) and, therefore, cells from these species are not sensitive to this prodrug. It is therefore relatively nontoxic in mouse cells and the increase in toxicity accompanying nitroreduction can be as much as 100,000-fold. The enormous increase in cytotoxicity following bioactivation of CB 1954, as well as the lack of requirement for DNA replication for cell killing, makes the NTR system an attractive proposition for inducible cell ablation (Drabek et al. 1997).

The gene encoding NTR has been cloned and in preliminary experiments this gene was introduced into mammalian cells in culture and shown to confer killing by CB 1954 (Clark et al. 1997). A conditionally immortalized human breast cell line (Stamps et al. 1994) was transfected with pR8NR comprising the NTR gene driven by the Rous sarcoma virus long terminal repeat. After 2 h of exposure to CB 1954 there was 100–1,000 times more susceptibility to killing by CB 1954 than in cells transfected with the vector alone. Importantly, cell killing was demonstrated at doses of CB 1954 that would be nontoxic in animals. These results therefore formed the basis for us to establish the use of NR for cell-specific ablation in transgenic animals. NTR-mediated sensitivity to CB 1954 for other mammalian cell types (NIH3T3, human melanoma, ovarian carcinoma, and mesothelioma) has been reported recently (Bridgewater et al. 1995). The detailed methods used have been previously described (Clark et al. 1997). Here we provide a summary of our findings.

Targeting of NTR Expression to the Mammary Gland in Transgenic Mice

Promoter sequences from the ovine β-lactoglobulin (BLG) gene were used to target NTR expression specifically to the mammary gland (Simons et al. 1987). We have previously shown that the BLG gene is expressed specifically and efficiently in the luminal cells of the mammary gland of transgenic mice (Simons et al. 1987; Harris et al. 1991) and that regulatory elements from this gene can be used to target the expression of a variety of heterologous gene sequences to this tissue (Archibald et al. 1990; Yull et al. 1995). Prokaryotic sequences such as *E.coli* NTR can be difficult to express in transgenic mice and, therefore, we cointegrated the BLG-NTR transgene with the unmodified BLG gene. This is the strategy that we have previously employed to enhance the efficiency of expression of otherwise poorly expressed gene constructs (Clark et al. 1992).

Transgene expression was demonstrated in lactating females from the selected transgenic line, using a combination of Western and Northern blotting of tissue extracts and immunostaining of pregnant, lactating, and control animals. By Northern analysis, NTR was not detected in the liver, spleen, or kidney although a trace of signal was evident in the salivary gland. The line exhibited high levels of BLG transgene mRNA in the mammary gland (Clark et al. 1992). NTR enzyme activity was confirmed using NADH menadione oxidoreductase (NMOR) activity and reduction of CB 1954. An equal proportion of the 2- and 4-hydroxylamines was observed in the active samples. NMOR activity was assayed by a spectrophotometric method as previously described (Anlezark et al. 1992), employing menadione as substrate at a concentration of 500 mM and cytochrome C as electron acceptor. Activity was defined as the cytochrome C reduction inhibited by 100 mM dicoumarol and expressed as nmol cytochrome C reduced/min per mg protein. CB 1954 reduction to the 2- and 4-hydroxylamino derivatives was determined by HPLC as previously described (Knox et al. 1992). In the liver, NMOR activity was similar in all the samples reflecting the endogenous enzyme DT diaphorase. In the mammary gland, virtually undetectable levels of NMOR-reducing activity were present in control samples whereas high levels of activity were detected in the samples from the transgenic line.

BLG and NTR antisera were used to localize the transgene products on sections of mammary gland tissue taken during gestation and pregnancy. Transgene expression was restricted to the luminal cells; however, for NTR a mosaic pattern of expression was observed. Within the patches of expressing cells the NTR staining was generally homogenous with high expression. The expression of BLG was uniformly positive in lobules with lipid accumulation or secretory activity in all the animals investigated. The morphology and general appearance of the mammary tissue from these animals were quite normal.

Tissue Ablation with NTR and CB 1954

CB 1954 was administered to both transgenic lines during late gestation when cell division is taking place and during early lactation when little cell division is taking place (Traurig 1967). No gross effects of the administration of CB 1954 on the whole animal were observed during late gestation either in the experimental or control animals. By contrast, lactation failed in a number of the transgenic mice given the prodrug at this stage, whereas no such effects were observed in the control mice. CB 1954 administration had no discernible effects on the overall structure and size of the mammary glands from control mice; by contrast, mammary glands from many of the transgenic mice were reduced in size. This effect was more marked with samples taken at lactation than it was with the samples taken at late gestation. Inspection of whole mounts of mammary gland taken from lactating mice showed that much of the alveolar tissue was destroyed in treated glands giving rise to a "moth-eaten" appearance, but the basic ductal structure was still evident. At the histological level this was seen as a combination of apoptotic and necrotic cell death in the luminal cells, in association with the NTR expression (see Clark et al. 1997). When an antibody to smooth muscle actin was used (to stain the myoepithelial cells), the cellular and structural collapse of the lobules with accentuation of the myoepithelial cells and the selective killing of the luminal cells was apparent (see Clark et al. 1997). The apoptotic cell death coincided with an upregulation of p53 expression. When the glands were examined 7 days after the last injection of CB 1954, there was no evidence of residual NTR expression and in the areas of cell death the myoepithelial cells remained, indicating that there was no evidence of a bystander effect. From all the available evidence the NTR-mediated killing of luminal cells by CB 1954 was quite specific to this cell type and the closely associated myoepithelial cells appeared unaffected. At the end of the death phase, when the luminal cells had been removed, the collapsed alveoli comprised little more than intact myoepithelial cells and there was no evidence that these cells were undergoing apoptosis even 7 days after the initial prodrug administration. This contrasts with previous reports of significant bystander effects observed in culture when CB 1954-treated Walker tumour cells were cultured with otherwise insensitive V79 (Knox et al. 1988) or NTR-expressing NIH3T3 cells were cocultured with nonexpressing cells (Bridgewater et al. 1995).

The effects of CB 1954 administration were dosage dependent. Lactating animals given single or triple doses of CB1954 at 50 mg/kg body weight (bw) exhibited considerably more cell death in the mammary gland than animals given a 10 mg/kg bw dosage, and at a dosage of 2 mg/kg bw little or no effect of the prodrug was observed. A single dose at 50 mg/kg was as effective as three doses on consecutive days.

Cell Ablation Is Independent of p53

In view of the increased expression of p53 on cellular ablation reported in Gusterson et al. 1997, we decided to investigate the role of p53 in nitroreductase–CB 1954 mediated cell ablation. By cross-breeding the BLG-NTR mice on a p53 null background we generated BLG-NTR transgenic mice on a p53 null background and tested cell ablation in these mice. The level of ablation in these mice was the same as in the p53 wild-type transgenic mice. Thus functional p53 is not required for ablation. In these experiments it was also shown that cell ablation occurred within 7 h of drug delivery.

Heterogeneous Transgene Expression

Variegated patterns of transgene expression have been noted in transgenic mice carrying fatty acid-binding protein fusion genes (Sweetser et al. 1988), tyrosinase fusion genes (Bradl et al. 1991), CD2 (Elliot et al. 1995), and α (Robertson et al. 1995) and β (Festenstein et al. 1996) globin-derived transgenes. We have also reported variegated expression of BLG transgenes in the mammary gland of certain lines of transgenic mice. In these mice the mosaic pattern of BLG was very similar to that observed for NTR in this present study and was correlated with variable levels of transgene expression within the ine. This pattern of expression appears to be a consequence of the chromosomal location and/or nature of the integration site (Dobie et al. 1996).

Advantages of NTR-CB 1954

The use of NTR for selective ablation of cells in transgenic mice may have significant advantages over the HSV-tk. In the luminal population of the mammary gland it is, clearly, very effective and widespread cell death was apparent only 48 h after the first inoculation. Efficient cell killing by CB 1954 does not require cell proliferation (Bridgewater et al. 1995). First, this was apparent in the present study by the fact that lactating cells, which have a very low mitotic index (Traurig 1967), are sensitive. This is not surprising since we know that activated CB 1954 cross-links DNA and we presume that this is the trigger for apoptosis and predict that any NTR-expressing cell will be sensitive irrespective of its metabolic or proliferative state. Secondly, no side-effects associated with carrying or expressing NTR were observed in the lines of transgenic mice generated and both sexes were fully fertile. Thirdly, the pharmacokinetics and toxicity in mice and other animals of CB 1954 are well established (Workman et al. 1986a, b). This compound readily crosses the blood–brain barrier and, therefore, we anticipate that it will be feasible to target specific cell types within the central nervous system (CNS), which to our knowledge has yet to be accomplished using HSV-tk. CB 1954 is readily administered by i.p. injection, whereas most ablation studies using HSV-tk have used minipumps.

Despite the fact that bystander effects have been observed with CB 1954 in cell culture (Bridgewater et al. 1995), it is interesting to note that our results in the mammary gland indicate that cell killing is quite specific and that in this tissue these effects are at a minimum.

Inducible Ablation of Astrocytes in the Adult Brain

Although our in vivo data are in variance with some of the in vitro data on bystander effect with this combination of enzyme and prodrug, we decided to further test the in vivo effects in another system and selected the ablation of astrocytes in the brain. In addition to providing potentially interesting biological information about the function of astrocytes, this would also enable us to test whether the prodrug could cross the blood–brain barrier.

Astrocytes are the most abundant glia in the central nervous system (CNS), yet their importance in CNS development and function has only been appreciated during the last decade. They display an almost complete set of CNS neurotransmitter receptors (Porter and McCarthy, 1997), express several ion channels (Largo et al. 1996), take up a number of neurotransmitters by means of specific transporters (Rothstein et al. 1994), and secrete several growth factors and cytokines (Traugott and Lebon 1988; Lindholm et al. 1992). It seems likely, therefore, that astrocytes participate in a variety of important physiological and pathological processes. Most of our current knowledge on astrocytes, however, is based on in vitro studies, and many aspects of their function in vivo remain unclear. For example, despite a large number of in vitro studies demonstrating that the survival of neurons is promoted by glia and vice versa (Lin et al. 1993; Raff et al. 1993; Baptista et al. 1994), there is little direct evidence of this in vivo (Delaney et al. 1996; Bush et al. 1999).

NTR-CB 1954 Can Conditionally Ablate Nonproliferative Cells in CNS of Adult Mice

We have recently used the NTR-CB 1954 combination successfully to ablate specific cell populations in the adult brain (Cui et al. 2001). We have conditionally ablated astrocytes in the brain of adult mice by targeting *E.coli* NTR gene expression to these cells with the GFAP promoter. The GFAP-NTR transgenic mice developed and bred normally until administration of the prodrug CB 1954. Immunohistochemistry and in situ hybridization showed that the expression of the NTR transgene was localized specifically to the glial cells, particularly in the hippocampus and the Bergmann glia in the cerebellum. Intraperitoneal injection of CB 1954 into these mice resulted in the complete elimination of the Bergmann glia.

Bergmann Glia Are Important for Survival of Granular Cells in Cerebellum

The loss of astrocytes in the brain after ablation was evaluated using NTR and GFAP immunostaining. In only one region of the brain, the Purkinje cell layer, was there any evidence of glial cell loss. In this layer, the so-called Bergmann glia were entirely eliminated. By contrast, there was no clear loss of astrocytes in other parts of the brain, and even an increase of GFAP-positive staining in some areas. One possible explanation for the result is that ablation itself may induce a reactive astrocytosis, a vigorous proliferative response to diverse neurologic insults (Eddleston and Mucke 1993).

The most striking changes in the ablated transgenic brain were seen in the cerebellar neurons. There was massive death of granular cells, disruption of the junction between granular cell layer and Purkinje cell layer, and degradation of the Purkinje cell dendrites. There was, however, no evidence of NTR transgene expression in the granular cells or Purkinje cells as shown by either in situ hybridization or NTR immunohistochemistry. Therefore, it was highly unlikely that the death of the granular cells was due to direct killing by activated CB 1954 unless a bystander effect occurred, in which cells not expressing the NTR transgene were killed by activated CB 1954 formed in neighbouring cells expressing the transgene. Bystander effects have been associated with NTR-CB 1954 system in cell culture (Green et al. 1997; Friedlos et al. 1998) but not as such in transgenic mice (Clark et al. 1997). The mechanism reported in cultured cells is thought to be due to a cell-permeable metabolite of CB 1954 (Bridgewater et al. 1997). If such bystander effects were the cause of death of the granular neurons in the GFAP-NTR mice, the damage to these cells would presumably have exhibited a gradient, in which the cells located near the Bergmann glia showed more severe effects than those further away, but in fact, the granular layer in which these neurons are located was uniformly disrupted. Therefore, the death of granular cells was more likely due to the elimination of the astrocytes, particularly Bergmann glia, and the effects on Purkinje cells must be either due to the loss of Bergmann glia or granular cells or both. From in vitro studies, it is known that cerebellar astrocytes increase Purkinje cell survival (Yuzaki et al. 1993) and that granular cells enhance the survival and dendritic development of these neurons (Baptista et al 1994; Morrison and Mason 1998). Nevertheless, we cannot exclude the possibility that the toxin exchange could occur out in the molecular layer where the processes of granular neurons and Bergmann glia are in intimate contact, even though there was no evidence of cell death in other neurons in the molecular layer.

Bergmann glia differentiate from radial glia. The cell bodies are located in a row around Purkinje cell somata and long radial fibres extend toward the pial surface. Bergmann glia are known to provide a scaffold for granular neuron migration during cerebellum development (Rakic 1971). In the adult brain, the function of Bergmann glia has not been reported. Using NTR-CB 1954 ablation in the GFAP-NTR mice, we have shown here that their elimination resulted in degeneration of granular neurons as well as disruption of Purkinje cell dendrites. These results suggest that Bergmann glia are critical to the survival of granular cells as well as Purkinje cells in the adult brain.

These results are similar to those observed by Delaney et al. (1997) in the developing brain of GFAP-tk transgenic mice after prodrug GCV treatment in their neonatal period. In those mice, however, no ablation was seen when GCV was administered to the adults. In another similar GFAP-tk transgenic mouse study (Bush et al. 1998, 1999), ablation effects were only observed in the adult brain after wounding, including depletion of astrocytes adjacent to the injury, increase of leucocyte infiltration, and degeneration of local neurons. Long-term treatment of GCV on these mice resulted in fulminating jejuno-ileitis.

This study demonstrates that, unlike the HSV-tk-mediated gangiclovir (GCV) system, which only ablates proliferating cells in the CNS, NTR-mediated CB 1954 ablation system is capable of destroying nondividing ells in the adult brain. As the blood–brain barrier may limit the concentration of CB 1954 in the brain (Workman et al. 1986), local delivery of the prodrug could achieve better ablation even with lower doses and reduce systemic side effects, such as temporary weight loss.

Reduced Glutamate Transport in Cerebellum May Account for Dysfunction of Motor Neurons

High concentrations of excitatory neurotransmitters are extremely toxic to neurons and glutamate is the predominant excitatory neurotransmitter in the mammalian central nerve system (Monaghan et al. 1989). The mechanism that maintains extracellular glutamate concentration below toxic levels is mediated by glutamate transporters, which terminate the synaptic transmission by removing the excitatory amino acid neurotransmitter from the synaptic cleft. Four subtypes of glutamate transporters have been cloned and characterized. Two of them, GLAST and GLT-1 are principally astrocyte-specific transporters and are expressed predominantly in the Bergmann glia of the cerebellum (Storck et al. 1992; Rothstain et al. 1994). Their presence in these cells supports the hypothesis that astrocytes are able to protect cultured neurons from the toxic effects of glutamate (Rosenberg and Aizenman 1989; Sugiyama et al. 1989; Rosenberg 1991).

After administration of CB 1954 in the GFAP-NTR transgenic mice, the levels of both GLAST and GLT-1 were decreased substantially. It has been reported previously that in vivo inactivation of these two transporters in the rats by antisense oligonucleotides resulted in elevated extracellular glutamate levels, neurodegeneration and progressive paralysis (Rothstein et al. 1996), a phenotype similar to the ablated GFAP-NTR transgenic mice described in this study. In another study, GLAST knockout mice showed impaired motor coordination and increased susceptibility to cerebellar injury (Watase et al. 1998). Therefore, the neuron degeneration effects we observed at the granular neurons and the Purkinje cells are consistent with a dramatic reduction in the expression of these transporters due to the ablation of the Bergmann glia.

CB 1954-treated GFAP-NTR transgenic mice did not show any clear histopathological abnormality in the neurons of the hippocampus. Nevertheless, glial cell death was detected by apoptosis TUNEL assay. Furthermore, a decrease of GLAST and GLT-1 expression was observed in the cerebrum after ablation, indicating that CB 1954 also ablated astrocytes in this general area of the brain. However, the number of GFAP- and NTR-positive cells was not decreased and, in fact, was slightly increased. This may result from a reactive astrocytosis, leading to an increased number of GFAP-expressing cells in response to neurological insult in the CNS and this may compensate for the loss of ablated astrocytes. Alternatively, granular neurons may be more susceptible to glutamate toxicity than other neurons, leading to histopathological abnormalities that were observed.

In conclusion, the NTR-CB 1954 system is able to effect ablation on a selected cell type in the CNS, regardless of the proliferative conditions. This system clearly has wider applications, such as in gene-direct enzyme prodrug therapy for brain tumours and for ablating specific neuronal type in the CNS. We have already used this system to ablate specifically the olfactory neurons (Isles et al. 2001). The GFAP-NTR transgenic mice generated in this study will provide a useful animal model to study the role of astrocytes in neurologic development and diseases, particularly as we have now shown that they are required for neuronal survival in the adult brain.

Inhibition of MYC-Dependent Tumour Formation of Transgenic Mice

We have recently published the ability of the NTR-CB1954 combination to inhibit tumour formation (Cui et al. 2002). The selective activation of CB 1954 and related prodrugs may offer the potential of novel anticancer strategies by gene-directed enzyme-producing therapy. In this regard transgenic mice carrying NTR transgenes should provide a powerful model to assess the efficacy of tumour cell killing in vivo. To test this hypothesis we have established transgenic mice in which the pro-oncogenes C-*myc* and NTR are fused to the internal ribosome entry site (IRES) sequences and coexpressed in luminal cells of the mammary gland and the control of the whey acidic protein (WAP) promoter. The expression of the C-*myc* disrupted normal cell cycle and induced tumour formation in the mammary gland of transgenic mice. The total number of carcinomas was strikingly reduced from 117 carcinomas in 14 non-ablated transgenics compared with 5 tumours in 14 treated animals. This clearly demonstrates the value of this model system to assess different prodrugs in vivo, a promising approach for cancer treatment. It is clear, however, that not every tumour cell appeared to stain with the nitroreductase antibody. Therefore, the high efficiency of tumour ablation observed in some mice could be due to a bystander effects. The results therefore demonstrate that NTR-CB 1954 has a considerable potential for GDEPT in the treatment of cancer in vivo. Moreover, this transgenic mouse strain provides an animal model to proceed to further studies on this enzyme prodrug system in tumour treatment. In particular, this is an excellent system in which to study the effects of different prodrugs and preclinical testing.

Summary and Applications in Chemoprevention

Targeted cell ablation is an important development in the process of engineering appropriate animal models to study both cell–cell interactions and in which to model enzyme/prodrug combinations for therapy. We have clearly demonstrated the utility of the NTR-CB1954 combination in both applications. This combination gives the potential to target any cell population at any time in development and in many different species from flies to mammals. The only limitation is the presence of an endogenous enzyme with the same activity.

In relation to chemoprevention of tumours, the main limitation with any animal model is the current lack of information concerning the target cell population for the environmental carcinogen or the genetic defect. At the present time we can set up "proof of principle" testing and can design more efficient and better targeted enzyme/prodrug combinations, but our ignorance in underlying mechanisms of cancer and understanding of the natural history is holding us back. The Annapolis meeting in 1999 (Cardiff et al. 2000) was a landmark event as it became clear that a single gene could direct the phenotype of the tumour produced in genetically engineered mice, but that this could be varied by the promoter, even if targeted to the mammary gland. Thus the phenotype of the tumour and developing a model of human disease will need to take into account the specific cell targeted, the ability of the target cell to differentiate, the specific changes produced by the targeted gene within that specific cellular background and additional features due to predisposition to secondary changes.

Acknowledgements. This work was supported by BBSCR, CRC and an MRC ROPA Award. Professor Gusterson's laboratory is supported by Breakthrough Breast Cancer.

References

Al-Shaw R, Burke J, Wallace H, Joes C, Harrison S, Buxton D, Maley S, Chandley A, Bishop J (1991) The herpes simplex virus type I thymidine kinase is expressed in the testes of transgenic mice under the control of a cryptic promoter. Mol Cell Biol 11:4207–4216

Anlezark GM, Melton RG, Sherwood RF, Coles B, Friedlos F, Knox RJ (1992) The bioactivation of 5-(aziridin-1-yl)-2,4-dinitrobenzamide (CB 1954). I. Purification and properties of a nitroreductase enzyme for *Escherichia coli*-a potential enzyme for antibody directed enzyme prodrug therapy (ADEPT). Biochem Pharmacol 44:2289–2295

Archibald AL, McClenaghan M, Hornsey V, Simons JP, Clark AJ (1990) Expression of biologically active human α1-antitrypsin in the milk of transgenic mice. Proc Natl Acad Sci USA 87:5178–5182

Baptista CA, Hatten ME, Blazeski R, Mason CA (1994) Cell-cell interactions influence survival and differentiation of purified Purkinje cells in vitro. Neuron 12:243–260

Behringer RR, Mathews LS, Palmiter RD, Brinster RL (1988) Dwarf mice produced by genetic ablation of growth hormone-expressing cells. Genes Dev 2:453–461

Bernstein A, Breitman M (1989) Genetic ablation in transgenic mice. Molecular Biol Med 6:523–530

Borrelli E, Heyman RA, Arias C, Sawchenko PE, Evans RM (1989) Transgenic mice with inducible dwarfism. Nature 339:538–541

Bradl M, Larue L, Mintz B (1991) Mosaic expression of a tyrosinase fusion gene in albino mice yields a heritable striped coat colour pattern in transgenic homozygotes. Proc Natl Acad Sci USA 88: 9643–9647

Bridgewater JA, Springer CJ, Knox RJ (1995) Expression of nitroreductase enzyme in mammalian cells renders them selectively sensitive to killing by the prodrug CB 1954. Eur J Cancer 31A:2362–2370

Bridgewater JA, Knox RJ, Pitts JD, Collins MK, Springer CJ (1997) The bystander effect of the nitroreductase/CB 1954 enzyme/prodrug system is due to a cell-permeable metabolite. Hum Gene Ther 8:709–717

Burrows HL, Birkmeier TS, Seasholtz AF, Camper SA (1996) Targeted ablation of cells in the pituitary primordia of transgenic mice. Mol Endocrinol 10:1467–1477

Bush TG, Savidge TC, Freeman TC, Cox HJ, Campbell EA, Micke L, Johnson MH, Sofroniew MV (1998) Fulminant jejuno-ileitis following ablation of enteric glia in adult transgenic mice. Cell 93:189–201

Bush TG, Puvanachandra N, Horner CH, Polito A, Ostenfeld T, Svendsen CN, Mucke L, Johnson MH, Sofroniew MV (1999) Leukocyte infiltration, neuronal degeneration and neurite outgrowth after ablation of scar-forming reactive astrocytes in adult transgenic mice. Neuron 23:297–308

Canfield V, West AB, Goldenring JR, Levenson R (1996) Genetic ablation of parietal cells in transgenic mice: a new model for analysing cell lineage relationship in the gastric mucosa. Proc Natl Acad Sci USA 93:2431–2435

Cardiff RD, Anver MR, Gusterson BA, Henninghausen L, Jensen RA, Merino MJ, Rehm S, Russo J, Tavassoli FT, Wakefield LM, Ward JM, Green JE (2000) The mammary pathology of genetically engineered mice: the consensus report and recommendations from the Annapolis meeting. Oncogene 19:968–988

Chen S, Knox R, Lewis AD, Friedlos F, Workman P, Deng PS, Fung M, Ebenstein D, Wu K, Tsai TM (1995) Catalytic properties of NAD(P):quinone acceptor oxidoreductase: study involving mouse, rat, human and mouse-rat-chimeric enzymes. Mol Pharmacol 44:2297–2301

Clark AJ, Cowper A, Wallace R, Wright G, Simons JP (1992) Rescuing transgene expression by cointegration. Biotechnology (NY) 10:1450–1454

Clark AJ, Iwobi M, Cui W, Crompton M, Harold G, Hobbs S, Kamalati R, Knox R, Neil C, Yull F, Gusterson B (1997) Selective cell ablation in transgenic mice express E.coli nitroreductase. Gene Ther 4:101–110

Collier RJ (1975) Diphtheria toxin: mode of action and structure. Bacteriol Rev 39:54–85

Cui W, Gusterson B, Clark AJ (1999) Nitroreductase-mediated cell ablation is very rapid and mediated by a p53-independent apoptotic pathway. Gene Ther 6:764–770

Cui W, Gusterson B, Clark AJ (2001) Inducible ablation of astrocytes shows that these cells are required for neuronal survival in the adult brain. Glia 34:272–282

Cui W, Gusterson B, Clark AJ (2002) Inhibition of MYC-dependent breast tumour formation in transgenic mice. Breast Cancer Res Treat 71:9–20

Delaney CL, Brenner M, Messing A (1996) Conditional ablation of cerebellar astrocytes in postnatal transgenic mice. J Neurosci 16:6908–6918

Dobie KW, Lee M, Fantes JA, Graham E, Clark AJ, Springbett A, Lathe RL, McClenaghan M (1996) Variegated expression in mouse mammary gland is determined by the transgene integration locus. Proc Natl Acad Sci U S A 93:6659–6664

Drabek D, Guy J, Craig R, Grosveld F (1997) The expression of bacterial nitroreductase in transgenic mice results in specific cell killing by the prodrug CB 1954. Gene Ther 4:93–100

Eddleston M, Mucke L (1993) Molecular profile of reactive astrocytes: implications for their role in neurologic disease. Neuroscience 54:15–36

Elliot JI, Festenstein R, Tolaini M, Kioussis D (1995) Random activation of a transgene under the control of a hybrid CD2 locus control region/Ig enhancer regulatory element. EMBO J 14:575–584

Festenstein R, Tolaini M, Corbella P, Mamalaki C, Parrington J, Fox M, Miliou A, Jones M, Kioussis D (1996) Locus control region function and heterochromatin induced position effect variegation. Science 271:1123–1125

Friedlos F, Court S, Ford M, Denny WA, Springer C (1998) Gene-directed enzyme prodrug therapy: quantitative bystander cytotoxicity and DNA damage induced by CB 1954 in cells expressing bacterial nitroreductase. Gene Ther 5:105–112

Green NK, Youngs DJ, Neoptolemos JP, Friedlos F, Knox RJ, Springer CJ, Anlezark GM, Michael NP, Melton RG, Ford MJ, Young LS, Kerr DJ, Searle PF (1997) Sensitization of colorectal and pancreatic cancer cell lines to the prodrug 5-(aziridin-1-yl)-2,4-dinitrobenzamide (CB 1954) by retroviral transduction and expression of the E. coli nitroreductase gene. Cancer Gene Ther 4:229–238

Gusterson B, Cui W, Iwobi M, Harold G, Hobbs S, Kamalati T, Knox R, Neil C, Howard B, Clark B (1997) selective cell ablation in the mammary gland of transgenic mice. Endocr Relat Cancer 4:67–74

Harris S, McClenaghan M, Simons JP, Ali S, Clark AJ (1991) Developmental regulation of the sheep β-lactoglobulin gene in the mammary gland of transgenic mice. Dev Genet 12:299–307

Isles AR, Ma D, Milsom C, Skynner M, Cui W, Clark J, Keverne EB, Allen ND (2001) A novel strategy for conditional ablation of neurons in transgenic mice. J Neurobiol 47:183–193

Knox RJ, Friedlos F, Jarman M, Roberts JJ (1988) A new cytotoxic agent DNA interstrand crosslinking agent 5' (aziridin-1-yl)-4-hydroxylamino-2-dinitrobenzamide (CB 1954) by a nitroreductase enzyme in Walker carcinoma cells. Biochem Pharmacol 37:4661–4669

Knox RJ, Friedlos F, Marchbank F, Roberts JJ (1992) The bioactivation of CB 1954. A comparison of an *Escherichia coli* nitroreductase and Walker DT diaphorase. Biochem Pharmacol 44: 2297–2301

Knox RJ, Friedlos F, Boland M (1993) The bioactivation of CB 1954 and its use as a prodrug in antibody directed enzyme pro-drug therapy. Cancer Metastasis Rev 12:195–212

Kuwada J, Goodman CS (1985) Neuronal determination during embryonic development of the grasshopper nervous system. Dev Biol 110:114–126

Lamb FI, Roberts LM, Lord MJ (19850 Nucleotide sequence of cloned cDNA coding for preporicin. Eur J Biochem 148:265–270

Landel CP, Zhao J, Bok D, Evans GA (1988) Lens-specific expression of recombinant ricin induces developmental defects in the eyes of transgenic mice. Genes Dev 2:1168–1178

Largo C, Cuevas P, Herreras O (1996) Is glia dysfunction the initial cause of neuronal death in ischemic penumbra? Neurol Res 18:445–448

Lin LF, Doherty DH, Lile JD, Bektesh S, Collins F (1993) GDNF: a glial cell line-derived neurotrophic factor for midbrain dopaminergic neurons. Science 260:1130–1132

Lindholm D, Castren E, Kiefer R, Zafra F, Thoenen H (1992) Transforming growth factor-beta 1 in the rat brain: increase after injury and inhibition of astrocyte proliferation. J Cell Biol 117:395–400

Lohs-Schardin M, Cremer C, Nusslein-Volhard C (1979) A fate map for the larval epidermis of *Drosophila melanogaster*: localized cuticle defects following irradiation of blastoderm with an ultraviolet laser microbeam. Dev Biol 73:239–255

Miller JP, Selverson AI (1979) Rapid killing of single neurons by irradiation of intracellularly injected dye. Science 206:702–704

Monaghan DT, Bridges RJ, Cotman CW (1989) The excitatory amino acid receptors: their classes, pharmacology and distinct properties in the function of the central nervous system. Annu Rev Pharmacol Toxicol 29:365–402

Morrison ME, Mason CA (1998) Granule neuron regulation of Purkinje cell development: striking a balance between neurotrophin and glutamate signaling. J Neurosci 18:3563–3573

Mulligan RC, Berg P (1980) Expression of a bacterial gene in mammalian cells. Science 209:1422–1427

Palmiter RD, Behringer RR, Quaife CJ, Maxwell F, Maxwell IH, Brinster RL (1987) Cell lineage ablation in transgenic mice by cell specific expression of a toxin gene. Cell 50: 435–443

Pappenheimer AM Jr (1977) Diphtheria toxin. Annu Rev Biochem 46:69–94

Porter JT, McCarthy KD (1997) Astrocytic neurotransmitter receptors in situ and in vivo. Prog Neurobiol 51:439–455

Raff MC, Barres BA, Burne JF, Coles HS, Ishizaki Y, Jacobson MD (1993) Programmed cell death and the control of cell survival: lesions from the nervous system. Science 262:695–700

Rakic P (1971) Neuron-glia relationship during granule cell migration in developing cerebellar cortex: a Golgi and electronmicroscopic study in Macacus Rhesus. J Comp Neurol 141:283–312

Robertson G, Garrick D, Wu W, Kearns M, Martin D, Whitelaw E (1995) Position-dependent variegation of globin transgene expression in mice. Proc Natl Acad Sci U S A 92:5371–5375

Rosenberg PA, Aizenman E (1989) Hundred-fold increase in neuronal vulnerability to glutamate toxicity in astrocyte-poor cultures of rat cerebral cortex. Neurosci Lett 103:162–168

Rosenberg PA (1991) Accumulation of extracellular glutamate and neuronal death in astrocyte-poor cortical cultures exposed to glutamine. Glia 4:91–100

Rothstein JD, Martin L, Levey AI, Dykes-Hoberg M, Jin L, Wu D, Nash N, Kuncl RW (1994) Localization of neuronal and glial glutamate transporters. Neuron 13:713–725

Rothstein JD, Dykes-Hoberg M, Pardo CA, Bristol LA, Jin L, Kuncl RW, Kanai Y, Hediger MA, Wang Y, Schielke JP, Welty DF (1996) Knockout of glutamate transporters reveals a major role for astroglial transport in excitotoxicity and clearance of glutamate. Neuron 16:675–686

Salomon B, Maury S, Loubiere L, Caruson M, Onclerq R, Klatzman D (1995) A truncated herpes simplex virus thymidine kinase phosphorylates thymidine and nucleoside analogues and does not cause sterility in transgenic mice. Mol Cell Biol 15:5322–5328

Simons JP, McClenaghan M, Clark AJ (1987) Alteration of the quality of milk by expression of sheep β-lactoglobulin in transgenic mice. Nature 328:530–532

Smith H (1989) Pattern regulation during the development of the ventral abdomen in the flesh fly Sarcophaga agryostoma. Development 105:35–342

Stamps AC, Davies SC, Burman J, O'Hare MJ (1994) Analysis of proviral integration in human mammary epithelial cell lines immortalized by retroviral infection with a temperature-sensitive SV40 T-antigen construct. Intl J Cancer 57:865–874

Storck T, Schulte S, Hofmann K, Stoffel W (1992) Structure, expression and functional analysis of a Na(+)-dependent glutamate/aspartate transporter from rat brain. Proc Natl Acad Sci U S A 89:10955–10959

Sugiyama K, Brunori A, Mayer ML (1989) Glial uptake of excitatory amino acids influences neuronal survival in cultures of mouse hippocampus. Neuroscience 32:779–791

Sweetser DA, Hauft SM, Hoppe PC, Birkenmeier EH, Gordon JI (1988) Transgenic mice containing intestinal fatty acid binding protein human growth hormone fusion gene exhibit correct regional and cell specific expression of the reporter gene in the intestine. Proc Natl Acad Sci U S A 85:9611–9615

Traugott U, Lebon P (1988) Multiple sclerosis: involvement of interferons in lesion pathogenesis. Ann Neurol 24:243–251

Traurig H (1967) A radioautographic study of cell proliferation in the mammary gland of the pregnant mouse. Anat Rec 159:239–248

Wallace H, Clarke AR, Harrison DJ, Hooper ML, Bishop JO (1996) Ganciclovir-induced ablation of non-proliferating thyrocytes expressing herpes virus thymidine kinase occurs by p53 independent apoptosis. Oncogene 13:55–61

Watase K, Hashimoto K, Kano M, Yamada K, Watanabe M, Inoue Y, Okuyama S, Sakagawa T, Ogawa S, Kawashima N, Hori S, Takimoto M, Wada K, Tanaka K (1998) Motor discoordination and increased susceptibility to cerebellar injury in GLAST mutant mice. Eur J Neurosci 10:976–988

Workman P, White RAS, Talbot K (1986a) CB 1954 revisited. I: disposition kinetics and metabolism. Cancer Chemother Pharmacol 16:1–8

Workman P, White RAS, Talbot K (1986b) CB 1954 revisited. II: toxicity and antitumour activity. Cancer Chemother Pharmacol 16:9–14

Yull F, Harold G, Cowper A, Percy J, Cottingham I, Clark AJ (1995) Fixing human factor IX (fIX): correction of a cryptic Rna splice enables the production of biologically active human factor IX in the mammary gland. Proc Natl Acad Sci U S A 92:10899–10903

Yuzaki M, Mikoshiba K, Kagawa Y (1993) Cerebellar astrocytes specifically support the survival of Purkinje cells in culture. Biochem Biophys Res Commun 197:123–129

Mouse Skin as a Model for Cancer Chemoprevention by Nonsteroidal Anti-Inflammatory Drugs

Friedrich Marks, Gerhard Fürstenberger, Gitta Neufang, Karin Müller-Decker

F. Marks · G. Fürstenberger (✉)
Research Program Tumor Cell Regulation,
Deutsches Krebsforschungszentrum (DKFZ), 69120 Heidelberg, Germany

Abstract

The mouse skin model of multistage carcinogenesis has demonstrated that cancer results from a synergism between genotoxic and nongenotoxic factors. The former induce irreversible genetic alterations, whereas the latter promote tumor development by favoring the clonal outgrowth of the genetically altered cells. While therapeutic gene repair is a still unrealized dream, tumor promotion provides an attractive target for cancer prevention. A key event in epithelial tumor development is an aberrant constitutive overexpression of cyclooxygenase-2 (COX-2), being detectable already in premalignant lesions and leading to an overproduction of prostaglandins. In the mouse skin model, prostaglandin $F_{2\alpha}$ has been identified as an endogenous tumor promoter. The well-established chemopreventive effect of nonsteroidal anti-inflammatory drugs seems to be mainly due to COX-2 inhibition. Targeted transgenic overexpression of COX-2 in mouse epidermis induces a preneoplastic phenotype and renders the tissue extremely sensitive to genotoxic carcinogens; i.e., for the induction of skin tumor development, tumor promoter treatment can be omitted in those animals. It is concluded that COX-2 acts as an endogenous tumor promoter and that its overexpression represents a first order risk factor for cancer development. Conversely, specific COX-2 inhibitors rank among the most promising agents for cancer chemoprevention.

Introduction

Mouse skin is the classical animal model of carcinogenesis. Better than any other tissue, it allows a clearcut experimental separation of tumor development into defined stages. This so-called multistage approach of carcinogenesis is based on the synergism between genotoxic carcinogens required for initiation and stepwise progression to malignancy, and nongenotoxic carcinogens acting as tumor promoters (DiGiovanni, 1992; Marks and Fürstenberger, 1995). While tumor promotion is mostly due to a permanent (but reversible) overstimulation of certain pathways of cellular signal processing (thereby creating a situation resembling tissue repair), the genotoxic effects lead to mutations of proto-oncogenes and tumor suppressor genes. The majority of these genes encode proteins (receptors, protein kinases, GTPases, transcription factors, etc.), which are constituents of the signal-processing network of cells. To repair such mutations is the – still unrealized – dream of cancer research. The mutations of proto-oncogenes and suppressor genes inevitably result, on the other hand, in a dysregulation of additional genes operating downstream. This dysregulation, if essential for tumor development, may be a potential therapeutic target. One of such downstream effector genes is *Ptgs-2* the product of which, cyclooxygenase-2 (COX-2), plays indeed a pivotal role in tumor promotion and has become most attractive for chemoprevention measures (Gupta and DuBois 2001; Marks and Fürstenberger 2000; Marks 2001). Today, cancer chemoprevention by cyclooxygenase inhibitors, i.e., nonsteroidal anti-inflammatory drugs (NSAIDs) is an established fact and has already gained access to medical practice (Giardiello et al. 1993; Winde et al. 1997; Steinbach et al. 2000; Rivers et al. 2002).

Cellular Targets of Nonsteroidal Anti-Inflammatory Drugs

The major cellular targets of NSAIDs are the cyclooxygenases (Vane et al. 1998). These enzymes catalyze the oxygenation of arachidonic acid and related C_{20} fatty acids to prostaglandin endoperoxide. This is the key reaction of prostanoid biosynthesis (Vane et al. 1998; Müller-Decker 1999). Other proteins which have been found to interact with Aspirin, salicylate and related drugs at least in vitro, include IκB kinase (Yin et al. 1998), stress-activated cJun-N-terminal kinase (JNK) (Schwenger et al. 1997), the transcription factors AP1 (Huang et al. 1997) and PPARδ (peroxisome proliferator-activated receptor delta) which are inhibited, and PPARα and -γ (Lehman et al. 1997) as well as the stress-activated protein kinase p38 (Schwenger et al. 1998) which become activated by NSAIDs or salicylate. NSAIDs also induce cell death in vitro along apparently COX-independent pathways (Zhang et al. 1999; Hanif et al. 1996; Williams et al. 2000). This effect, in particular, has been proposed to explain the antineoplastic activity of NSAIDs. However, the doses required are much higher than those sufficient for cancer chemoprevention in vivo (Gupta and DuBois 2001). In fact, the cyclooxygenases are the most sensitive NSAID targets both in vivo and in vitro. Moreover, a wide variety of tumor types have been shown to exhibit elevated prostaglandin levels together with increased COX activities. Therefore, and despite some ongoing controversy (Rigas and Shiff 2000; Tegeder et al. 2001), most investigators arrived at the conclusion that the antineoplastic effect of NSAIDs is *mainly* due to an inhibition of COX-catalyzed prostaglandin synthesis.

Table 1. Aberrant constitutive expression of cyclooxygenase-2 in human neoplasias and preneoplastic disorders

Colon carcinoma (Hao et al. 1999; Müller-Decker et al. 1999b)
Morbus Crohn and ulcerative colitis (Hendel et al. 1997; Singer et al. 1999; Müller-Decker et al. 1999b)
Stomach carcinoma (Ristimäki et al. 1997)
Helicobacter pylori infection (Sawaoka et al. 1998)
Esophagus carcinoma (Zimmermann et al. 1999; Ratnasinghe et al. 1999)
Barrett's esophagus (Wilson et al. 1998)
Primary hepatocellular carcinoma (Koga et al. 1999; Shiota et al. 1999)
Bile duct carcinoma (Chariyalertsak et al. 2001)
Mammary gland carcinoma (Hwang et al. 1998)
Squamous cell carcinoma of skin (Buckman et al. 1998; Müller-Decker et al. 1999a)
Actinic keratosis of skin (Buckman et al. 1998; Müller-Decker et al. 1999a)
Squamous cell carcinoma of head and neck (Chan et al. 1999)
Non-small cell lung carcinoma (Watkins et al. 1999; Wolff et al. 1998)
Pancreas carcinoma (Tucker et al. 1999)
Cervix carcinoma (Kulkarni et al. 2001)
Prostate carcinoma (Yoshimura et al. 2000)
Urinary bladder carcinoma (Ristimäki et al. 2001)
Desmoid tumor (Poon et al. 2001)
Glioma (Shono et al. 2001)

The human genome obviously encodes two COX isoforms (Vane et al. 1998). While the isoform COX-1 is a house-keeping enzyme found to be ubiquitously and constitutively expressed, COX-2 may be looked upon as an "emergency enzyme" which undergoes strong but reversible expression in most tissues only when an increased supply of prostanoids is required, i.e., upon hormonal stimulation or environmental stress as, for example, in the course of inflammatory processes and tissue repair. In fact, *Ptgs-2* is considered to be a proinflammatory immediate–early gene. The *Ptgs-2* gene promoter contains numerous responsive elements, enabling the gene to respond to a wide variety of exogenous and endogenous factors, including hormones (such as the gonadotropins), growth factors, cytokines, and oncogenes (Tsuji et al. 2001), as well as tumor promoters such as the phorbol esters in the skin (Müller-Decker et al. 1995) or secondary bile acids in the intestine (Zhang et al. 1998). On the molecular level the *Ptgs-2* gene is targeted by the 3 MAPkinase cascades known, but also by the NFκB cascade and other signal transducing pathways, thus explaining the enormous variability of stimulatory effects (for a review see Marks and Fürstenberger 2000).

Aberrant Expression of Cyclooxygenase-2 in Neoplastic Lesions

An aberrant constitutive COX-2 expression has been shown to be a consistent feature of a wide variety of neoplastic tissues as well as of preneoplastic states (Table 1). In most cases no such correlation has been found for COX-1 (see, for instance, Chariyalertsak et al. 2001). There is no evidence for a mutation of the *Ptgs-2* gene or its regulatory sequences in neoplastic cells (Tsuji et al. 2001). Instead, the constitutive overexpression of COX-2 in tumors seems to be due to autocrine dysregulation mediated by growth factors and prostaglandins and being a consequence of mutations of proto-oncogenes and tumor suppressor genes. Thus, in mouse skin tumors carrying an oncogenic *H-ras* mutation COX-2 has been found to be overexpressed while in intestinal cells a similar situation is brought about by a deletion of the *APC* tumor suppressor gene, i.e., the major initiating event in intestinal cancer. The H-Ras-induced COX-2 expression most probably occurs along the Ras-Raf-MAPkinase (Erk) pathway (Marks et al. 1999), whereas the causal relationship between APC deletion and COX-2 expression is still unclear since the APC-regulated β-catenin signaling pathway apparently does not target the *Ptgs-2* gene directly (Howe et al. 2001; for a review see Marks and Fürstenberger 2000).

The discovery of the proneoplastic role of COX-2 can be traced back to accidental observations showing that NSAIDs such as Aspirin prevent tumor development. For man this chemopreventive effect has been firmly established for colorectal cancer (reviewed by Gupta and DuBois 2001; Jänne and Mayer 2000) and partially proven for breast cancer (Sharpe et al. 2000), while in animal models a wide variety of epithelial neoplasias has been found to be NSAID-susceptible (Smalley and DuBois 1997; Marks and Fürstenberger 2000).

Prostaglandins as Endogenous Mediators of Tumor Promotion

Mouse skin was one of the very first animal models for which the antineoplastic effects of NSAIDs was described and unequivocally related to tumor promotion. The application of the prototypical skin tumor promoter phorbol ester TPA (12-O-tetradecanoylphorbol-13-acetate) results in a complex pattern of prostaglandin accumulation in epidermal cells which is inhibited by topical application of NSAIDs such as indomethacin (Fürstenberger et al. 1989). Indomethacin also suppresses tumor promotion when applied together with TPA. This inhibitory effect could be specifically overcome by local application of prostaglandin $F_{2\alpha}$ ($PGF_{2\alpha}$) rather than by any other prostaglandin type (Fürstenberger et al. 1989). To date, this result provides the only case where an antineoplastic effect of an NSAID could be causally related to the formation of a distinct prostaglandin species (Marks et al. 1999).

Only one type of cellular $PGF_{2\alpha}$ receptor has been described (for reviews see Narumiya et al. 1999; Marks 1999). This so-called FP receptor stimulates G_q proteins leading to a release of the second messengers diacylglycerol, a PKC activator, and inositol-1.4.5-trisphosphate (IP_3), a Ca^{2+}-mobilizing factor. The activation of such a signaling pathway is expected to exert a promitogenic, proangiogenic, and anti-apoptotic effect and could, thus, easily explain prostaglandin-mediated tumor promotion. In intestinal epithelium PGE_2 instead of $PGF_{2\alpha}$ seems to promote tumor development (Gupta and DuBois

2001). PGE_2 interacts with at least four receptor types (EP1 to EP4) stimulating either G_q-controlled DAG/IP_3-release or G_s-controlled cyclic AMP signaling. While genetic and pharmacological studies on chemically induced large bowel cancer in mice and rats indicate the G_q-activating EP1 receptor (Watanabe et al. 1999, 2000) or the G_s-activating EP4 receptor (Mutoh et al. 2002) to be involved, in mice carrying a deleted *APC* tumor suppressor gene the G_s-activating EP2 receptor has been found to play a critical role in small-intestinal tumorigenesis (Sonoshita et al. 2001). Some prostaglandins do not only stimulate cellular signaling cascades but can, in addition, directly activate PPARs, a family of ligand-controlled nuclear transcription factors. PPAR-subtypes have been found to be activated by prostacyclin (PGI_2) and 15-deoxy $\Delta^{12,14}$-prostaglandin J_2, as well as by some other arachidonic acid metabolites (reviewed by Marks 1999; Gupta and DuBois 2001; Marks and Fürstenberger 2000). Whether or not effects on PPARs are involved in the antineoplastic effect of NSAIDs is, however, still unknown.

Prostaglandins and other prostanoids are short-lived tissue hormones that coordinate and modulate the interactions between different cell types and tissue compartments in the course of a physiological reaction such as, for instance, an inflammatory and tissue repair response. As far as their role in neoplastic development is concerned, prostaglandins are thought to enhance tumorigenesis by stimulating cell proliferation and angiogenesis and inhibiting apoptosis and terminal differentiation, i.e., along pathways which normally play a critical role in the course of both fetal tissue development and wound repair. In fact, COX-2 has been found to be constitutively expressed in embryonic mouse skin, becoming downregulated immediately after birth. Moreover, skin wounding exerts a strong stimulus on COX-2 expression (Müller-Decker et al. 2002a). Since wounding has a substantial tumor-promoting effect of its own, the latter observation supports the notion of a close relationship between tumor promotion and wound healing (Marks and Fürstenberger 1995), i.e., that "a tumor resembles a wound that does not heal."

Like most other tissues, untreated mouse epidermis expresses COX-1 but almost no COX-2 (Scholz et al. 1995). However, upon tumor promoter application or wounding, COX-2 expression becomes induced whereby its expression coincides with $PGF_{2\alpha}$ accumulation thus providing additional evidence for the role of this prostaglandin type in skin tumor promotion (Müller-Decker et al. 1995). A causal relationship between COX-2 expression and tumor development is strongly supported by experiments with specific COX-2 inhibitors. Such inhibitors have been recently developed as antirheumatic drugs being more or less devoid of those well-known side effects of conventional NSAIDs which are thought to be due to COX-1 inhibition (reviewed by Marnett and Kalgutkar 1999). In animal models COX-2 inhibitors have been found to be extremely powerful anticancer agents (Table 2), and presently several clinical trials are going on to prove their clinical applicability for the chemoprevention of human cancer. The preliminary data of one of these trials carried out with familial adenomatous polyposis patients give reason for optimism (Steinbach et al. 2000).

Table 2. Inhibition of experimental tumorigenesis by COX-2-specific NSAIDs

Species	Tumor	Treatment	Maximal inhibition observed (%)	Reference
Mouse	Papilloma and squamous cell carcinoma of skin	DMBA/TPA	50	Müller-Decker et al. 1998; 2002b
		UV	60–90	Pentland et al. 1999; Fischer et al. 1999
Rat	Colon carcinoma	Azoxymethane	96	Kawamori et al. 1998; Reddy et al. 2000
Rat	Mammary carcinoma	DMBA	85	Harris et al. 2000
Rat	Urinary bladder carcinoma	Nitrosamine	95	Grubbs et al. 2001
Rat	Tongue carcinoma	4-Nitroquinoline-1-oxide	90	Shiotani et al. 2001
Mouse	Intestinal adenoma	APC-mutation	70	Jacoby et al. 2000
Mouse	Intestinal adenoma	APC-mutation	80	Oshima et al. 2001
Nude mouse	Human head and neck carcinoma	Xenograft	90	Nishimura et al. 1999
Nude mouse	Human lung and colon carcinoma cell lines	Xenograft	95	Masferrer et al. 2000

Decreased Sensitivity for Carcinogenesis upon Genetic "Knockout" of COX

COX-knockout mice were generated and tested for carcinogen sensitivity using the two-stage approach of skin carcinogenesis. An about 75% inhibition of skin tumor development was reported for either COX-1- or COX-2-deficient mice. This result would indicate that both COX isotypes contribute to carcinogenesis (Tiano et al. 1998, 2000; Langenbach et al. 1999). Additional evidence for a causal relationship between a genetic knockout of COX-2, in particular, and an impairment of tumor development has been provided for intestinal adenoma formation in mice lacking the APC tumor suppressor gene (Oshima et al. 1996) and for teratocarcinoma formation upon injection of embryonic stem cells into syngeneic mice (Zhang et al. 2000).

Increased Sensitivity for Carcinogenesis upon Transgenic Overexpression of COX-2

To investigate the consequences of aberrant constitutive COX-2 expression on normal and pathological skin development we have produced transgenic mice carrying the full-length COX-2 cDNA under the control of the keratin-5 promoter (Neufang et al. 2001). This resulted in a selective expression of the transgene in the basal cell compartment of stratified epithelia. The heterozygous transgenic animals were viable and fertile, although some of them died from pancreatitis at the age of about 10 months. The tissue and blood levels of prostaglandins were about 3–5 times higher than in wild-type mice. Hair follicle development was impaired, resulting in a sparse hair coat, and sebaceous gland hyperplasia led to a strongly increased secretion of sebum, giving the animals a greasy and shaggy appearance.

The epidermis of the transgenics exhibited a dysplastic morphology characterized by hyperplasia and hyperkeratosis, loss of cell polarity, an irregular occurrence of proliferative cells in suprabasal cell layers, the formation of horn pearls, and endophytic papillary growth into the underlying dermis. The dysplasia was due to a delay of terminal differentiation rather than increased cellular proliferation, as shown by immunohistochemical analysis of markers of proliferation (Ki67) and differentiation (keratin-10, involucrin, loricrin). Treatment with a COX-2 inhibitor prevented the development of this phenotype (Müller-Decker et al. 2002b). In addition, as compared to wild-type animals, an almost threefold higher blood vessel density was found in the skin, indicating an angiogenic effect of the COX-2 transgene (unpublished results). This transgenic phenotype widely corresponds to preneoplastic changes observed in the course of a two-stage carcinogenesis experiment and could be suppressed again by treating the animals with a specific COX-2 inhibitor starting immediately after birth.

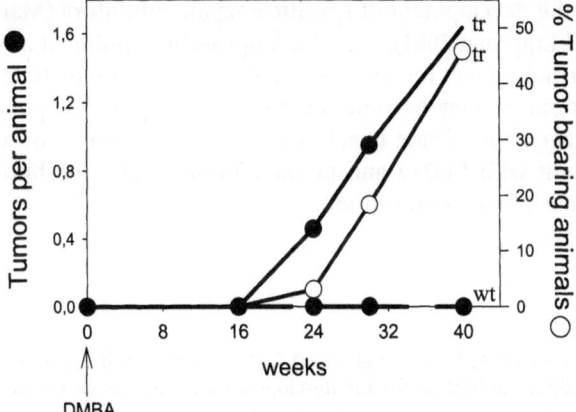

Fig. 1. Skin tumor promotion by a keratin-5 cyclooxygenase-2 transgene. Tumor initiator dimethyl-benz[a]anthracene (DMBA) was topically applied at zero time as a single dose of 100 nmole. In the absence of any other treatment, wild-type animals (*broken line*) did not develop skin tumors, whereas transgenic animals (*solid lines*) exhibited a strong tumor response (papillomas, carcinomas, sebaceous gland adenomas). The *left ordinate* represents the average number of tumors per surviving animal (●), the *right ordinate* the percentage of tumor bearing animals (○); 20 animals per group

In a two-stage carcinogenesis experiment using a "subthreshold dose" of dimethylbenz[a]anthracene (DMBA) as an initiator, wild-type animals developed skin papillomas and carcinomas only when subsequently treated with the tumor promoter TPA for several weeks. In contrast, TPA treatment was not required for tumor growth when the experiment was carried out with heterozygous transgenic mice (Fig. 1). However, DMBA-treatment was obligatory, i.e., transgenic animals not initiated with DMBA did not develop tumors. This result shows that the COX-2 transgene acts as an endogenous tumor promoter, i.e., that COX-2, when overexpressed, dramatically sensitizes a tissue for genotoxic carcinogens (Müller-Decker et al. 2002b). Recently, a high rate of mammary gland carcinomasgenesis was found for animals carrying the COX-2 transgene under the control of the mouse mammary tumor virus promoter (Liu et al. 2001).

Conclusion and Outlook

A constitutive overexpression of COX-2, such as that found in preneoplastic disorders (Table 1), has to be considered to be a high risk factor for cancer mainly due to a strong synergism with the generally rather low doses of genotoxic carcinogens in the environment. Specific inhibition of COX-2 is supposed, therefore, to provide a promising means of future cancer chemoprevention. In addition to COX-2, several lipoxygenases, another group of arachidonic acid-metabolizing enzymes, seem to be critically involved in tumorigenesis, and may provide additional targets of cancer chemoprevention depending on the development of specific enzyme inhibitors (Marks et al. 1999; Shureiqi and Lippman 2001). Whether approaches aiming at a blockade of eicosanoid formation will remain restricted to certain tumor types and to high-risk populations or may become more generally applied depends, first of all, on the management of side-effects which are expected to occur upon long-term treatment with COX-2 and perhaps lipoxygenase inhibitors, as it is required for cancer chemoprevention.

References

Buckman SY, Gresham A, Hale P, et al (1998) COX-2 expression is induced by UVB exposure in human skin: implication for the development of skin cancer. Carcinogenesis 19:723–729

Chan G, Boyle JO, Yang EK, et al (1999) Cyclooxygenase-2 expression is upregulated in squamous cell carcinoma of the head and the neck. Cancer Res 59:991–994

Chariyalertsak S, Sirikulchajanonta V, Mayer D, et al (2001) Aberrant cyclooxygenase isozyme expression in human intrahepatic cholangiocarcinoma. Gut 48:80–86

DiGiovanni J (1992) Multistage carcinogenesis in mouse skin. Pharmacol Ther 54:63–128

Fischer SM, Lo HH, Gordon GB, et al (1999) Chemopreventive activity of Celecoxib, a specific cyclooxygenase-2 inhibitor, and indomethacin against ultraviolet light-induced skin carcinogenesis. Mol Carcinog 25:231–240

Fürstenberger G, Gross M, Marks F (1989) Eicosanoids and multistage carcinogenesis in NMRI mouse skin: role of prostaglandins E and F in conversion (first stage of tumor promotion) and promotion (second stage of tumor promotion). Carcinogenesis 10:91–96

Giardiello F, Hamilton SR, Krush AJ, et al (1993) Treatment of colonic and rectal adenomas with sulindac in familial adenomatous polyposis. N Engl J Med 328:1313–1316

Grubbs CJ, Lubet RA, Koki AT, et al (2000) Celecoxib inhibits N-butyl-N-(4-hydroxybutyl)-nitrosamine-induced urinary bladder cancers in male B6D2F1 mice and female Fischer-344 rats. Cancer Res 60:5599–5602

Gupta RA, DuBois RN (2001) Colorectal cancer prevention and treatment by inhibition of cyclooxygenase-2. Nature Rev Cancer 1:11–21

Hanif R, Pittas A, Feng Y, et al (1996) Effects of nonsteroidal anti-inflammatory drugs on proliferation and on induction of apoptosis in colon cancer cells by prostaglandin-independent pathway. Biochem Pharmacol 62:237–246

Hao Y, Bishop AE, Wallace M, et al (1999) Early expression of cyclooxygenase-2 during sporadic colorectal carcinogenesis. J Pathol 187:295–301

Harris RE, Alshafie GA, Abov-Issa H, et al (2000) Chemoprevention of breast cancer in rats by Celecoxib, a cyclooxygenase-2 inhibitor. Cancer Res 60:2101–2103

Hendel J, Nielsen OH (1997) Expression of cyclooxygenase-2 mRNA in active inflammatory bowel disease. Am J Gastroenterol 92:1170–1173

Howe LR, Crawford HC, Subbaramaiah K, et al (2001) PEA3 is up-regulated in response to Wnt1 and activates the expression of cyclooxygenase-2. J Biol Chem 276:20108–20115

Huang C, Ma WY, Hahnenberger D, Cleary MP, Bowden GT, Dong Z (1997) Inhibition of ultraviolet B-induced activator protein-1 (AP-1) activity by aspirin in AP-1-luciferase transgenic mice. J Biol Chem 272:26325–26331

Hwang D, Scollard D, Byrne J, et al (1998) Expression of cyclooxygenase-1 and cyclooxygenase-2 in human breast cancer. J Natl Cancer Inst 90:455–460

Jacoby RF, Seibert K, Cole CE, et al (2000) The cyclooxygenase-2 inhibitor Celecoxib is a potent preventive and therapeutic agent in the Min mouse model of adenomatous polyposis. Cancer Res 60:5040–5044

Jänne PA, Mayer RJ (2000) Chemoprevention of colorectal cancer. New Engl J Med 342:1960–1968

Kawamori T, Rao CV, Seibert K, et al (1998) Chemopreventive activity of Celecoxib, a specific cyclooxygenase-2 inhibitor, against colon carcinogenesis. Cancer Res 58:409–412

Koga H, Sakisaka S, Ohishi M, et al (1999) Expression of cyclooxygenase-2 in hepatocellular carcinoma: relevance to tumor dedifferentiation. Hepatology 29:688–696

Kulkarni S, Rader JS, Zhang F, et al (2001) Cyclooxygenase-2 is overexpressed in human cervical cancer. Clin Cancer Res 7:429–434

Langenbach R, Loftin C, Lee C, et al (1999) Cyclooxygenase knockout mice. Biochem Pharmacol 58:1237–1246

Lehman JM, Lenhard JM, Oliver BB, et al (1997) Peroxisome proliferator-activated receptors α and γ are activated by indomethacin and other nonsteroidal anti-inflammatory drugs. J Biol Chem 272:3406–3410

Liu CH, Chang SH, Narko K, et al (2001) Overexpression of cyclooxygenase-2 is sufficient to induce tumorigenesis in transgenic mice. J Biol Chem 276:18563–18569

Marks F (1999) Arachidonic acid and companions: an abundant source of biological signals. In: Marks F, Fürstenberger G (eds) Prostaglandins, leukotrienes, and other eicosanoids: Wiley-VCH, Weinheim, pp 1–46

Marks F. (2001) Krebs- und Alzheimer-Prävention mit nicht-steroidalen Entzündungshemmern. Dtsch Med Wschr 126:308–313

Marks F, Fürstenberger G (2000) Cancer chemoprevention through interruption of multistage carcinogenesis: the lessons learnt by comparing mouse skin carcinogenesis and human large bowel cancer. Eur J Cancer 36:314–29

Marks F, Fürstenberger G (1999) Eicosanoids and cancer. In: Marks F, Fürstenberger G (eds) Prostaglandins, leukotrienes, and other eicosanoids. Wiley-VCH, Weinheim, pp 303–330

Marks F, Fürstenberger G (1995) Tumor promotion in skin. In: Arcos CE, Arcos MF, Woo Y-T (eds) Chemical induction of cancer. Birkhäuser, Boston, pp 125–160

Marks F, Fürstenberger G, Müller-Decker K (1999) Metabolic targets of cancer chemoprevention: interruption of tumor development by inhibitors of arachidonic acid metabolism. In: Senn JH, Costa A, Jordan VC (eds) Chemoprevention of cancer. Springer, Berlin, pp 45–67

Marnett LJ, Kalgutkar AS (1999) Cyclooxygenase-2 inhibitors: discovery, selectivity and the future. Trends Pharmacol Sci 20:465–469

Masferrer JL, Leahy KM, Koki AT, et al (2000) Anti-angiogenic and antitumor activities of cyclooxygenase-2 inhibitors. Cancer Res 60:1306–1311

Müller-Decker K (1999) Cyclooxygenases. In: Marks F, Fürstenberger G (eds) Prostaglandins, leukotrienes and other eicosanoids. VCH-Wiley, Weinheim pp 65–88

Müller-Decker K, Scholz K, Marks F, et al (1995) Differential expression of prostaglandin H synthase isozymes during multistage carcinogenesis in mouse epidermis. Mol Carcinog 12:31–41

Müller-Decker K, Kopp-Schneider A, Marks F, et al (1998) Localization of prostaglandin H synthase isozymes in murine epidermal tumors: suppression of skin tumor promotion by PGHS-2 inhibition. Mol Carcinog 23:36–44

Müller-Decker K, Reinerth G, Krieg P, et al (1999a) Expression of prostaglandin-H synthase isozymes in normal human skin and epidermal neoplasias. Int J Cancer 80:648–656

Müller-Decker K, Albert C, Lukanov T, et al (1999b) Cellular localization of cyclooxygenase isozymes in Crohn's disease and colorectal cancer. Int J Colorectal Dis 14:212–218

Müller-Decker K, Hirschner W, Marks F, et al (2002a) The effects of cyclooxygenase isozyme inhibition on incisional wound healing in mouse skin. J Invest Dermatol 119:1189–1195

Müller-Decker K, Neufang G, Berger I, et al (2002b) Transgenic cyclooxygenase-2 overexpression sensitizes mouse skin for carcinogenesis. Proc Natl Acad Sci USA 99:12483–12488

Mutoh M, Watanabe K, Kitamura T, et al (2002) Involvement of prostaglandin E receptor subtype EP(4) in colon carcinogenesis. Cancer Res 62:28–32

Narumiya S, Sugimoto J, Ushikubi F (1999) Prostanoid receptors: structures, properties, and function. Pharmacol Rev 79:1193–1226.

Neufang G, Fürstenberger G, Heidt M, et al (2001) Abnormal differentiation of epidermis in transgenic mice constitutively expressing cyclooxygenase-2 in skin. Proc Natl Acad Sci USA 98:7629–7634

Nishimura G, Yanoma S, Mizuno H, et al (1999) A selective cyclooxygenase-2 inhibitor suppresses tumor growth in nude mouse xenografted with human head and neck squamous carcinoma cells. Jpn J Cancer Res 90:1152–1162

Oshima M, Dinchuk JE, Kargman SL, et al (1996) Suppression of intestinal polyposis in APC$^{\delta716}$ knockout mice by inhibition of cyclooxygenase-2 (COX-2). Cell 67:803–809

Oshima M, Murai N, Kargman S, et al (2001) Chemoprevention of intestinal polyposis in the APC$^{\Delta716}$ mouse by Rofecoxib, a specific cyclooxygenase-2 inhibitor. Cancer Res 61:1733–1740

Pentland AP, Schoggins JW, Scott GA, et al (1999) Reduction of UV-induced skin tumors in hairless mice by selective COX-2 inhibition. Carcinogenesis 20:1939–1944

Poon R, Smits R, Li C, et al (2001) Cyclooxygenase-2 modulates proliferation in aggressive fibromatosis (desmoid tumor). Oncogene 20:451–460

Ratnasinghe D, Tanrea J, Roth MJ, et al (1999) Expression of cyclooxygenase-2 in human squamous cell carcinoma of the esophagus: an immunohistochemical study. Anticancer Res 19:171–174

Reddy BS, Hirose Y, Lubet R, et al (2000) Chemoprevention of colon cancer by specific cyclooxygenase-2 inhibitor, Celecoxib, administered during different stages of carcinogenesis. Cancer Res 60:293–297

Rigas B, Shiff SJ (2000) Is inhibition of cycloxygenase required for the chemopreventive effect of NSAIDs in colon cancer? A model reconciling the current contradiction. Med Hypotheses 54:210–215

Ristimäki A, Honkanen N, Jänkälä H, et al (1997) Expression of cyclooxygenase-2 in human gastric carcinoma. Cancer Res 57:1270–1280

Ristimäki A, Nieminen O, Saukkonen K, et al (2001) Expression of cyclooxygenase-2 in human transitional cell carcinoma of the urinary bladder. Am J Pathol 158:849–853

Rivers JK, Arlette J, Shear N, et al (2002) Topical treatment of actinic keratoses with 3.0% diclofenac in 2.5% hyaluronan gel. Brit J Dermatol 146:1–7

Sawaoka H, Kawano S, Tsujii S, et al (1998) Helicobacter pylori infection induces cyclooxygenase-2 expression in human gastric mucosa. Prostaglandins Leukot Essent Fatty Acids 59:313–316

Scholz K, Fürstenberger G, Müller-Decker K, et al (1995) Differential expression of prostaglandin-H synthase isoenzymes in normal and activated keratinocytes in vivo and in vitro. Biochem J 309:263–269

Schwenger P, Alpert D, Skolnik EY, et al (1998) Activation of p38 mitogen-activated protein kinase by sodium salicylate leads to inhibition of tumor necrosis factor-induced IkappaB alpha phosphorylation and degradation. Mol Cell Biol 18:78–84

Schwenger P, Bellosta P, Victor I, et al (1997) Sodium salicylate inhibits apoptosis via p38 mitogene-activated protein kinase but inhibits TNFα-induced cJun N-terminal kinase/stress-activated protein kinase activation. Proc Natl Acad Sci 94:2869–2873

Sharpe CR, Collet J-P, McNurr M, et al (2000) Nested case-control study of the effects of nonsteroidal anti-inflammatory drugs on breast cancer risk and stage. Br J Cancer 83:112–120

Shiota G, Okubo M, Noumi T, et al (1999) Cyclooxygenase-2 expression in hepato-cellular carcinoma. Hepatogastroenterology 46:407–412

Shiotani H, Denda A, Yamamota K, et al (2001) Increased expression of cyclooxygenase-2 protein in 4-nitroquinoline-1-oxide-induced rat tongue carcinomas and chemopreventive efficacy of a specific inhibitor, Nimesulide. Cancer Res 61:1451–1456

Shono T, Tofilon PJ, Bruner JM, et al (2001) Cyclooxygenase-2 expression in human gliomas: prognostic significance and molecular correlations. Cancer Res 61:4375–4381

Shureiqi I, Lippman SM (2001) Lipoxygenase modulation to reverse carcinogenesis. Cancer Res 61:6307–6312

Singer II, Kawka DW, Schloemann S, et al (1999) Cyclooxygenase-2 is induced in colonic epithelial cells in inflammatory bowel disease. Gastroenterology 115:297–306

Smalley WE, DuBois RN (1997) Colorectal cancer and nonsteroidal anti-inflammatory drugs. Adv Pharmacol 39:1–20

Sonoshita, M, Takaku K, Sasaki N, et al (2001) Acceleration of intestinal polyposis through prostaglandin receptor EP2 in *Apc* Δ^{716} knockout mice. Nature Med 9:1048–1051

Steinbach G, Lynch PM, Phillips RKS, et al (2000) The effect of Celecoxib, a cyclooxygenase-2 inhibitor, in familial adenomatous polyposis. New Engl J Med 342:1946–1952

Tegeder I, Pfeilschifter J, Geisslinger G (2001) Cyclooxygenase-independent actions of cyclo-oxygenase inhibitors. FASEB J 15:2057–2072

Tiano HF, Chulada PC, Spalding J, et al (1998) Effects of cyclooxygenase deficiency on inflammation and papilloma formation in mouse skin. Proc Am Assoc Cancer Res 38:253

Tiano HF, Loftin CD, Akunda J, et al (2002) Deficiency of either cyclooxygenase COX-1 or COX-2 alters epidermal differentiation and reduces mouse skin tumorigenesis. Cancer Res 62:3395–3401

Tsuji S, Tsujii M, Kawano S, et al (2001) Cyclooxygenase-2 upregulation as a perigenetic change in carcinogenesis. J Exp Clin Cancer Res 20:117–129

Tucker ON, Dannenberg AJ, Yang EK, et al (1999) Cyclooxygenase expression is up-regulated in human pancreatic cancer. Cancer Res 59:987–990

Vane JR, Bakhle YS (1998) Botting RM Cycloxygenase 1 and 2. Annu Rev Pharmacol Toxicol 38:97–120

Watanabe K, Kawamori T, Nakatsugi S, et al (1999) Role of the prostaglandin E receptor subtype EP1 in colon carcinogenesis. Cancer Res 59:5093–5096

Watanabe K, Kawamori T, Nakatsugi S, et al (2000) Inhibitory effect of a prostaglandin E receptor subtype E1 selective antagonist. ONO-8713, on development of azoxymethane-induced aberrant crypt foci in mice. Cancer Lett 156:57–61

Watkins DN, Lenzo JC, Segal A, et al (1999) Expression and localization of cyclo-oxygenase isoforms in nonsmall cell lung cancer. Eur Respir J 11:412–418

Williams GS, Watson AJ, Sheng H, et al (2000) Celecoxib prevents tumor growth in vivo without toxicity to normal gut: lack of correlation between in vitro and in vivo models. Cancer Res 60:8045–8051

Wilson KT, Fu S, Ramanujam KS, et al (1998) Increased expression of inducible nitric oxide synthase and cyclooxygenase-2 in Barrett's esophagus and associated adenocarcinomas. Cancer Res 58:2929–2934

Winde G, Schmid KW, Brandt B, et al (1997) Clinical and genomic influence of sulindac on retal mucosa in familial adenomatous polyposis. Dis Colon Rectum 40:1156–1169

Wolff H, Saukonen K, Anttila S, et al (1998) Expression of cyclooxygenase-2 in human lung carcinoma. Cancer Res 58:4997–5001

Yin MY, Yamamoto Y, Gaynor RB (1998) The anti-inflammatory agents aspirin and salicylate inhibit the activity of I kappa B kinase-beta. Nature 396:77–80

Yoshimura R, Sano H, Masuda C, et al (2000) Expression of cyclooxygenase-2 in prostate carcinoma. Cancer 89:589–596

Zhang F, Subbaramaiah K, Altorki N, Dannenberg AJ (1998) Dihydroxy bile acids activate the transcription of cyclooxygenase-2. J Biol Chem 273:2424–2436

Zhang X, Morham SG, Langenbach R, Young DA (1999) Malignant transformation and antineoplastic actions of nonsteroidal antiinflammatory drugs (NSAIDs) on cyclooxygenase-null embryo fibroblasts. J Exp Med 190:451–459

Zhang X, Morham SG, Langenbach R, et al (2000) Lack of cyclooxygenase-2 inhibits growth of teratocarcinomas in mice. Exp Cell Res 254:232–240

Zimmermann KC, Sarbi M, Weber AA et al (1999) Cyclooxygenase-2 expression in human esophageal carcinoma. Cancer Res 59:198–204

Preclinical Models for Chemoprevention of Colon Cancer

Eugene W. Gerner, Natalia A. Ignatenko, David G. Besselsen

E.W. Gerner (✉)
Arizona Radiation Oncology, The University of Arizona, 1515 N Campbell, P.O. Box 240524, Tucson, AZ 85724, USA

Abstract

Colon cancer is the second leading cause of cancer incidence and death in the USA in 2002. Specific genetic defects have been identified which cause hereditary colon cancers in humans. In addition, a number of intestinal luminal risk factors for colon cancer have been described. This information has been exploited to develop experimental cell and rodent models which recapitulate features of human colon cancer. In this chapter, we will discuss the strengths and limitations of these models to further our understanding of basic mechanisms of colon carcinogenesis and to develop strategies for colon cancer chemoprevention.

Keywords Cell and rodent models · Colon cancer · Chemoprevention · Inherited intestinal cancer syndromes

Abbreviations APC, adenomatous polyposis coli; CEA, carcinoembryonic antigen; COX-2, cyclooxygenase-2; DFMO, difluoromethylornithine; EGFR, epidermal growth factor receptor; EP_2, a cell-surface receptor of PGE_2; FAP, familial adenomatous polyposis; HNPCC, hereditary nonpolyposis colon cancer; LOH, loss of heterozygosity; Min, multiple intestinal neoplasia; MMR, mismatch repair; MUC2, mucin-2; NOS2, nitric oxide synthase 2; NSAID, nonsteroidal anti-inflammatory drugs; ODC, ornithine decarboxylase; PGE_2, prostaglandin E_2.

Introduction

Genes involved in several inherited intestinal cancer syndromes in humans have been identified over the past 15 years. These include the adenomatous polyposis coli (APC) tumor suppressor gene in familial adenomatous polypo-

Recent Results in Cancer Research, Vol. 163
© Springer-Verlag Berlin Heidelberg 2003

sis (FAP) (Groden et al. 1991; Kinzler et al. 1991), several mismatch repair (MMR) genes in hereditary nonpolyposis colon cancer (HNPCC) (Fishel et al. 1993; Nicolaides et al. 1994; Papadopoulos et al. 1994), and the transforming growth factor (TGF)-β signaling gene SMAD4 in juvenile polyposis (Howe et al. 1998).

One of these genes, APC, seems to be especially relevant in sporadic, or nonheritable, colon cancers in the USA. While FAP accounts for less than 2% of colon cancers in the USA, single allele mutations in the APC tumor suppressor gene have been detected in greater than 90% of somatic cells in sporadic colon polyps and colon cancers in humans (Iwamoto et al. 2000). This result suggests that the process of colon carcinogenesis in humans selects for APC mutations. Since APC mutations are detected in both small and large polyps, it appears that APC mutation is an early event in this disease process.

Since APC is mutated in essentially all colon polyps, it is a rational target for colon cancer chemoprevention strategies. Restoring loss of function of APC in somatic intestinal mucosal cells is not currently readily achievable. Alternatively, identifying downstream mediators of APC may uncover "gain of function" gene products which might be more tractable targets for chemoprevention strategies. Preclinical models, exploiting known genetic and intestinal luminal risk factors in human colon carcinogenesis, provide important tools to develop rational approaches to colon cancer chemoprevention. Pathophysiological targets, such as APC, can be investigated along with potential modifier genes. Potential gene–environment interactions can be investigated in preclinical models.

During the last decade, several clinical lung cancer chemoprevention trials were discontinued early due to the unexpected induction of excess cancers by the interventions (Albanes et al. 1996; Omenn et al. 1996). A general consensus was that a more complete understanding of relevant biological mechanisms, using appropriate preclinical models, should have been obtained prior to conducting these large-scale clinical trials (Pryor et al. 2000). These lung cancer chemoprevention studies underscore the importance of preclinical studies in experimental models to extensively evaluate the biological mechanisms involved in any specific chemoprevention strategy.

Preclinical Models Should Recapitulate Features of Human Colon Cancer

It is generally agreed that human colon carcinogenesis proceeds by a step-wise progression of normal mucosa to noninvasive colon polyps to invasive, and finally metastatic, adenocarcinomas (Kronborg and Fenger 1999). Preclinical models should recapitulate features of this process. Human colon cancer is influenced by specific genetic and intestinal luminal risk factors. Preclinical models should be able to incorporate these risk factors in experiments designed to evaluate specific chemoprevention strategies. Human colon carcinogenesis is influenced by interactions between colonic epithelial cells and stro-

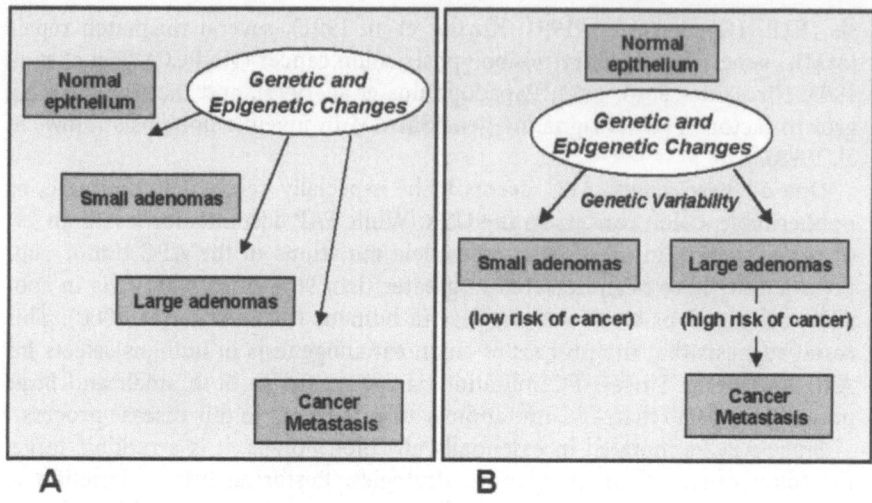

Fig. 1A, B. Molecular genetic models of colon carcinogenesis. Panel **A** predicts a step-wise progression from normal mucosa to small adenomas to large adenomas and finally invasive cancer and metastases (Fearon and Vogelstein 1990) This progression is mediated by both genetic and epigenetic changes in the colorectal mucosa. Panel **B** is a modification of this model. The same genetic and epigenetic changes associated with the progression from normal to neoplastic colonic tissue are included in this model, but genetic variability in these alterations, or in downstream mediators of these early genetic/ epigenetic alterations, is predicted to be an important determinant in this progression

ma (Bosman et al. 1993). Inflammation may be involved in this disease process (Katori and Majima 2000).

It is well recognized that not all colon polyps will progress to invasive cancers in humans (Kronborg and Fenger 1999). A recent analysis from Martinez et al. (Martinez et al. 2001) of a large polyp prevention trial, conducted at the Arizona Cancer Center and affiliated institutions, found that recurrent polyp size and risk of colon cancer was strongly related to polyp size determined at entry into the trial. This finding suggests a modification to the widely accepted view of the molecular processes involved in the polyp-carcinoma sequence, as proposed by Fearon and Vogelstein (Fearon and Vogelstein 1990) and depicted in Fig. 1. Given the bulk of evidence for monoclonal derivation of cancer, and understanding that the neoplastic cells in the initial polyp were removed at the entry colonoscopy, it would be expected that recurrent polyp size would be normally distributed to reflect stocastic events in carcinogenesis and be independent of initial polyp size. The boundary conditions, that APC is mutated in essentially all polyps (Iwamoto et al. 2000) and recurrent polyp size is related to initial polyp size, fit the model (also shown in Fig. 1) that APC is an early genetic alteration in colon carcinogenesis and that subsequent cancer risk is influenced by variability in APC or other genetic factors. This model predicts that carcinogenesis resulting from certain initiating events (e.g., chemical carcinogens, genetic risk factors) will be influenced by genetic variability of downstream mediators of these initiators. Second, the model predicts that responses to some chemoprevention strategies may be influenced by genetic variability among individuals. Evidence exists to support both of these predictions, as will be discussed later in this chapter.

Classes of Preclinical Models for Colon Cancer Chemoprevention

Three general classes of preclinical models have proven useful in studies of chemoprevention strategies. These classes include chemical carcinogen-treated rodents, genetically altered cell lines and genetically altered rodents. Each class of preclinical models has strengths and weaknesses.

Carcinogen-treated rodents have been used for some time. Table 1 lists a number of chemicals which induce colon carcinogenesis in rodents. A strength of the carcinogen-treated rodent model of colon carcinogenesis is that these animals develop cancer via the adenoma-carcinoma sequence in a similar manner as that observed in human colon carcinogenesis (Thurnherr et al. 1973; Maskens and Dujardin-Loits 1981). Both benign colonic adenomas and invasive adenocarcinomas, which develop in dimethylhydrazine- or azoxymethane-treated rodents, contain mutated genes, such as APC and K-ras, which are also found to be mutated in human colon tumors (Erdman et al. 1997; Maltzman et al. 1997). These models have been useful in identifying biochemical changes in both stromal and epithelial cells during colon carcinogenesis (Takahashi et al. 2000). This model has been widely used to evaluate the efficacy of chemopreventive agents (Reddy 2000; Wargovich et al. 2000). Chemical carcinogen-treated rodents were used to identify the efficacy of both calcium supplementation (Sitrin et al. 1991) and COX-2 inhibitors (Kawamori et al. 1998) to inhibit colon carcinogenesis. The utility of these preclinical models was highlighted by subsequent clinical trials in humans, which found that calcium supplementation inhibited colon polyp recurrence (Baron et al. 1999) and one COX-2 inhibitor suppressed polyp formation in FAP patients (Steinbach et al. 2000).

A weakness of this model is that exposure to chemical carcinogens, and specifically dimethyhydrazine or azoxymethane, is not generally associated with human colon cancers. Further, these carcinogens cause mutations in many genes which may or may not be involved in human colon carcinogene-

Table 1. Chemical carcinogens inducing colon tumors in rodents

Chemical carcinogen	Reference
1,2-dimethylhydrazine	Thurnherr et al. 1973
Azoxymethane	Reddy et al. 1975
N-methyl-N-nitrosourea (instilled intrarectally)	Cohen et al. 1982
2-Amino-3,4-dimethylimidazo[4,5-f] quinoline (MeIQ)	Fujita et al. 1999
1-Hydroxyanthraquinone (1-HA) plus methylazoxymethanol (MAM) acetate	Suzui et al. 2001 (Suzui, Sugie, et al. 2001)

sis. Carcinogen-treatment also damages cells and tissues other than those that may be involved in colon carcinogenesis in humans. These unintended effects of the chemical carcinogens could impair processes involved in responses to certain chemoprevention strategies.

Genetically altered cells have also proven to be useful preclinical models in chemoprevention studies. Genetically altered cells can be used to assess mechanisms, which may be relevant in clinical trials in humans. The role of activated K-ras in responses to the nonsteroidal anti-inflammatory drug (NSAID) Sulindac was evaluated in rodent cells, expressing a normal K-ras, transfected with a mutant K-ras (Arber et al. 1997). The activated K-ras was found to confer resistance to Sulindac. This finding has been recently corroborated in molecular studies humans with FAP, which suggest that K-ras mutations are associated with Sulindac resistance in these patients (Keller et al. 2001).

Genetically Altered Mouse Models of Colon Carcinogenesis

An important class of preclinical models includes genetically altered rodents. An ever-expanding list of genetically altered mouse strains has been developed to evaluate the role of specific genes and their modifiers in colon carcinogenesis. Mice with genetically altered APC have been widely studied (Table 2). The first mouse model with a genetic defect in APC (stop codon at codon 850) was the *Min* (multiple intestinal neoplasia) mouse, developed by Moser et al. (Moser et al. 1990). The strength of this model is that the genotype (mutant APC) is associated with a relevant phenotype (intestinal tumors) (Su et al. 1992). A weakness of this model is that the animals develop benign, but not invasive, intestinal cancers (Fig. 2).

Histologically, adenomas in the C57BL/6 Min mouse are composed of well-delineated, tubular and/or villous structures that are lined by dysplastic mucosal epithelium. The degree of dysplasia is characterized as low (retaining basal nuclear polarity and low N/C ratio) or high (loss of nuclear polarity and high N/C ratio). Invasion beyond the muscularis mucosa and desmoplasia are not observed.

Human FAP has also been studied using the mouse strain $APC^{\Delta716}$ (Oshima et al. 1995). The $APC^{\Delta716}$ animals have a knockout mutation in one of the APC alleles. These animals develop numerous polyps in the intestinal tract as early as 3 weeks of age due to loss of the remaining wild-type APC allele in the proliferative zone cells [i.e., loss of heterozygosity (LOH)] by the second hit. Conversely, polyps could arise in FAP patients as a result of heterozygosity for an APC mutation with minimal genetic changes (Miyaki et al. 1990). Additional studies should explain this discrepancy, since APC gene LOH is not the only mechanism in human FAP. The $APC^{\Delta716}$ mutant mouse strain provides a useful model system for analyzing various carcinogens and evaluating anticancer and chemopreventive agents (Oshima et al. 1995, 1996).

Genetic alteration of other genes, either in combination with mutated APC or alone, have also been reported to affect formation of invasive colon cancers

Table 2. Genetically altered mouse models of intestinal carcinogenesis

Genotype	Phenotype	Reference
Min (APC stop codon 850), phenotype selected from carcinogen-treated pregnant mice	Multiple noninvasive intestinal tumors (primarily small intestinal)	Moser et al. 1990; Su et al. 1992
APC (1638N)	Same as above, but fewer small intestinal tumors, colonic tumors persist	Fodde et al. 1994
APC (delta 716)	Same as above, but more small intestinal tumors	Oshima et al. 1995
Min × Ptgs-1 (COX-1) knockout	Fewer intestinal tumors	Chulada et al. 2000
Min or APC (delta 716) × Ptgs2 (COX-2) knockout	Fewer intestinal tumors	Oshima et al. 1996; Chulada et al. 2000
Min × MMP7 (matrilysin) knockout	Fewer intestinal tumors	Wilson et al.
Min × Pla2g4 knockout (group II secretory phospholypase)	Fewer intestinal tumors	Cormier et al. 1997, 2000
Min × NOS2 knockout	Fewer intestinal tumors	Ahn and Ohshima, 2001
Min × NOS2 knockout	More intestinal tumors	Scott et al. 2001
Min × Mlh1 knockout	More tumors, but no increase in size or invasion	Shoemaker et al. 2000
Min × Mlh2 knockout	more small intestinal and colonic tumors	Lal et al. 2001
Min × p53 targeted disruption	More tumors, increase in invasion	Halberg et al. 2000
Min × Dnmt1 $^{N/+}$	Decreases tumor multiplicity	Cormier and Dove 2000
PI3Kγ p110 catalytic subunit knockout	Invasive colon cancers	Sasaki et al. 2000
APC (delta 716) × SMAD4 knockout (+/-)	Bigger tumors	Takaku et al. 1998
APC (1638N) × H-2K^b transgenic	Invasive colon tumors	Horig et al. 2001
APC (delta 716) × EP$_2$ knockout	Fewer intestinal tumors	Sonoshita et al. 2001
APC (1638N) × MUC2 knockout	Invasive colon cancers	Velcich et al. 2002

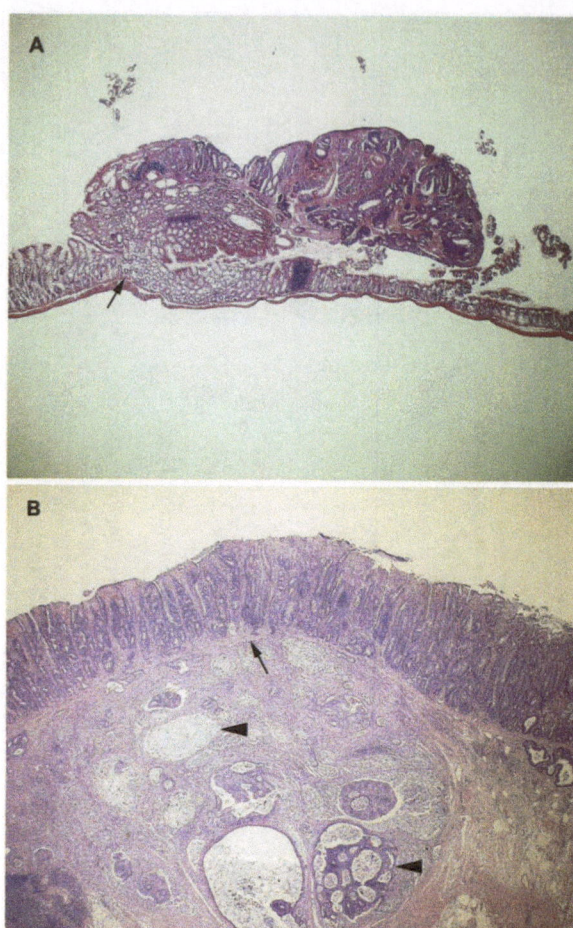

Fig. 2A, B. Histologic appearances of (**A**) a colonic adenoma in a Min mouse and (**B**) a colonic adeno-carcinoma from an AOM-treated mouse (Courtesy Mouse Models of Human Cancer Consortium). Note lack of invasion through the muscularis mucosa (*arrow*) in the Min mouse adenoma. Extensive invasion beyond the muscularis mucosa (*arrow*) with formation of mucinous lakes and islands of neoplastic tubular structures (*arrowheads*) are observed in the AOM-treated mouse. H&E, ×6.6

and may be better models of sporadic colon carcinogenesis in humans (Table 2). Several combined models were developed based on the APC$^{\Delta716}$ mouse model. A knockout mutation of the COX-2 gene (*Ptgs2*) was introduced into the APC$^{\Delta716}$ knockout mice to assess the role of COX-2 in colorectal tumorigenesis (Dinchuk et al. 1995). It has been found that expression of COX-2 is markedly elevated in the polyp stromal cells, and that inhibition of the COX-2 gene can suppress intestinal polyposis, either by introduction of a COX-2 gene knockout mutation or by treatment of the APC$^{\Delta716}$ mice with COX-2 inhibitors (Oshima et al. 1996). This mouse model helped establish the rationale for treating colonic polyposis in FAP patients with COX-2 inhibitors (Taketo 1998; Steinbach et al. 2000). APC$^{\Delta716}$ mice combined with mice carrying homozygous deletion of the gene encoding EP$_2$ (a cell-surface receptor of PGE$_2$) were employed to determine the mechanism of the Cox-2 metabolite prostaglandin E$_2$ (PGE$_2$) induction in tissues of intestinal adenoma and colon cancer. The APC$^{\Delta716}$ EP$_2$($^{-/-}$) mice develop smaller number and size of intestinal polyps, a phenotype similar to the COX-2 gene compound mice (Sonoshita et al. 2001).

The APC$^{\Delta716}$ mouse model was also crossed with a mutation in *Smad4*, a gene involved in the TGF-β signaling. Compound mutant mice develop very invasive adenocarcinomas that are much larger than the APC$^{\Delta716}$ polyp adenomas (Takaku et al. 1998). The APC$^{\Delta716}$ model and its crosses with *Ptgs2*, *Smad4* and EP$_2$ knockouts have been used recently to investigate angiogenesis during intestinal polyp development (Seno et al. 2002).

Besides stop codon mutations 716 and 850, other APC mouse mutations (1638N, 1638T, 1572T) have been developed to study chromosomal instability in the adenoma-carcinoma sequence process. As seen in Table 2, mutations in APC occurring in the mutation cluster region for humans (e.g., 1638N) result in fewer small intestinal, but persistent colon tumors (Fodde et al. 1994), a phenotype more characteristic of human colon carcinogenesis. A set of APC mouse mutations (850, 1638N, 1638T, 1572T) is characterized by different degrees of β-catenin signaling defects for both in vitro and in vivo studies (Fodde and Smits 2001). Using mouse models with these APC mutations, Fodde and his research team (unpublished data) were able to show that APC regulates the differentiation number of stem cells in the colonic crypt and that loss of APC function may result in growth of crypt stem cell population. These strengths and weaknesses suggest that the Min mouse is a reasonable model for early stages of FAP, before invasive intestinal tumors develop, recapitulating the intestinal tumor phenotype of human FAP patients.

Mouse models that have been reported to develop invasive colon cancers include Min mice carrying the p53 deficiency (Halberg et al. 2000), APC (1638N) mice crossed with transgenic mice expressing the human carcinoembryonic antigen (CEA) (Horig et al. 2001), and knockout mice failing to express the p110 subunit of the P(I)3 γ kinase (Sasaki et al. 2000) or the mucin-2 (MUC2) gene (Velcich et al. 2002). The APC 1638N mouse model was also bred with a recently generated transgenic mouse Tg-K-ras^{V12G} (encoding for the human K-ras gene mutated at codon 12 under the control of the intestine-specific villin promoter). The APC1638N/TG-K-ras^{V12G} animals develop 10 times more intestinal tumors then APC1638N mice, and these tumors have the ability to invade (Fodde et al. 2002). Intestinal tumors from these animals exhibit an increased chromosomal instability level when compared to original APC 1638N tumors. These animals are suitable for studying downstream effectors, which are responsible for both tumor initiation and progression in the gastrointestinal tract. Convincing documentation of the invasive colon tumor phenotype remains to be reported for some of these genetic mouse models of colon carcinogenesis.

In general, various APC knockout mice are limited by their lack of large numbers of colonic adenomas and aberrant crypt foci. Several studies have conducted genetic analysis of the human MMR system. Mutations in human MMR genes are associated with increased cancer risk and result in hereditary nonpolyposis coli (HNPCC). On the molecular level, HNPCC tumors exhibit a replication error phenotype that is reflected in genetic instability. The majority of HNPCC patients have mutations in *MSH2* and *MLH1* genes which are the mammalian homologs of the *E.coli mutS* and *mutL* genes. Mouse lines with knockouts of these genes have been generated (de Wind et al. 1995; Reitmair et al. 1996). These mouse lines provide excellent model systems to study the individual roles of the mammalian MutS homologs in MMR and to determine their importance for cancer suppression. Lal et al. reports of a combined DNA mismatch-repair-deficient Min mouse model ($Apc^{\Delta716}$ -$Msh2^{-/-}$) that has genetic features of both FAP and HNPCC and develops numerous small and large-intestinal adenomas, as well as colonic aberrant crypt foci (Lal et al. 2001). Loss of function of the other two mismatch repair proteins, MSH3 and MSH6, which form heterodimeric protein complexes MSH2-MSH3 and MSH2-MSH6 necessary for mismatch recognition in humans, causes a partial MMR defect (Edelmann et al. 1997, 2000). MSH3 and MSH6 knockout mice that also carry the APC 1638N allele acquire an accelerated rate of intestinal tumor formation and increased morbidity (Kuraguchi et al. 2001).

It appears that knowledge coming from different rodent models offers an effective way of studying tumorigenesis and testing clinical chemopreventive agents.

Downstream Mediators of APC: Relevant Pathophysiological Targets in Colon Cancer Chemoprevention

A variety of genes have been identified which confer phenotypes, including colonic neoplasia in rodents (Table 2). APC has been implicated in intestinal neoplasia in rodents and humans (Iwamoto et al. 2000). Thus, APC is a rational pathophysiological target for colon cancer chemoprevention. Methods to restore APC loss of function, targeting APC directly, are not obvious. However, APC is known to regulate the expression of a number of genes (He et al. 1998). Some of the genes, whose expression is altered by loss of APC function, are upregulated. These "gain of function" downstream mediators of loss of APC function are also rational targets for colon cancer chemoprevention (Fig. 3). Further, targeting these downstream mediators may prove to be more feasible than targeting APC itself.

COX-2 is upregulated by loss of APC function in human colon tumor-derived cells (Hsi et al. 1999). Ornithine decarboxylase (ODC), the first enzyme in polyamine synthesis, is also upregulated in this human cell model (Fultz and Gerner 2002) and in Min mice (Erdman et al. 1999). Genetic studies discussed above indicate that elimination of COX-2 alleles in mice suppress APC-dependent intestinal carcinogenesis. Selective inhibitors of COX-2 (Jacoby et

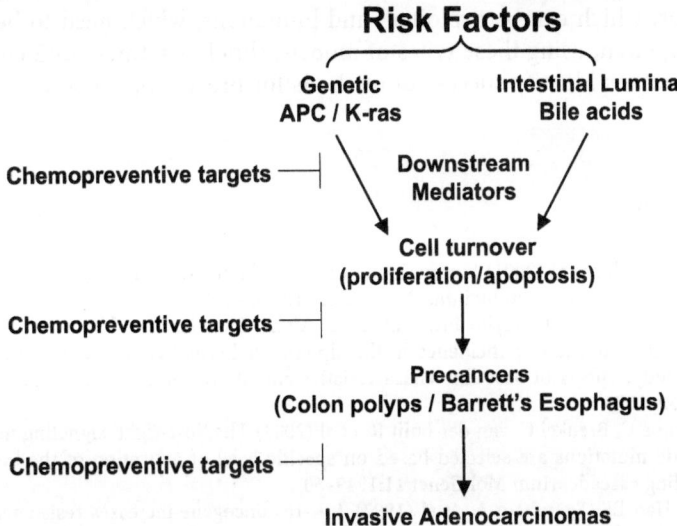

Fig. 3. Identification of downstream mediators of genetic and/or intestinal luminal risk factors as rational targets for chemoprevention strategies. Restoring loss of function of inactivated tumor suppressor genes is currently not technically feasible. As indicated in this model, loss of tumor suppressor gene functions can be associated with gain of function of downstream mediators of the tumor suppressor gene. These gain of function genes may be better targets for chemoprevention strategies

al. 2000) and ODC (Erdman et al. 1999) suppress intestinal tumor number in Min mice. These observations have provided the rationale for combination chemoprevention trials in humans using inhibitors of COX-2 and ODC (Meyskens and Gerner 1999).

The idea of combination chemoprevention was proposed over 20 years ago (Sporn 1980). A variety of other combination chemoprevention strategies for colon carcinogenesis may be successful in humans. As shown in Table 2, knockouts of several genes suppress APC-dependent intestinal carcinogenesis. EGFR (epidermal growth factor receptor) may also be a rational target for colon cancer chemoprevention (Torrance et al. 2000; Roberts et al. 2002).

Genetically altered rodent models have also been used to assess the role of specific genes in responses to chemopreventive agents. Halberg et al. (Halberg et al. 2000) constructed Min x p53 knockout mice to investigate the role of the p53 tumor suppressor gene in responses to inhibitors of ODC and COX-2. The tumor suppressing activities of piroxicam and DFMO were found to be independent of p53 function in this model.

Conclusions

At least three major types of preclinical models of colon carcinogenesis have been shown to contribute to the development and implementation of colon cancer chemoprevention strategies in humans. Each model has specific strengths, which can be exploited, and limitations, which need to be considered. Research, using these types of models, should continue until clinical trials in humans identify successful methods for preventing colon cancer in humans.

References

Ahn B and Ohshima H (2001) Suppression of intestinal polyposis in Apc(Min/+) mice by inhibiting nitric oxide production. Cancer Res 61:8357–8360

Albanes D, Heinonen OP, Taylor PR, et al (1996) Alpha-Tocopherol and beta-carotene supplements and lung cancer incidence in the alpha-tocopherol, beta-carotene cancer prevention study: effects of base-line characteristics and study compliance. J Natl Cancer Inst 88:1560–1570

Albuquerque C, Breukel C, van der Luijt R, et al (2002) The 'just-right' signaling model: APC somatic mutations are selected based on specific level of activation of the beta-catenin signaling cascade. Hum Mol Genet 11:1549–60

Arber N, Han EK, Sgambato A, et al (1997) A K-ras oncogene increases resistance to sulindac-induced apoptosis in rat enterocytes. Gastroenterology 113:1892–1900

Baron JA, Beach M, Mandel JS, et al (1999) Calcium supplements for the prevention of colorectal adenomas. Calcium Polyp Prevention Study Group. N Engl J Med 340:101–107

Bosman FT, de Bruine A, Flohil C, et al (1993) Epithelial-stromal interactions in colon cancer. Int J Dev Biol 37:203–211

Chulada PC, Thompson MB, Mahler JF, et al (2000) Genetic disruption of Ptgs-1, as well as Ptgs-2, reduces intestinal tumorigenesis in Min mice. Cancer Res 60:4705–4708

Cohen BI, Raicht RF, Mahler JF, et al (1982) Reduction of N-methyl-N-nitrosourea-induced colon tumors in the rat by cholesterol. Cancer Res 42:5050–5052

Cormier RT and Dove WF (2000) Dnmt1 N/+ reduces the net growth rate and multiplicity of intestinal adenomas in C57BL/6-multiple intestinal neoplasia (Min)/+ mice independently of p53 but demonstrates strong synergy with the modifier of Min 1(AKR) resistance allele. Cancer Res 60:3965–3970

Cormier RT, Hong KH, Halberg RB, et al (1997) Secretory phospholipase Pla2g2a confers resistance to intestinal tumorigenesis. Nat Genet 17:88–91

de Wind N, Dekker M, Bernset A, et al (1995) Inactivation of the mouse Msh2 gene results in mismatch repair deficiency, methylation tolerance, hyperrecombination, and predisposition to cancer. Cell 82:321–330

Dinchuk JE, Car BD, Focht RJ, et al (1995) Renal abnormalities and an altered inflammatory response in mice lacking cyclooxygenase II. Nature 378:406–409

Edelmann W, Umar A, Yang K, et al (2000) The DNA mismatch repair genes Msh3 and Msh6 cooperate in intestinal tumor suppression. Cancer Res 60:803–807

Edelmann W, Yang K, Umar A, et al (1997) Mutation in the mismatch repair gene Msh6 causes cancer susceptibility. Cell 91:467–477

Erdman SH, Ignatenko NA, Powell MB, et al (1999) APC-dependent changes in expression of genes influencing polyamine metabolism, and consequences for gastrointestinal carcinogenesis, in the Min mouse. Carcinogenesis 20:1709–1713

Erdman SH, Wu HD, Hixson LJ, et al (1997) Assessment of mutations in Ki-ras and p53 in colon cancers from azoxymethane- and dimethylhydrazine-treated rats. Mol Carcinog 19:137–144

Fearon ER and Vogelstein B (1990) A genetic model for colorectal tumorigenesis. Cell 61:759–767

Fishel R, Lescoe MK, Rao MR, et al (1993) The human mutator gene homolog MSH2 and its association with hereditary nonpolyposis colon cancer. Cell 75:1027–1038

Fodde R, Edelmann W, Yang K, et al (1994) A targeted chain-termination mutation in the mouse Apc gene results in multiple intestinal tumors. Proc Natl Acad Sci USA 91:8969–8973

Fodde R and Smits R (2001) Disease model: familial adenomatous polyposis. Trends Mol Med 7:369–373

Fujita T, Hara A, Yamazaki Y, et al (1999) The value of acute-phase protein measurements after curative gastric cancer surgery. Arch Surg 134:73–75

Fultz KE and Gerner EW (2002) APC-regulation of ornithine decarboxylase in human colon tumor cells. Mol Carcinog 34:10–18

Groden J, Thliveris A, Samowitz W, et al (1991) Identification and characterization of the familial adenomatous polyposis coli gene. Cell 66:589–600

Halberg RB, Katzung DS, Hoff PD, et al (2000) Tumorigenesis in the multiple intestinal neoplasia mouse: redundancy of negative regulators and specificity of modifiers. Proc Natl Acad Sci USA 97:3461–3466

He TC, Sparks AB, Rago C, et al (1998) Identification of c-MYC as a target of the APC pathway. Science 281:1509–1512

Horig H, Wainstein A, Long L, et al (2001) A new mouse model for evaluating the immunotherapy of human colorectal cancer. Cancer Res 61:8520–8526

Howe JR, Roth S, Ringold JC, et al (1998) Mutations in the SMAD4/DPC4 gene in juvenile polyposis. Science 280:1086–1088

Hsi LC, Angerman-Stewart J, Eling TE, et al (1999) Introduction of full-length APC modulates cyclooxygenase-2 expression in HT-29 human colorectal carcinoma cells at the translational level. Carcinogenesis 20:2045–2049

Iwamoto M, Ahnen DJ, Franklin WA, et al (2000) Expression of beta-catenin and full-length APC protein in normal and neoplastic colonic tissues. Carcinogenesis 21:1935–1940

Jacoby RF, Seibert K, Cole CE, et al (2000) The cyclooxygenase-2 inhibitor celecoxib is a potent preventive and therapeutic agent in the min mouse model of adenomatous polyposis. Cancer Res 60:5040–5044

Katori M, Majima M (2000) Cyclooxygenase-2: its rich diversity of roles and possible application of its selective inhibitors. Inflamm Res 49:367–392

Kawamori T, Rao CV, Seibert K, et al (1998) Chemopreventive activity of celecoxib, a specific cyclooxygenase-2 inhibitor, against colon carcinogenesis. Cancer Res 58:409–412

Keller JJ, Offerhaus GJ, Drillenburg P, et al (2001) Molecular analysis of Sulindac-resistant adenomas in familial adenomatous polyposis. Clin Cancer Res 7:4000–4007

Kinzler KW, Nilbert MC, Vogelstein B, et al (1991) Identification of a gene located at chromosome 5q21 that is mutated in colorectal cancers. Science 251:1366–1370

Kronborg O and Fenger C (1999) Clinical evidence for the adenoma-carcinoma sequence. Eur J Cancer Prev 1:73–86

Kuraguchi M, Yang K, Wong E, et al (2001) The distinct spectra of tumor-associated Apc mutations in mismatch repair-deficient Apc1638N mice define the roles of MSH3 and MSH6 in DNA repair and intestinal tumorigenesis. Cancer Res 61:7934–7942

Lal G, Ash C, Hay K, et al (2001) Suppression of intestinal polyps in Msh2-deficient and non-Msh2-deficient multiple intestinal neoplasia mice by a specific cyclooxygenase-2 inhibitor and by a dual cyclooxygenase-1/2 inhibitor. Cancer Res 61:6131–6136

Maltzman T, Whittington J, Driggers L, et al (1997) AOM-induced mouse colon tumors do not express full-length APC protein. Carcinogenesis 18:2435–2439

Martinez ME, Sampliner R, Marshall JR, et al (2001) Adenoma characteristics as risk factors for recurrence of advanced adenomas. Gastroenterology 120:1077–1083

Maskens AP, Dujardin-Loits RM (1981) Experimental adenomas and carcinomas of the large intestine behave as distinct entities: most carcinomas arise de novo in flat mucosa. Cancer 47:81–89

Meyskens FL Jr, Gerner EW (1999) Development of difluoromethylornithine (DFMO) as a chemoprevention agent. Clin Cancer Res 5:945–951

Miyaki M, Seki M, Okamoto M, et al (1990) Genetic changes and histopathological types in colorectal tumors from patients with familial adenomatous polyposis. Cancer Res 50:7166–7173

Moser AR, Pitot HC, Dove WF, et al (1990) A dominant mutation that predisposes to multiple intestinal neoplasia in the mouse. Science 247:322–324

Nicolaides NC, Papadopoulos N, Liu B, et al (1994) Mutations of two PMS homologues in hereditary nonpolyposis colon cancer. Nature 371:75–80

Omenn GS, Goodman GE, Thornquist MD, et al (1996) Risk factors for lung cancer and for intervention effects in CARET, the Beta-Carotene and Retinol Efficacy Trial. J Natl Cancer Inst 88:1550–1559

Oshima M, Dinchuk JE, Kargman SL, et al (1996) Suppression of intestinal polyposis in Apc delta716 knockout mice by inhibition of cyclooxygenase 2 (COX-2) Cell 87:803–809

Oshima M, Oshima H, Kitigawa K, et al (1995) Loss of Apc heterozygosity and abnormal tissue building in nascent intestinal polyps in mice carrying a truncated Apc gene. Proc Natl Acad Sci U S A 92:4482–4486

Oshima M, Oshima H, Tsutsumi M, et al (1996) Effects of 2-amino-1-methyl-6-phenylimidazo[4,5-b]pyridine on intestinal polyp development in Apc delta 716 knockout mice. Mol Carcinog 15:11–17

Oshima M, Takahashi M, Oshima H, et al (1995) Effects of docosahexaenoic acid (DHA) on intestinal polyp development in Apc delta 716 knockout mice. Carcinogenesis 16:2605–2607

Papadopoulos N, Nicolaides NC, Wei YF, et al (1994) Mutation of a mutL homolog in hereditary colon cancer. Science 263:1625–1629

Pryor WA, Stahl W, Rock CL, et al (2000) Beta carotene: from biochemistry to clinical trials. Nutr Rev 58:39–53

Reddy BS (2000) The Fourth DeWitt S Goodman lecture. Novel approaches to the prevention of colon cancer by nutritional manipulation and chemoprevention. Cancer Epidemiol Biomarkers Prev 9:239–247

Reddy BS, Narisawa T, Wright P, et al (1975) Colon carcinogenesis with azoxymethane and dimethylhydrazine in germ- free rats. Cancer Res 35:287–290

Reitmair AH, Redston M, Cai JC, et al (1996) Spontaneous intestinal carcinomas and skin neoplasms in Msh2-deficient mice. Cancer Res 56:3842–3849

Roberts RB, Min L, Washington MK, et al (2002) Importance of epidermal growth factor receptor signaling in establishment of adenomas and maintenance of carcinomas during intestinal tumorigenesis. Proc Natl Acad Sci U S A 99:1521–1526

Sasaki T, Irie-Sasaki J, Horie Y, et al (2000) Colorectal carcinomas in mice lacking the catalytic subunit of PI(3)Kgamma. Nature 406:897–902

Scott DJ, Hull MA, Cartwright EJ, et al (2001) Lack of inducible nitric oxide synthase promotes intestinal tumorigenesis in the Apc(Min/+) mouse. Gastroenterology 121:889–899

Seno H, Oshima M, Ishikawa TO, et al (2002) Cyclooxygenase 2- and prostaglandin E(2) receptor EP(2)-dependent angiogenesis in Apc(Delta716) mouse intestinal polyps. Cancer Res 62:506–511

Shoemaker AR, Haigis KM, Baker SM, et al (2000) Mlh1 deficiency enhances several phenotypes of Apc(Min)/+ mice. Oncogene 19:2774–2779

Sitrin MD, Halline AG, Abrahams C, et al (1991) Dietary calcium and vitamin D modulate 1,2-dimethylhydrazine-induced colonic carcinogenesis in the rat. Cancer Res 51:5608–5613

Sonoshita M, Takaku K, Sasaki N, et al (2001) Acceleration of intestinal polyposis through prostaglandin receptor EP2 in Apc(Delta 716) knockout mice. Nat Med 7:1048–1051

Sporn MB (1980) Combination chemoprevention of cancer. Nature 287:107–108

Steinbach G, Lynch PM, Phillips RK, et al (2000) The effect of celecoxib, a cyclooxygenase-2 inhibitor, in familial adenomatous polyposis. N Engl J Med 342:1946–1952

Su LK, Kinzler KW, Vogelstein B, et al (1992) Multiple intestinal neoplasia caused by a mutation in the murine homolog of the APC gene. Science 256:668–670

Suzui M, Sugie S, Mori H, et al (2001) Different mutation status of the beta-catenin gene in carcinogen-induced colon, brain, and oral tumors in rats. Mol Carcinog 32:206–212

Takahashi M, Mutoh M, Hatmaker AR, et al (2000) Altered expression of beta-catenin, inducible nitric oxide synthase and cyclooxygenase-2 in azoxymethane-induced rat colon carcinogenesis. Carcinogenesis 21:1319–1327

Takaku K, Oshima M, Miyoshi H, et al (1998) Intestinal tumorigenesis in compound mutant mice of both Dpc4 (Smad4) and Apc genes. Cell 92:645–656

Taketo MM (1998) Cyclooxygenase-2 inhibitors in tumorigenesis (part I). J Natl Cancer Inst 90:1529–1536

Taketo MM (1998) Cyclooxygenase-2 inhibitors in tumorigenesis (Part II). J Natl Cancer Inst 90:1609–1620

Thurnherr N, Deschner EE, Stonehill EH, et al (1973) Induction of adenocarcinomas of the colon in mice by weekly injections of 1,2-dimethylhydrazine. Cancer Res 33:940–945

Torrance CJ, Jackson PE, Montgomery E, et al (2000) Combinatorial chemoprevention of intestinal neoplasia. Nat Med 6:1024–1028

Velcich A, Yang W, Heyer J, et al (2002) Colorectal cancer in mice genetically deficient in the mucin Muc2. Science 295:1726–1729

Wargovich MJ, Jimenez A, McKee K, et al (2000) Efficacy of potential chemopreventive agents on rat colon aberrant crypt formation and progression. Carcinogenesis 21:1149–1155

Wilson CL, Heppner KJ, Labosky PA, et al (1997) Intestinal tumorigenesis is suppressed in mice lacking the metalloproteinase matrilysin. Proc Natl Acad Sci USA 94:1402–1407

New Cancer Biomarkers Deriving from NCI Early Detection Research

Mukesh Verma, Sudhir Srivastava

S. Srivastava (✉)
Cancer Biomarkers Research Group, Division of Cancer Prevention,
National Cancer Institute, National Institute of Health,
6130 Executive Boulevard, EPN-3142, Rockville, MD 20852-7346, USA

Abstract

Cancer is not a single disease but an accumulation of several events, genetic and epigenetic, arising in a single cell over a long time interval. A high priority in the cancer field is to identify these events. This can be achieved by characterizing cancer-associated genes and their protein products. Identifying the molecular alterations that distinguish any particular cancer cell from a normal cell will ultimately help to define the nature and predict the pathologic behavior of that cancer cell. It will also indicate the responsiveness to treatment of that particular tumor. Understanding the profile of molecular changes in any particular cancer will be extremely useful as it will become possible to correlate the resulting phenotype of that cancer with molecular events. Achieving these goals and knowledge will provide an opportunity for discovering new biomarkers for early cancer detection and developing prevention approaches. This will also help us identify new targets for therapeutic development. Advancement in technology includes methods and tools that enable research including, but not limited to, instrumentation, techniques, devices, and analysis tools (e.g., computer software). Resources such as databases, reagents, and tissue repositories are different than technologies. The identification and definition of the molecular profiles of cancer will require the development and dissemination of high-throughput molecular analysis technologies, as well as elucidation of all of the molecular species embedded in the genome of cancer and normal cells. The main challenge in cancer control and prevention is to detect the cancer early. This could then enable effective interventions and therapies contributing to reduction in mortality and morbidity. At a specific time, biomarkers serve as molecular signposts of the physiologic state of a cell. These signposts are the result of genes, their products (proteins) and other organic chemicals made by the cell. Biomarkers could prove to be vital for the identification of early cancer and subjects at risk of developing cancer as a normal cell progresses through the complex process of transformation to a cancerous state. This chapter discusses ongoing research in genetic and proteomic approaches to identify molecular signatures such as protein profiles, microsatellite instability, hypermethylation, and single nucleotide polymorphisms. Other topics covered here include the use of genomics and proteomics as high-throughput technology platforms to facilitate biomarker-aided detection of early cancer. Other areas covered include issues surrounding the analysis, validation, and predictive value of biomarkers using such technologies. Recent advances in noninvasive techniques, such as buccal cell isolates serving as viable sources of biomarkers, complementary to traditional sources such as serum or plasma, are also presented. The review also brings attention to the efforts of the Early Detection Research Network (EDRN) at the National Cancer Institute (NCI), in bringing together scientific expertise from leading national and international institutions, to identify and validate biomarkers for the detection of precancerous and cancerous cells in determining risk for developing cancer. The network's serious determined efforts in linking discovery to process development, resulting in early detection tests and clinical assessment, are also discussed.

Introduction

Multiple, sequential, and interconnected changes in cellular processes that override normal biological regulation result in cancer that causes a cell to become neoplastic and invasive. It has been a challenging task to detect these changes during the early stages of cancer. We would be able to suppress the mortality due to cancer if we could detect it at the incipient stage and prevent it by established procedures. Biomarkers are important in this regard. Biomarkers are cellular indicators of physiologic state and also of change during a disease process. Biomarkers are unique identifiers called the "molecular signature" of a cell that may reflect genotoxicity, hyperproliferation, altered pattern of gene expression (with or without mutation), hyperplasia, inflammation, aberrant crypt foci; and enzymatic, biochemical, physiological, and immunological alterations that are responses to inherited, acquired, and environmental causes of cancer. Novel technologies with high-throughput are developed to investigate the molecular machinery within human cells and might enable us to overcome the challenges in early detection and prevention.

The EDRN brings together national and international expertise to promote the discovery of biomarkers, through emerging technologies, to help in early detection of cancer. This network includes experts from the academic as well as the industrial community, with the goal of translating research discovery into substantial benefits that can be implemented in the clinic or the population setting. To help facilitate this, Biomarkers Developmental Laboratories (BVL), Biomarkers Validation Laboratories (BVL), Clinical and Epidemiologic Centers (CEC), and Data Management and Coordinating Center (DMCC) are organized into the network. We expect to have exciting information from such a collaborative effort, which can be applied in screening respective populations.

Microscopic examination of tissue detects the disease after a disease is developed. This is important in forecasting tumor behavior and prognosis but additional procedures are essential for early detection. The inherent property and utility of a biomarker lies in its ability to provide an early indication of the progression of the disease. Biomarkers should be easy to detect, measurable across populations, and suitable to use in detection at an early stage, identification of high-risk individuals, early detection of recurrence, and/or serve as an intermediate endpoint in chemoprevention. Since the inception of the EDRN, a number of markers have been identified. In this chapter, we have described those biomarkers and the future directions of their clinical implication.

Biomarkers of Lung Cancer

Methylation of the promoter region is an epigenetic process that is attracting increasing attention, both because of its potential significance to our basic understanding of cancer pathogenesis, and because of its possible use to improve cancer detection. Aberrant methylation of genes has been linked to the development of cancer. Methylation commences early during the lengthy preneoplastic process, and thus may be a marker for risk assessment. The UT Southwestern Medical Center has observed abnormal methylation of a panel of genes in samples from high-risk lung cancer subjects: DAP kinase, APC, RASSF1, FHIT, GSTP1, CASP8, CDH1, CDH13, RAR-beta, MGMT, and p16 (Virmani et al. 2002). Methylation of these genes is being validated in other EDRN-supported institutes (such as the Johns Hopkins University, University of South Florida, University of Colorado). They studied methylation of p16, RAR-beta, and RSSF1 in sputum and bronchial brush samples from subjects heavily exposed to smoking damage without cancer. RAR-beta and p16 were positive in one-fifth of brushes and to a lesser extent in sputum specimens. Correlation between paired brushes and sputum samples was more than 80%. Allelic loss at chromosomal regions 3p and 9p, and microsatellite alterations have also been observed as early markers of lung cancer. Sequential changes during lung cancer pathogenesis have been reported by this group recently (Hirsch et al. 2001).

Efforts at the Johns Hopkins University indicate the overexpression of PGP9.5 and mitochondrial mutations (located in the D-loop) in lung cancer using Serial Analysis of Gene Expression (SAGE); these investigators have cataloged genes that have increased expression in lung cancer samples as compared to normal.

At the University of Michigan, the focus of the research is on the detection and identification of protein antigens that induce humoral response and on proteins secreted by tumor cells in lung cancer. Tumor proteins may induce a humoral response as a result of their overexpression, increased turnover, posttranslational modification, or other unique processing in neoplastic cells. There is evidence that a humoral response to such protein antigens may predate the diagnosis of cancer, indicating the utility of assays for specific tumor protein antigens or antibodies in serum or biological fluids for the early detection of cancer. A large number of proteins of interest have been characterized and their derived information has been entered into a database. Several lung cancer specific protein markers have been identified and are being characterized (Hanash et al. 2001; Oh et al. 2001).

Biomarkers of Prostate Cancer

The Eastern Virginia Medical School (EVMS) Biomarker Developmental Laboratory is employing the SELDI MS (surface enhanced laser desorption/ionization mass spectrometry) system to discover prostate cancer (PCA). In the past, they reported SELDI-based approaches for detecting known prostate cancer biomarkers, such as prostate specific antigen (PSA), prostate acid phosphatase (PAP) and prostate specific membrane antigen (PSMA) in cell lysates from laser capture microdissected (LCM) cells, seminal plasma, and serum (Banks et al. 1999; Fung et al. 2000; Wright et al. 1999). Studies from this group are directed at the systematic development of biomarkers for prostate cancer and refining the assays. Easily collectable biofluids (seminal plasma and serum) and microdissected tissue samples were subjected to SELDI MS analysis to identify patterns of peptides that can discriminate noncancer from cancer samples. Normal cells were collected from the same subject as microdissection allows this opportunity to adopt for sample collection (few cells). The analysis identified three differentially expressed proteins which were overexpressed in PCA cells compared to benign and normal epithelial cells. Using a ratio of peak intensity of these proteins, the cancer population could be clearly differentiated from the benign and normal cell populations. In the same tissue sample, normal cells had higher level of the PSA compare to the cancer cells. Four very low molecular proteins have been identified to date that can discriminate preneoplastic lesions from the normal (Verma et al. 2001). Validation of these proteins in a larger number of samples is being accomplished. Same markers are also being analyzed in body fluids to know whether these markers are restricted to tissue sample or can be obtained in body fluids also. If the tissue markers turn out to be equally good in body fluids also, microdissection of cells would not be needed.

For a brief background of the technology, SELDI allows the simultaneous analysis of multiple proteins to establish peptide profiles that discriminate cancer from noncancer. Seminal plasma and serum from normal age-matched men, and from patients diagnosed with benign prostate hyperplasia (BPH) or PCA were subjected to this analysis. The raw time-of-flight (TOF) data were analyzed using two different learning algorithms developed by investigators at the EDRN Data Management Coordinating Center (DMCC). The Binary Combinations algorithm resulted in 88% sensitivity and 89% specificity. This protein profiling algorithm correctly "diagnosed" cancers, BPH, and normal subjects. Similarly, sera from PCA patients and normal age-matched men were used to train the Wavelet algorithm. The analyses of 11 protein masses resulted in a specificity of 100% and a sensitivity of 97% for the training set. These are preliminary data that are being tested for a large number of samples which may lead to innovative clinical assay for the early detection/diagnosis of prostate and bladder cancers. With the SELDI approach, protein identification and characterization may not be necessary for development of clinical assays and only SELDI protein profile should be sufficient for screening a population. By the same token, if a specific protein is identified during the process, it can be further characterized in terms of its composition and other properties.

Biomarkers of Gastrointestinal Tract Cancer

At the University of Maryland hypermethylation of the p14(ARF) gene in ulcerative colitis-associated colorectal carcinogenesis has been investigated recently (Sato et al. 2002). This protein degrades p53 via an intermediate step of inhibiting MDM-2, an oncoprotein. This group demonstrated that p14(ARF) expression is downregulated, in colorectal cancer, by p14(ARF) via epigenetic mechanism that involves hypermethylation of this gene. Four stages of ulcerative colitis were selected to determine whether p14(ARF) inactivation was involved in the process of carcinogenesis. The frequency and timing of p14(ARF) methylation, using methylation specific PCR and bisulfite sequencing, was followed in this study. Results indicated methylation of p14(ARF) in 50% adenocarcinomas, one-third dysplasia and more than half nonneoplastic UC mucosae. The level of methylation in normal tissue was extremely low. In this region of the gene, more than 25 CpG islands were present (as confirmed by sequencing) and the number of methylated CpGs ranged from 0 to 4, 0 to 20, and 0 to 28 in the normal, dysplastic, and carcinomatous samples, respectively. Another remarkable observation was that densely methylated alleles were detected only in carcinomas.

Results from this study suggest that methylation of p14(ARF) is a relatively common early event in UC-associated carcinogenesis, and p14(ARF) could be used as a biomarker for the early detection of cancer or dysplasia in UC. The analyses of p14(ARF) methylation in other organs should explore frank cancers and other premalignant lesions. This group has also developed an artificial neural network (ANN) that distinguishes among subtypes of neoplastic colorectal lesions (Selaru et al. 2002). There is a clear distinction between sporadic colorectal adenomas and cancers (SAC) and inflammatory bowel disease (IBD)-associated dysplasias and cancers. This distinction is clinically important because sporadic adenomas are usually managed by polypectomy alone, whereas IBD-related high-grade dysplasias mandate subtotal colectomy. The investigators at the University of Maryland evaluated the ability of ANN based on complementary DNA (cDNA) microarray data to discriminate between these two types of colorectal lesions. They hybridized cDNA microarrays, each containing more than 8000 cDNA clones, to RNAs derived from more than 30 colorectal neoplastic specimens. Hierarchical clustering based on these clones failed to correctly categorize the SACs and IBDNs. However, the ANN correctly diagnosed more than ten blinded samples in a test set. Furthermore, using an iterative process based on the computer programs GeneFinder, Cluster, and MATLAB, they reduced the number of clones. Even with this reduced clone set, the ANN retained its capacity for correct diagnosis. The cluster analysis performed with small number of clones separated the two types of lesions and results indicated that ANNs had the potential to discriminate among different clinical entities, such as IBDNs and SACs. This can be used to identify gene subsets having the power to make these diagnostic distinctions and should be useful to apply for screening of high-risk populations.

Biomarkers of Ovarian and Cervical Cancers

At Northwestern University and the US Food and Drug Administration (FDA) Laboratories, proteomic spectra were generated by SELDI MS (Petricoin et al. 2002). In this approach the focus is not on single marker (peptide) but a pattern of several hundred peptides, mostly of low molecular weight, generated during the procedure. Serum samples were collected from 50 unaffected women and 50 ovarian cancer patients to generate a preliminary training set spectra. An interactive searching algorithm analyzed SELDI MS data and identified normal and cancer patient with 100% accuracy. The template pattern was further utilized to analyze more serum samples from women with ovarian cancer, unaffected women, or those with nonmalignant disorders. More than 100 such samples were successfully classified in this EDRN collaborative study. Thus, the algorithm generated in this study specified a cluster pattern that, in the training set, completely distinguished cancer from noncancer (normal). The judicious discriminatory pattern identified all ovarian cancer cases in the blind samples tested to date, including all stage I cases. Of all the nonmalignant disease results, more than half were recognized as not cancer. Final results indicated 100% sensitivity and 95% specificity, which is the best example of ovarian cancer-related analysis completed to date. This study also established that proteomic pattern analysis can be used as a prospective population-based assessment for screening of different stages of ovarian cancer in different populations. The main importance of the technology is that a very small amount of sample is needed for the analysis and validation of results.

Methylation of selected genes was tested for detecting cervical cancer also. Using a panel of five genes (p16, RAR-beta, GSTP1, MGMT, and FHIT) a methylation profile of cervical cancer was developed for women without cancer. These women were divided into those without dysplasia or with CIN 1, and those with high-grade dysplasia CIN 2 or CIN3. There was a progressive increase in the methylation index with increasing severity of disease. These findings from the UT Southwestern Medical Center suggest that the aberrant methylation may predict which women are at highest risk of progressing to high-grade dysplasia or cancer.

Biomarkers of Bladder Cancer

Like the EVMS team, investigators at the M. D. Anderson Cancer Center have also discovered differentially expressed proteins in urine from patients with bladder cancer using SELDI. Most of these proteins are of low molecular mass. Analysis of the urine from patients with bladder squamous cell carcinoma (SSC) has found a number of significant differentiation markers, such as the presence of keratins 10, 13, 15, and 19, and loss of a number of proteins, including glutathione-S-transferase. Another putative urinary SCC marker, psoriasin, a calcium-binding protein which is widely expressed in tissues containing stratified squamous epithelium, has also been studied.

At Johns Hopkins University, investigators have developed a microsatellite-based assay to detect bladder cancer by utilizing urine samples from the patients. In future, this marker will be validated in the EDRN validation laboratories.

Biomarkers of Breast Cancer

By utilizing the "secretory trap technology" involving MaRX recombinase-based excision system, Mao retrovirus system, and LinX packaging cells, EDRN investigators from Genetica Inc. have identified a breast cancer specific marker. This marker is expressed by a novel gene which is overexpressed in breast cancer. It shows 50% homology with lysosomal protein α-L-fucosidase and probably involved in glycosylation of proteins. The trap technology has the capability to identify differentially expressed proteins from samples isolated at early stages of the disease development. A variety of samples, such as serum, tissues, breast nipple aspirate, and breast lavage from the preneoplastic tissues, were used for this research. Attempts are being made to make this procedure automatic. By design, this technique traps a breast tumor library that has not been normalized. Therefore, signal sequences that emerge, especially signal sequences that were recovered multiple times, are likely to represent abundant mRNAs in tumors.

Research by EDRN investigators at the Georgetown University Lombardi Cancer Center and Johns Hopkins University aims to characterize differences in protein signatures between foci of normal breast epithelium, ductal carcinoma in situ (DCIS), and invasive cancer from fresh surgical specimens; to determine whether differences identified above can be detected in nipple aspirate fluid (NAF) samples from women without breast abnormalities, with DCIS, or with early invasive breast cancer; and to determine whether differentially expressed proteins can be detected in serum samples from women with different stages of breast cancer development. A number of potential candidates have been identified using LCM and SELDI-based approaches.

Biomarkers of Liver Cancer

Individuals chronically infected with hepatitis B or C virus (HBV, HCV) are at high risk for the development of hepatocellular carcinoma (HCC), with disease progression occurring relentlessly over many years (Steel et al. 2001). The diagnosis of HCC usually occurs at late stages in the disease when there are few effective treatment options and the prognosis for patients with HCC is very poor. The long latency period, as long as 20 years, together with clearly identified at-risk populations, provides opportunities for earlier detection that will allow more timely and effective treatment of this devastating cancer. Investigators at Thomas Jefferson University are using a proteomic approach (two-dimensional gel electrophoresis) to test the hypothesis that changes in the amount of certain serum polypeptides, or changes in their posttranslational modifications, can be used to predict the onset of HCC. Advances in the standardization of two dimensional gel electrophoresis (2DE) coupled with computerized image analysis, and automation of critical steps now permit the reproducible resolution of thousands of polypeptides per run. Serum polypeptides from individuals at different stages in the disease continuum are being resolved by 2DE to identify those that change with disease progression. Polypeptides found by this method can be further characterized by mass spectrometry (MS). In addition, the potential for changes in the glycan structure of certain polypeptides to serve as a marker for disease progression is being investigated.

To identify the best indicators or biomarkers of the progression of the disease (HCC) the proteomic approach is expected to liberate us from the need to guess and enable us to analyze data. Information may also be obtained about the pathobiology of the disease process. The same group has also demonstrated inhibition of hepatitis B virus DNA replication by imino sugars without the inhibition of the DNA polymerase (Mehta et al. 2001). Previously, in the woodchuck model of chronic hepatitis B virus (HBV) infection, it was demonstrated that the imino sugar inhibitor of N-linked glycan processing, N-nonyl-deoxynojirimycin (N-nonyl-DNJ), had antiviral activity. To shed light on understanding the mechanism of action of this compound, it was demonstrated that imino sugars could inhibit HBV secretion without inhibiting N-linked glycoprocessing. Although N-nonyl-DNJ is an inhibitor of the endoplasmic reticulum (ER) glucosidase, these studies established that N-nonyl-DNJ retained antiviral activity at concentrations that had no significant impact on ER glucosidase function. Taken together, results suggested that N-nonyl-DNJ contained an antiviral activity designated to a function other than an impact on glycoprocessing. This idea was tested with experiments showing that N-nonyl-deoxygalactojirimycin (N-nonyl-DGJ), an alkyl derivative of galactose with no impact on glycoprocessing, retains anti-HBV activity. The data suggested that N-nonyl-DGJ exerted its antiviral action at a point before viral was encapsulated and might prevent the proper infectivity of the HBV pregenomic RNA (Mehta et al. 2001).

Other Biomarkers

At the University of Maryland, plasma telomerase assay has been developed that shows great promise in identification of cancer in the early stages. Although this marker is not specific to any specific cancer, it will be useful to include this marker with other markers for screening high-risk populations.

Tumor markers shed into the serum have been sought to identify individuals at risk for developing cancer. An alteration in the oligosaccharides associated with glycoproteins is one of the many molecular changes that accompany malignant transformations (Hakomori 1996; Kobata 1998; Verma and Davidson 1999; Verma et al. 1999). However, the methodology used to assess these alterations has been hindered by a number of factors, for example, insensitive techniques requiring large sample amounts, poor quantitation, and no truly accurate information about the relative quantitation of all the oligosaccharides present. As a result of this a systematic and thorough structural analysis of all the oligosaccharides associated with particular proteins from cancer patient/ tissue has not been carried out. Since specific alterations in oligosaccharides are typically used in histology studies to differentiate between cancer and noncancerous cells, the potential for oligosaccharides to serve as biomarkers in noninvasive methodologies remains a promising but unexploited area. Attempts are being made to explore oligosaccharide structure and disease state relationships using a new robust technology platform, employing fluorescent HPLC (high-pressure liquid chromatography) analysis of sugars, which can

Table 1. Biomarkers for early cancer detection

Cancer type	Putative biomarkers
Lung	DAP kinase, APC, RASSF1, FHIT, GSTP1, CASP8, CDH1, CDH13, RARbeta, MGMT, p16, chromosomal instability, mitochondrial DNA mutation, annexin I, annexin II, pGP9.5
Prostate	Peptide profile of low molecular mass (33 kDa, 8.5 kDa, and 9.5 kDa)
Gastrointestinal tract	P14(ARF), peptide profile of low molecular mass
Ovarian and cervical cancer	Peptide profile of low molecular mass, p16, RARβ, MGMT, FHIT
Bladder cancer	Keratin 10, 13, 15, 19; microsatellite instability, STK/BTAK kinase
Breast cancer	Breast cancer specific protein, peptide profile of low molecular mass
Liver cancer	Glycosylated proteins

APC, adenomatous polyposis coli; DAP Kinase, death associated protein kinase; FHIT, fragile histidine triad; GSTP1, glutathione-S-transferase gene GSTP1 in prostate cancer tissue; CASP8, caspase 8; CDH1, E-cadherin; CDH13, H-cadherin; MGMT, O6-methylguanine-DNA-methyltransferase; RARbeta, retinoic acid receptor ß; RASSF1, RAS associated domain family protein 1a (RAS effector homolog); STK/BTAK, Bruton's tyrosine kinase.

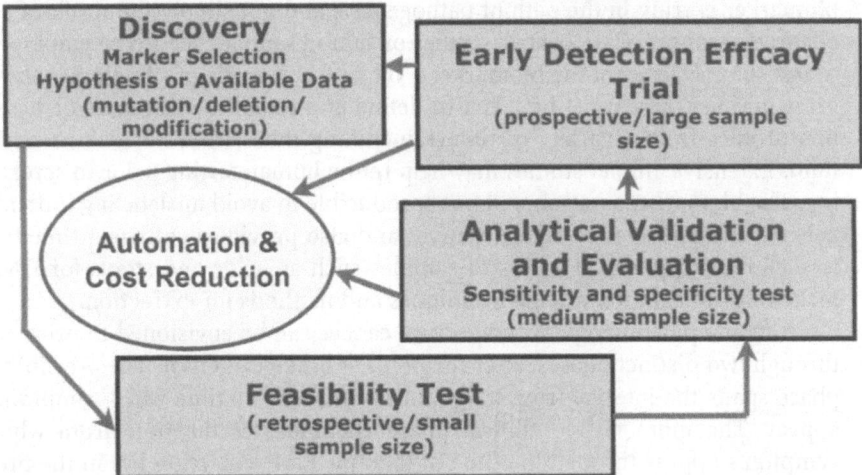

Fig. 1. General steps needed to take a biomarker from the bench (laboratory) to the bedside (patient)

quantitate every oligosaccharide present (abundance of >0.1% in the total glycan pool) in protein samples (Mattu et al. 2000). Some of the markers identified to date, such as fucosylated glycoform of α fetoprotein, have altered glycosylation patterns in the disease state (Ando et al. 2001; Dwek et al. 2001).

Thus, a number of potential biomarkers have been identified by EDRN investigators (Table 1), which will be validated in different laboratories using a large number of samples (Fig. 1). If validated, these markers would be extremely valuable for screening populations at high risk for cancer and developing prevention strategies for a variety of cancers.

Validation of Biomarkers

A biomarker should be tested in the intended population for ultimate use since a test for early detection often requires higher specificity than a test in the clinical diagnosis. An intelligent approach for early detection and developing prevention strategies should be to screen for a cluster or pattern of markers from biological samples for substantial accuracy in performing risk assessment. The positive predictive value of a test and minimize labeling individuals as either false positives or false negatives can be achieved by using a panel of biomarkers.

Novel biomarkers have to be validated prior to their general use. Sensitivity, specificity, and predictive value have to be determined through the use of body fluids, paired tumors, and surrounding tissue from a wide variety of cancers. A large number of samples from individuals with known characteristics should be processed to minimize the problems of confounding and avoiding forged associations. Prior to field testing, it should be established that the biomarker is truly in the path of pathogenesis and not simply the result of an adaptive response. Case control studies on stored samples should be employed to test the efficiency of the biomarkers. While the emerging technologies show great promise, care must be taken to define and establish references or baseline profiles from a variety of tissues including those from normal, or body fluid. Extensive animal studies may help refine human testing prior to screening. The biomarker assay should be reproducible to avoid mislabeling individuals as false positives or false negatives and also provide a sufficient time before clinical diagnosis. Sources of samples such as urine and stools for DNA make it significant to evaluate techniques and methods for extraction.

From an epidemiological perspective, cancer can be envisioned to progress through two distinct phases, after the point of biological onset. The preclinical phase spans the interval from the point of onset to the time when symptoms appear. The more visible clinical phase encompasses the time from when symptoms appear through the time of therapy. Early detection lies in the preclinical phase of this continuum and biomarkers, predictive of this phase, hold the greatest promise in helping design effective interventions to stop or possibly reverse progression.

Conclusion: Future Directions

The promise of biomarkers in cancer detection and diagnosis to detect cancer at the earliest stage has never been better. Knowledge of molecular events during the early stages of cancer has advanced at a rapid pace. This advancement has been aided by the development of new high-throughput technologies enabling the detection of molecular changes at genomic and proteomic levels. Applications of biomarker detection in clinical practice, however, have been limited to single entity quantitation or the use of small panels of tests that can identify changes in proteins whose presence or absence signifies an important event. However, as the number of new discoveries of biomarkers increases, it is becoming evident that no single marker will provide the information necessary to make the best decision in detection and diagnosis. The NCI's Early Detection Research Network is promoting a multiparametric, multimarkers approach to biomarkers development. High-density oligonucleotide and cDNA arrays are generating information to predict and understand the disease state that can be used to develop novel sentinel endpoints for chemopreventive interventions. In contrast, proteomic-based approaches, such as a SELDI-TOF and matrixes-assisted laser desorption ionization time of flight (MALDI-TOF) are enabling rapid ascertainment of diseased status directly from human body fluids, such as serum, nipple aspirate, and seminal plasma. These potentially new models for diagnostic technologies are rapid (within minutes), require small samples inputs (less than 1 μl) and, most important, are sensitive and accurate in predicting the disease state.

The focus of future research in the EDRN is on analytical and clinical validation of the potential biomarkers identified to date. As biomarkers are discovered early in the preclinical phase of the disease, caution will be exercised in validation since diagnosis lies in the future and there may be no clear "gold standard." While the emerging technologies show great promise, care will be taken to define and establish a reference baseline profile from normal tissue, cell, or body fluid. One of the EDRN validation laboratories, National Institute of Standard and Technology, has started analytical validation of mitochondrial mutations in clinical samples collected at Johns Hopkins Medical Center. In future, we expect to conduct clinical validation of biomarkers for their efficacy in screening high-risk individuals.

References

Ando S, Kimura H, Iwai M, et al (2001) Optimal combination of seven tumor markers in prediction of advanced stage at first examination of patients with nonsmall cell lung cancer. Anticancer Res 21:3085–3092

Banks RE, Dunn MJ, Forbes MA, et al (1999) The potential use of laser capture microdissection to selectively obtain distinct populations of cells for proteomic analysis-preliminary findings. Electrophoresis 20:689–700

Dwek MV, Ross HA, Leathem AJ (2001) Proteome and glycosylation mapping identifies posttranslational modifications associated with aggressive breast cancer. Proteomics 6:756–762

Fung ET, Wright GL, Dalmasso EA (2000) Proteomic strategies for biomarker identification: progress and challenges. Curr Opin Mol Ther 2:643–650

Hakomori S (1996) Tumor malignancy defined by aberrant glycosylation and sphingo(glyco)lipid metabolism. Cancer Res 56:5309–5318

Hanash S, Brichory F, Beer D (2001) A proteomic approach to the identification of lung cancer markers. Dis Markers 17:295–300

Hirsch FR, Franklin WA, Gazdar AF, Bunn PA (2001) Early detection of lung cancer: clinical perspectives of recent advances in biology and radiology. Clin Cancer Res 7:5–22

Kobata A (1998) A retrospective and prospective view of glycopathology. Glycoconj J 15:323–331

Mattu TS, Royle L, Langridge J, et al (2000) O-glycan analysis of natural human neutrophil gelatinase B using a combination of normal phase-HPLC and online tandem mass spectrometry: implications for the domain organization of the enzyme. Biochemistry 39:15695–15704

Mehta A, Carrouee S, Conyers B, et al (2001) Inhibition of hepatitis B virus DNA replication by imino sugars without the inhibition of the DNA polymerase: therapeutic implications. Hepatology 33:1488–1495

Oh JM, Brichory F, Puravs E, et al (2001) A database of protein expression in lung cancer. Proteomics 1:1303–1319

Petricoin EF, Ardekani AM, Hitt BA, et al (2002) Use of proteomic patterns in serum to identify ovarian cancer. Lancet 359:572–577

Sato F, Harpaz N, Shibata D, et al (2002) Hypermethylation of the p14(ARF) gene in ulcerative colitis-associated colorectal carcinogenesis. Cancer Res 62:1148–1151

Selaru FM, Xu Y, Yin J, et al (2002) Artificial neural networks distinguish among subtypes of neoplastic colorectal lesions. Gastroenterology 122:606–613

Steel LF, Mattu TS, Mehta A, et al (2001) A proteomic approach for the discovery of early detection markers of hepatocellular carcinoma. Dis Markers 17:179–189

Verma M, Baraniuk J, Blass C, et al (1999) CFTR antisense phosphorothioate oligodeoxynucleotides (S-ODNs) induce tracheo-bronchial mucin (TBM) mRNA expression in human airways mucosa. Glycoconj J 16:7–11

Verma M, Davidson EA (1999) MUC1 upregulation by ethanol. Cancer Biochem Biophys 17:1–11

Verma M, Wright G L, Hanash SM, et al (2001) Proteomic approaches within the NCI Early Detection Research Network for the discovery and identification of cancer biomarkers. Ann N Y Acad Sci 945:103–115

Virmani AK, Tsou JA, Siegmund KD, et al (2002) Hierarchical clustering of lung cancer cell lines using DNA methylation markers. Cancer Epidemiol Biomarkers Prev 11:291–297

Wright GL, Cazares LH, Leung SM, et al (1999) ProteinChip surface enhanced laser desorption/ionization (SELDI) mass spectrometry: A novel protein biochip technology for detection of prostate cancer biomarkers in complex protein mixtures. Prostate Cancer Prostatic Dis 2: 264–276

Update in Chemoprevention 3
of Breast Cancer

Tamoxifen's Impact as a Preventive Agent in Clinical Practice and an Update on the STAR Trial

D. Lawrence Wickerham

D.L. Wickerham (✉)
NSABP Operations Center, East Commons Professional Building,
Four Allegheny Center, 5th Floor, Pittsburgh, PA 15212, USA

Abstract

Tamoxifen has long been an established adjuvant treatment in the management of advanced breast cancer. Studies carried out by the National Surgical Adjuvant Breast and Bowel Project (NSABP) and other groups also established its use in the treatment of early breast cancer and subsequently as a risk-reducing agent for the development of contralateral breast cancer in breast cancer patients. The NSABP began its investigation of tamoxifen as a preventive agent in the early 1990s in women who had never had the disease with its Breast Cancer Prevention Trial (P-1). Its second prevention study, the STAR trial, is currently under way.

Keywords National Surgical Adjuvant Breast and Bowel Project ·
Tamoxifen · Breast cancer · Chemoprevention

Introduction

The National Surgical Adjuvant Breast and Bowel Project (NSABP), established in 1958, is a cooperative trials group sponsored by the National Cancer Institute (NCI) of the United States. In its history, more than 50,000 patients have entered NSABP trials evaluating new treatments for both primary breast and bowel cancer. The group has conducted tamoxifen treatment trials since the late 1970s, initially in node-positive breast cancer but subsequently in node-negative, receptor-positive disease, as well as studies of ductal carcinoma in situ (DCIS) (Fisher et al. 1987, 1999, 2001). In NSABP studies and other adjuvant trials, women who received tamoxifen as adjuvant treatment for invasive breast cancer were shown to have a significant reduction in contralateral breast cancer (Scottish BCTC 1987; CRC Adjuvant Breast Trial Working Party 1988; Rutqvist et al. 1991; Fisher and Redmond 1991). Evaluating the use of tamoxifen in the prevention of primary breast cancer was a logical next step.

Recent Results in Cancer Research, Vol. 163
© Springer-Verlag Berlin Heidelberg 2003

In 1992 the group undertook its first cancer chemoprevention trial, now referred to as "P-1." That trial was designed to evaluate tamoxifen for the reduction of risk of primary breast cancer in women at increased risk for the disease (Fisher et al. 1998).

NSABP P-1

Between 1 June 1992, and 30 September 1997, 13,388 women age 35 years and older entered the P-1 trial and were randomly assigned to receive either tamoxifen 20 mg per day or placebo. The initial results published in 1998 demonstrated a highly significant reduction in invasive breast cancers for those women who received the drug: 175 cases of invasive breast cancer in the placebo group and 89 in the tamoxifen group [risk ratio (RR) 0.51, 95% confidence interval (CI) 0.39–0.66, $p<0.0001$]. The annual event rate for invasive breast cancer among the women who took tamoxifen was 3.4 per 1,000, compared with 6.8 per 1,000 for those who took placebo (Table 1). Tamoxifen reduced the risk of developing invasive breast cancer in all age groups in the trial and among all risk groups. A striking benefit was also seen for women with a history of lobular carcinoma in situ (LCIS), (RR 0.44, 95%, CI 0.16–1.06), and for women with a history of either atypical lobular or ductal hyperplasia, 0.4 (95% CI 0.03–0.47). In addition, there was a 50% reduction in noninvasive breast cancer shown with tamoxifen (69 cases in the placebo group and 35 in the tamoxifen group [RR 0.50 (95% CI 0.33–0.77) $p<.002$], and a recent report demonstrates a reduction in benign breast biopsies as well for those women who received tamoxifen (Tan-Chiu et al. 2001). Tamoxifen therapy resulted in fewer breast biopsies of benign lesions, and the proliferative nature of the biopsies was also reduced by this therapy.

The distribution of primary tumor size and pathologic involvement of axillary lymph nodes was not markedly different between women who took tamoxifen and women who took placebo. There was a substantial difference, however, in the number of estrogen receptor-(ER)-positive tumors that occurred in the two groups. The incidence rate of ER-positive breast cancers was 5 per 1,000 in the placebo group and only 1.6 per 1,000 in the tamoxifen-treated group, a 69% reduction. The rates of ER-negative tumors were not significantly different between the two groups.

Other Endpoints

Of the women in P-1, 955 experienced bone fractures. The incidence of osteoporotic fracture events involving the hips, spine, or lower radius was reduced 19% among women who received tamoxifen. There were 137 events in the placebo group versus 111 events in the tamoxifen-treated group. Most notable was a 45% reduction in fractures of the hip.

Table 1. Average annual rates for outcomes in the Breast Cancer Prevention Trial (P-1) (from Fisher et al. 1998)

Cancer outcomes	Rate per 1,000 women		Risk ratio (95% confidence interval)
	Tamoxifen	Placebo	
Invasive breast cancer	3.4	6.8	0.51 (0.39–0.66)
Noninvasive breast cancer	1.4	2.7	0.50 (0.33–0.77)
Invasive BrCa by patient characteristic			
Age (years)			
≤49	3.8	6.7	0.56 (0.37–0.85)
50–59	3.1	6.3	0.49 (0.29–0.81)
≥60	3.3	7.3	0.45 (0.27–0.74)
History of LCIS			
Yes	5.7	13.0	0.44 (0.16–1.06)
No	3.3	6.4	0.51 (0.39–0.68)
History of atypical hyperplasia			
Yes	1.4	10.1	0.14 (0.03–0.47)
No	3.6	6.4	0.56 (0.42–0.73)
Number of 1st-degree relatives with BrCa			
0	3.0	6.4	0.46 (0.24–0.84)
1	3.0	6.0	0.51 (0.35–0.73)
2	4.8	8.7	0.55 (0.30–0.97)
≥3	7.0	13.7	0.51 (0.15–1.55)
Risk of BrCa within 5 years (%)			
≤2	2.1	5.5	0.37 (0.18–0.72)
2.01–3.0	3.5	5.2	0.68 (0.41–1.11)
3.01–5.0	3.9	5.9	0.66 (0.39–1.09)
≥5.01	4.5	13.3	0.34 (0.19–0.58)
Invasive endometrial cancer			
Age (years)			
≤49	1.3	1.1	1.21 (0.41–3.60)
≥50	3.0	0.8	4.01 (1.70–10.90)
Fractures			
Hip	0.5	0.8	0.55 (0.25–1.15)
Hip, spine, lower radius combined	4.3	5.3	0.81 (0.63–1.05)
Thromboembolic events			
Stroke	1.4	0.9	1.59 (0.93–2.77)
Transient ischemic attack	0.7	1.0	0.76 (0.40–1.44)
Pulmonary embolism	0.7	0.2	3.01 (1.15–9.27)
Deep vein thrombosis	1.3	0.8	1.60 (0.91–2.86)

Despite a well-known reduction in total cholesterol that occurs with tamoxifen treatment (which ranges from 12% to 20% in different series), there was no demonstrable difference in cardiovascular outcomes between the tamoxifen- and placebo-treated groups. Even in those women who entered the P-1 trial with a preexisting history of cardiovascular disease, no substantial improvement in outcome could be identified (Reis et al 2001).

Toxicities

Women who received tamoxifen in the P-1 trial had a 2.5 times greater risk of developing invasive endometrial cancer than did women who received placebo; the average annual rates of endometrial cancer were 0.9 per 1,000 women in the placebo group and 2.3 per 1,000 in the tamoxifen-treated group. The excess risk was almost exclusively in postmenopausal women (defined as those aged 50 years and older at the time of randomization).

There was also an increase in the number of thromboembolic vascular events among those who took tamoxifen in P-1 (Table 1). While only the rate of pulmonary emboli reached statistical significance, there were also somewhat increased event rates for stroke or transient ischemic attack and deep vein thrombosis in those aged 50 years and older who took tamoxifen. In addition, there was a marginal increase in the rate of cataract development among women who took tamoxifen, a toxicity that had been reported in an earlier NSABP study (Gorin et al. 1998). Bothersome hot flashes were reported by 46% of the women in the tamoxifen-treated group compared with 29% in the placebo group. Vaginal discharge was also reported more frequently in the tamoxifen group (29% versus 13% in the placebo group).

Incorporation into Routine Practice

In December 1998, the U.S. Food and Drug Administration (FDA) approved tamoxifen for reduction in breast cancer incidence in high-risk women. "High risk" was defined as women at least 35 years of age, with a 5-year predicted risk of breast cancer $\geq 1.67\%$ as calculated by the Gail Model. Physicians were also instructed, "After an assessment of the risk of developing breast cancer, the decision regarding therapy with tamoxifen for the reduction in breast cancer incidence should be based upon an individual assessment of the benefits and risks of tamoxifen therapy." The NCI estimated that there were as many as 29,000,000 women in the United States who were potential candidates for tamoxifen based on these indications.

Precise data on the use of tamoxifen for prevention/risk reduction are not available. AstraZeneca, the manufacturer of tamoxifen in the United States, has seen an increase of 5%–10% in the sales of the drug, but this is unlikely to be due exclusively to its use in prevention. During the same time period, tamoxifen was approved for the adjuvant therapy of ductal carcinoma in situ (DCIS), and the 10-year Oxford overview results were published demonstrating the appropriateness of using tamoxifen for a 5-year period for the treatment of invasive breast cancer. However, even if all the increased use were attributed to prevention, this would still indicate that substantially fewer women than the estimated 29 million potential candidates are receiving the drug.

Why would so few women be receiving tamoxifen for breast cancer prevention? It is likely that there are many reasons, none of them dominant. Although tamoxifen provided substantial benefit in reducing the number of both invasive and noninvasive breast cancers, as well as fracture reduction, it was also associated, as noted above, with increased risk for several serious conditions including endometrial cancer, thromboembolic events, and cataracts. The decision to use this therapy is complex and requires a thorough evaluation of both benefit and risk.

Breast cancer risk in the P-1 trial was determined using a modification of the model developed by Gail et al. based on data from the Breast Cancer Detection Demonstration Project (Gail et al. 1989). This model has been validated and shown to be a very accurate predictor of breast cancer risk on a population basis (Costantino et al. 1999). In an effort to make the model available to health care professionals and the general public, the NCI began to distribute its Breast Cancer Risk Assessment Tool in both IBM and MAC formats. A web-based version of the program was also posted – http://bcra.nci.nih.gov/brc/ and AstraZeneca distributed a version of the model on a hand-held calculator.

At the same time, physicians and potential tamoxifen users were receiving mixed messages about tamoxifen's usefulness in prevention. Not long after the announcement of the NSABP P-1 results, two European trials were published in *Lancet* that also compared tamoxifen to placebo in a high-risk population (Veronesi et al. 1998; Powles et al. 1998). Neither of these trials demonstrated benefit from tamoxifen in the reduction of invasive breast cancers, and many individuals, including breast cancer advocates, expressed concern about the drug's potential toxicities and what they described as "mixed trial results." Although none of the studies was designed to evaluate survival as a primary endpoint, the lack of a documented survival benefit was widely discussed as a reason not to use tamoxifen.

Gail et al. have also described in great detail a method by which to assess benefit and risk with the goal of identifying appropriate candidates for tamoxifen preventive therapy (Gail et al. 1999). Their methods are extremely complex and impractical for most routine clinical use. Anecdotal reports suggest that clinicians have adopted tamoxifen with increasing frequency for two general groups of individuals: (1) women with biopsy-proven risk factors (LCIS or atypical hyperplasia of the breast), which are known to substantially increase the risk for future breast cancer; and (2) premenopausal women with substantial risk of future breast cancer who, based on the P-1 data, have little or no risk of endometrial cancer or thromboembolic disease resulting from tamoxifen. Women who have had a hysterectomy and thus have no risk of endometrial cancer are also more likely to be prescribed tamoxifen than those who have not had a hysterectomy.

The Study of Tamoxifen and Raloxifene (STAR)

Although P-1 has demonstrated that tamoxifen is effective in reducing the incidence of breast cancer, the drug's toxicities are a barrier to its routine use in this patient population. Identifying more effective agents with less toxicity is an appropriate goal, and the NSABP has initiated the next step in that direction.

Raloxifene is a benzothiophene serum that has been shown to increase bone density in postmenopausal women and is approved in the United States for both the treatment and the prevention of osteoporosis. Of all the newer SERMs, raloxifene has received the most attention with regard to its potential use for breast cancer chemoprevention.

MORE Trial

The Multiple Outcomes of Raloxifene Evaluation (MORE) Trial was a randomized, placebo-controlled, double-blinded study designed to determine whether raloxifene would reduce the risk of fracture in postmenopausal women with osteoporosis (Cummings et al. 1999; Cauley et al. 2001). Each of the 7,704 women enrolled (mean age, 66.5 years), was assigned to receive either 60 mg of raloxifene, 120 mg of raloxifene, or a placebo. The development of breast cancer was a secondary endpoint of the trial, and women were not selected because of their breast cancer risk. The 4-year results of the trial demonstrated a 72% risk reduction with raloxifene (RR 0.28, 95% CI 0.17–0.46). This drug also reduced the risk of ER-positive invasive breast cancer by 84% (RR 0.16, 95% CI 0.09–0.30). Thromboembolic disease occurred more frequently in the raloxifene-treated group than in the placebo-treated group, (p=0.003), but there was no excess risk of endometrial cancer among raloxifene-treated women.

STAR Trial

In July 1999, the NSABP began accrual to its second breast cancer prevention trial, *The Study of Tamoxifen and Raloxifene (STAR)*. This is a randomized, double-blinded trial to compare the proven benefits of tamoxifen to the promising results identified with raloxifene (Fig. 1). Eligible participants are postmenopausal women at increased risk for the future development of breast cancer based on a 5-year breast cancer risk estimate from the Gail Model $\geq$ 1.67%. Participants will be assigned to receive 20 mg of tamoxifen plus a placebo or 60 mg of raloxifene plus a placebo daily for 5 years. They will undergo breast examinations every 6 months as well as yearly mammograms, gynecologic examinations, and screening blood work. The goal is to determine whether raloxifene is as good as or better than tamoxifen in preventing

NSABP Protocol P-2 Schema

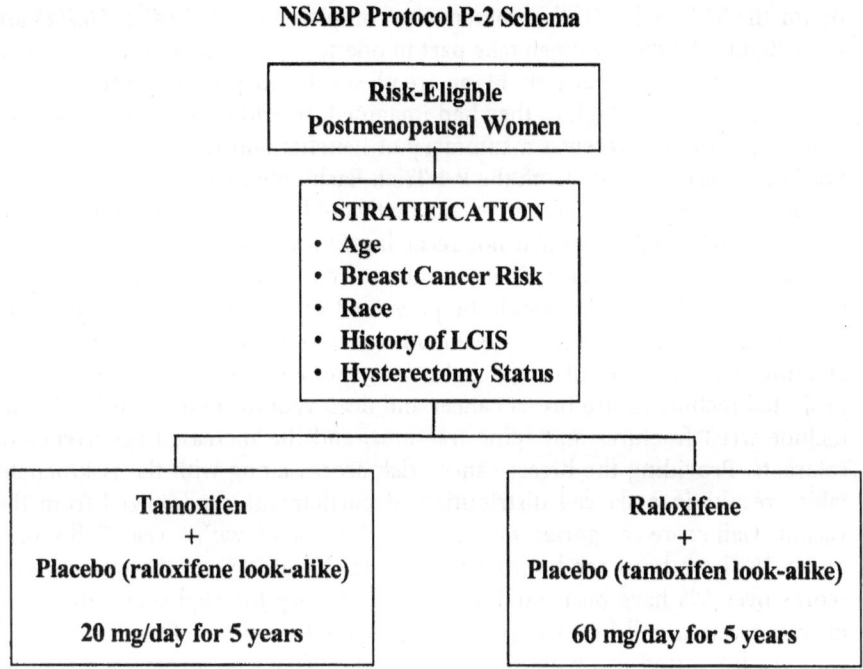

Fig. 1. Schema of the Study of Tamoxifen and Raloxifene (STAR) trial

breast cancer with fewer side effects. The sample size required to complete the study is 22,000 women.

There are currently 500 sites participating in the STAR Trial in the United States, Canada, and Puerto Rico. As of 31 January 2002, 12,387 participants had been randomized into the trial, which represents 56.2% of the sample size. Accrual at present is limited to postmenopausal women; raloxifene has not been evaluated extensively in premenopausal women, and there are no safety or efficacy data available for the drug in such women. The age distribution of current participants reflects this postmenopausal group: 10% of the population is under the age of 50, 50% is 50–59, and 40% is 60 years of age or older. Eleven percent of the women have a 5-year breast cancer risk as estimated by the Gail Model of less than 2%. Sixty-two percent have an estimated risk between 2% and 4.9%, and 27% have a 5-year breast cancer risk estimate of ≥5%. Of the participants randomized, 1,033 or 8.3% have a history of lobular carcinoma in situ, and 19.2% (2,377 participants) have a history of breast biopsy demonstrating atypical hyperplasia. Seventy-five percent of the participants have one or more first-degree relatives with breast cancer (mother, sister, or daughter). More than half (52.5%) have histories of hysterectomy with or without oophorectomy; this is more than the 37% of women in the P-1 trial who had had a hysterectomy prior to entry.

More than 105,000 women have filled out NSABP Risk Assessment Forms (RAF) to determine their Gail Model scores and to establish their risk eligibility for the STAR trial. Of the women who completed RAFs, 59,472 (56.2%) are risk-eligible. All these women take part in one-to-one discussions about breast cancer and breast cancer risk. Many are pleasantly surprised that their breast cancer risk is not as high as they had imagined. In addition to the Gail Model score, each woman receives a summary of benefits and risks associated with SERM use based on data from the P-1 Trial. Each potential participant also receives a table that shows certain events that would be expected during the next 5 years among 10,000 women not receiving SERM therapy, matched by age, race, and breast cancer risk. These numbers are then compared with the number of expected cases that would be prevented or caused by 5 years of SERM use. Life-threatening events listed include invasive breast cancer, hip fracture, endometrial cancer, stroke, and pulmonary embolus; severe events that are projected include in situ breast cancer and deep vein thrombosis; other events include wrist fractures and spine fractures, and the increased occurrence of cataracts. Providing the breast cancer risk scores along with the risk/benefit tables results in a skewed distribution of participants randomized from the various Gail score categories: only 2.3% of the women with 5-year Gail scores under 2% have been randomized into the trial, but 35% of the women with scores over 5% have been randomized. The higher the Gail score, the more likely a woman will be to have a more favorable risk/benefit ratio. Women who are interested in obtaining their breast cancer risk assessment and the risk/benefit projection will find a list of participating STAR sites at www.ns-abp.pitt.edu/STAR/index.html.

Summary

The NSABP breast cancer prevention trial P-1 is a large first step toward the final goal of true breast cancer prevention, but it is only a step. It does provide proof of principle that the incidence of breast cancer can be reduced, and reduced dramatically, through the use of pharmaceutical agents. Outside clinical trials, tamoxifen is being incorporated cautiously for breast cancer prevention, with many physicians apparently targeting high-risk groups of patients in whom the perceived benefit-to-risk ratio is the greatest. The STAR trial has entered over 50% of its required sample size in 30 months and is on track to enroll the required 22,000 postmenopausal participants who are at increased risk for breast cancer in the projected 5-year period.

References

Adjuvant tamoxifen in the management of operable breast cancer: The Scottish Trial. Report from the Breast Cancer Trials Committee (1987) Scottish Cancer Trials Office (MRC), Edinburgh. Lancet 2:171–175

Costantino JP, Gail MH, Pee D, et al (1999) Validation studies for models to project the risk of invasive and total breast cancer incidence. J Natl Cancer Inst 91:1541–1548

CRC Adjuvant Breast Trial Working Party (1988) Cyclophosphamide and tamoxifen as adjuvant therapies in the management of breast cancer. Br J Cancer 57:604–607

Cummings SR, Eckert S, Krueger KA, et al (1999) The effects of raloxifene on the risk of breast cancer in postmenopausal women: results from the MORE randomized trial. Multiple outcomes of raloxifene evaluation. JAMA 281:2189–2197

Fisher B, Brown A, Wolmark N, et al (1987) Prolonging tamoxifen therapy for primary breast cancer: findings from the National Surgical Adjuvant Breast and Bowel Project clinical trial. Ann Int Med 106:649–654

Fisher B, Redmond C (1991) New perspective on cancer of the contralateral breast: a marker for assessing tamoxifen as a preventive agent [editorial]. J Natl Cancer Inst 83:1278–1280

Fisher B, Costantino JP, Wickerham DL, et al (1998) Tamoxifen for prevention of breast cancer: report of the National Surgical Adjuvant Breast and Bowel Project P-1 study. J Natl Cancer Inst 18:1371–1388

Fisher B, Dignam J, Wolmark N, et al (1999) Tamoxifen in treatment of intraductal breast cancer: National Surgical Adjuvant Breast and Bowel Project B-24 randomised controlled trial. Lancet 353:1993–2000

Fisher B, Dignam J, Bryant J, Wolmark N (2001) Five versus more than five years of tamoxifen for lymph node-negative breast cancer: updated findings from the National Surgical Adjuvant Breast and Bowel Project B-14 randomized trial. J Natl Cancer Inst 93:684–690

Gail MH, Brinton LA, Byar DP, et al (1989) Projecting individualized probabilities of developing breast cancer for white females who are being examined annually. J Natl Cancer Inst 81:1879–1886

Gail MH, Costantino JP, Bryant J, et al (1999) Weighing the risk and benefits of tamoxifen for preventing breast cancer. J Natl Cancer Inst 91:1829–1846

Gorin MB, Day R, Costantino JP, et al (1998) Long-term tamoxifen citrate use and potential ocular toxicity. Am J Ophthalmol 125:493–501

Powles T, Eeles R, Ashley S, et al (1998) Interim analysis of the incidence of breast cancer in the Royal Marsden Hospital tamoxifen randomised chemoprevention trial. Lancet 352:98–101

Reis SE, Costantino JP, Wickerham DL, et al (2001) Cardiovascular effects of tamoxifen in women with and without heart disease: Breast cancer prevention trial. J Natl Cancer Inst 93:16–21

Rutqvist LE, Cedermark B, Glas U, et al (1991) Contralateral primary tumors in breast cancer patients in a randomized trial of adjuvant tamoxifen therapy. J Natl Cancer Inst 83:1299–1306

Tan-Chiu E, Costantino J, Wang J, et al (2001) The effect of tamoxifen on benign breast disease. Findings from the National Surgical Adjuvant Breast and Bowel Project (NSABP) Breast Cancer Prevention Trial (BCPT). Proc Ann San Antonio Breast Cancer Symposium 69:210

Veronesi U, Maisonneuve P, Costa A, et al (1998) Prevention of breast cancer with tamoxifen: preliminary findings from the Italian randomised trial among hysterectomised women. Lancet 352:93–97

Aromatase Inhibitors in Prevention – Data from the ATAC (Arimidex, Tamoxifen Alone or in Combination) Trial and the Design of IBIS-II (the Second International Breast Cancer Intervention Study)

Jack Cuzick

J. Cuzick (✉)
Cancer Research UK, Department of Epidemiology,
Mathematics and Statistics, Wolfson Institute of Preventive Medicine,
Charterhouse Square, London ECIM 6BQ

Abstract

Current prevention trials have shown that tamoxifen can reduce the incidence of breast cancer by about 30%–40% in high-risk women, but that the risk of thromboembolic disease and endometrial cancer are increased about twofold. An alternative approach for postmenopausal women is to use an aromatase inhibitor to reduce oestrogen to very low levels. Data from the ATAC adjuvant trial indicate that the aromatase inhibitor anastrozole is more effective than tamoxifen in reducing recurrence and preventing new contralateral tumours, and also has a more favourable side-effect profile. This has led us to launch a new prevention trial – IBIS-II – in 6,000 high-risk postmenopausal women comparing anastrozole against placebo. A parallel trial will compare anastrozole against tamoxifen in 4,000 women with locally excised DCIS.

Abbreviations ATAC, arimidex, tamoxifen alone or in combination; BMD, bone mineral density; BRCA1, breast cancer gene 1; CI, confidence interval; DCIS, ductal carcinoma in situ; DXA, dual x-ray absorptiometry; EBCC, European Breast Cancer Conference; HR, hazard ratio; IBIS, International Breast Cancer Intervention Study; OR, odds ratio; RMH, Royal Marsden Hospital; SERMs, selective oestrogen receptor modulators.

Introduction

Why Use Aromatase Inhibitors in Prevention?

In the prevention of breast cancer, there are currently two possible strategies: (1) the effects of oestrogen may be blocked using selective oestrogen receptor modulators (SERMs) such as tamoxifen; (2) alternatively, the oestrogen stimulus may be reduced using aromatase inhibitors. Four studies have now reported on the use of tamoxifen in the prevention of breast cancer and jointly support a 30%–40% reduction in new breast cancers (Powles 1998: Fisher 1998; Veronesi 1998; Cuzick 2000; IBIS 2002). Although no preventative studies have compared tamoxifen with aromatase inhibitors to date, the third-generation aromatase inhibitors anastrozole and letrozole have shown greater efficacy than tamoxifen as first-line therapy for postmenopausal women with advanced breast cancer (Bonneterre et al. 2000, 2001; Nabholtz et al. 2000; Mouridsen et al. 2001). In addition, anastrozole is a more effective adjuvant therapy than tamoxifen in postmenopausal women with early breast cancer, as demonstrated by the findings of the ATAC trial (ATAC 2002). These studies suggest that aromatase inhibitors may provide a superior approach to chemoprevention of breast cancer in postmenopausal women than tamoxifen.

In terms of tolerability and side effects, treatment with aromatase inhibitors has been shown to reduce the incidence of vascular events, stroke, endometrial cancer, hot flushes, and vaginal symptoms compared with tamoxifen (Bonneterre et al. 2000, 2001; Nabholtz et al. 2000; Mouridsen et al. 2001; ATAC Trial Group 2002). However, there are remaining concerns about the use of aromatase inhibitors in healthy postmenopausal women due to the very low levels of oestrogen achieved by these agents. The primary concern is with bone loss, but other potential concerns include cognitive function.

The first results of the ATAC trial in the treatment of early breast cancer are now available. A new trial, IBIS-II (the second International Breast cancer Intervention Study), has been designed to investigate whether the superiority of anastrozole over tamoxifen seen in the ATAC trial will translate into the prevention setting and thereby offer more choice to those patients living with the threat of breast cancer. Postmenopausal women who have had proven completely excised ductal carcinoma in situ (DCIS) or increased risk of breast cancer will be recruited into the study, which is due to be launched in November, 2002. This paper aims to discuss how the recent results of the ATAC trial support the case for conducting the IBIS-II prevention trial.

The ATAC Trial

The ATAC trial compared tamoxifen (20 mg/day) with anastrozole (1 mg/day) alone and with the combination of anastrozole plus tamoxifen as adjuvant treatment for women with early breast cancer.

Study Design

The trial was designed as a randomized, double-blind, multicentre study. Postmenopausal women with invasive breast cancer who had completed their primary therapy were recruited from 381 centres in 21 countries between July 1996 and March 2000; 9,366 patients entered the trial. These patients were ran-

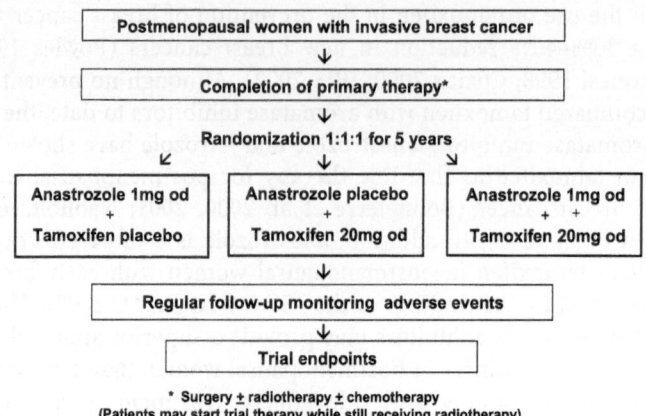

Fig. 1. ATAC trial design

domized equally between three treatment arms (Fig. 1) and they were followed up regularly and monitored for adverse events.

Study Endpoints

The primary endpoint of the ATAC trial was disease-free survival (defined as time to locoregional or distant tumour recurrence, new primary breast cancer, or death). Tolerability was also a primary concern. Secondary endpoints were time to recurrence or new breast cancer (censoring deaths before recurrence), time to distant recurrence of the tumour, incidence of new breast (contralateral) primaries, and survival.

Outcomes

Anastrozole was found to be superior to tamoxifen in terms of disease-free survival in the overall population [HR=0.83, 95% CI (0.71–0.96), P=0.013]. A larger 21% reduction was seen for breast cancer events [HR=0.79, 95% CI (0.67–0.94), P=0.008] and this increased still further to 27% when restricted to ER-positive patients [HR=0.73, 95% CI (0.59–0.90), P=0.003].

In addition, the incidence of contralateral breast cancer in the overall population was 58% lower (14 versus 33 new cancers) in patients treated with anastrozole compared to tamoxifen, [95% CI (21%–78%), P=0.007]. When only invasive contralateral tumours were considered, a 70% reduction was seen [9 versus 30, 95% CI (35%–88%), P=0.0008]. Given that tamoxifen itself is associated with a 40% reduction in new contralateral tumours, the overall reduction associated with anastrozole could be as high as 80%.

All treatments were generally well tolerated. Anastrozole was significantly better than tamoxifen with respect to incidence of endometrial cancer (3 versus 13 cases, $P=0.02$), vaginal bleeding (4.5% versus 8.1%, respectively, $P<0.0001$), vaginal discharge (2.8% versus 11.4%, respectively, $P<0.0001$), ischaemic cerebrovascular events (1.0% versus 2.1%, respectively, $P=0.0006$), venous thrombolic events (2.1% versus 3.5%, respectively, $P=0.0006$) and hot flushes (34.3% versus 39.7%, respectively, $P<0.0001$). Tamoxifen was better tolerated than anastrozole with respect to the incidence of musculoskeletal disorders (27.8% versus 21.3%, respectively, $P<0.0001$) and fractures (5.9% versus 3.7%, respectively, $P<0.0001$).

In all respects (i.e., for both efficacy and side effects), the combination of tamoxifen and anastrozole behaved very much like tamoxifen alone, indicating that the agonist properties of tamoxifen become dominant at the low oestrogen levels achieved by treatment with anastrozole, and that this limits the ultimate efficacy of tamoxifen. Thus the combined treatment does not appear promising, either in prevention or treatment of breast cancer.

However, these findings do show anastrozole to be an effective and well-tolerated endocrine option for the treatment of postmenopausal women with early breast cancer and provide justification and optimism about its potential role in prevention.

The IBIS-II Study

The IBIS-II study is a large, multicentre, randomized, double-blind controlled study comparing placebo with tamoxifen with anastrozole in postmenopausal women with DCIS or at increased risk of breast cancer.

Study Design

The study will be conducted in two strata. The first stratum will involve women at increased risk of breast cancer. These women will be randomized 1:1 into a trial to compare placebo with anastrozole over 5 years (Fig. 2). The target sample size for this study is 6,000.

In the second stratum of the trial, women who have had proven completely excised DCIS will be randomized 1:1 into a two-arm trial that will compare tamoxifen with anastrozole (Fig. 3). The target sample size for this study is 4,000.

Entry Requirements

To enter the trial, candidates must be postmenopausal women with an increased risk of developing breast cancer. They should have had a baseline dual x-ray absorptiometry (DXA) scan and a spinal radiograph to rule out osteoporosis; a blood sample will also be taken for marker studies. Women with evidence of osteoporosis will only be eligible if they join the bone subprotocol

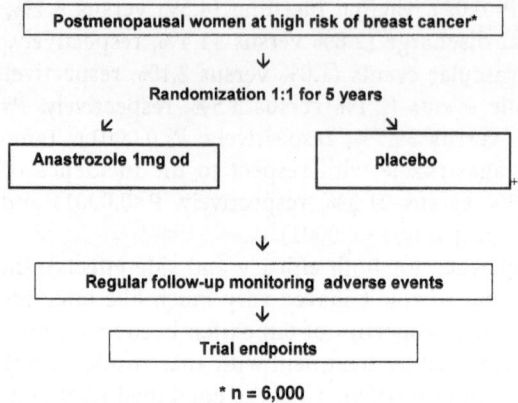

Fig. 2. IBIS-II study summary for patients at high risk

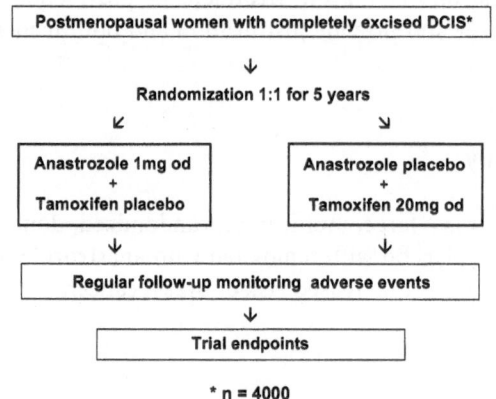

Fig. 3. IBIS-II study summary for patients in the DCIS arm

and take a bisphosphonate. In the prevention stratum, a baseline mammogram will be required to rule out breast cancer. For women entering the DCIS stratum, diagnostic histopathological blocks/samples will be requested for review of the diagnosis and additional marker studies.

Entry Criteria

Women Aged 45–70 Years

The entry criteria are based on a relative risk of at least twofold. At least one of the following must be satisfied. Patients must:

a. Have either a first-degree relative who developed breast cancer at age 50 or less; a first-degree relative who developed bilateral breast cancer; two or more first- or second-degree relatives who developed breast cancer or ovarian cancer (if both relatives are second-degree and on opposite sides of the family, then at least one must have been diagnosed at age 50 or less)

b. Be nulliparous (or first birth at age 30 or above) and have a first-degree relative who developed breast cancer

c. Have a benign biopsy with proliferative disease and a first-degree relative who developed breast cancer

d. Show increased mammographic density covering at least 50% of the breast

Women Aged 60–70 Years

Because of their higher baseline risk, women aged 60–70 years can enter the study with a smaller baseline risk and need only have one or more of the following risk factors. They need to have either a first-degree relative with breast cancer at any age; to have been aged 55 years or older at menopause; or to be nulliparous (or first birth at age 30 years or more).

Women Aged 40–44 Years

Women aged 40–44 years who are postmenopausal (usually because of a bilateral oophorectomy) are eligible if they satisfy one or more of the following criteria, which confer an approximately fourfold or greater risk. They should:

a. Have two or more first or second-degree relatives who developed breast cancer or ovarian cancer at age 50 or less

b. Have a first-degree relative with bilateral breast cancer who developed the first breast cancer at age 50 or less

c. Be nulliparous and a have first-degree relative who developed breast cancer at age 40 or less

d. Have a benign biopsy with proliferative disease and a first degree relative who developed breast cancer at age 40 or less

Women Aged 40–70 Years

Women who have had certain breast conditions will also be eligible. These conditions are lobular carcinoma in situ, atypical ductal or lobular hyperplasia in a benign lesion and DCIS treated by mastectomy.

Study Recruitment

Recruitment is planned to begin in November 2002 when the trial is launched. Patients will be recruited from Europe, Asia, Australasia and South America.

Study Endpoints

The primary endpoint for the trial is the incidence of breast cancer. A range of secondary endpoints will also be examined including fracture rates, other cancers, and cause-specific mortality.

Supplementary Studies

To investigate the tolerability issues associated with aromatase inhibitor therapy, there will be three prospectively planned subprotocol studies focusing on bone mineral density (BMD) and bone biomarkers, cognitive function, and DCIS pathology.

IBIS-II Bone Subprotocol

A total of 1,000 postmenopausal women with increased risk of breast cancer will be recruited into this subprotocol. Baseline DXA scans will be taken and then follow-up scans will be taken 1, 3, 5, and 7 years later. Of these women, 300 will have T-scores in the osteoporotic range (T<−2.5) and will be required to take a bisphosphonate. Another 400 will be in the osteopenic range (−1.5>T>−2.5) and will be randomized to a bisphosphonate or not, and the remaining 300 will range T-scores greater than −1.5 and will be monitored but not treated.

IBIS-II Timeline

Subject to final regulatory and funding approval, IBIS-II is scheduled to be launched in December 2002. The timeline leading up to the trial launch is shown in Fig. 4.

IBIS II- Time Line

• April 2001	ICRF Scientific Approval
• June 2001	MREC Approval
• December 2001	ATAC Results Announced
• March 2002	IBIS-I Results Announced
• June 2002	Funding Approval by UK Charities
• September 2002	MREC Approval for amended trial
• October 2002	MCA Regulatory Approval (CTC)
• November 2002	Trial Launch

Fig. 4. The IBIS-II timeline prior to trial launch

Conclusions

Based on the results from the ATAC trial presented above, the prospects for the use of anastrozole in prevention look very favourable. However, the use of this drug is relatively recent and very little long-term experience is available. Important concerns still remain, especially in terms of bone loss, and a major challenge will be to learn how to minimize and effectively manage this concern. Undoubtedly greater use of DXA scans will be required along with selective use of bisphosphonates when bone mineral declines below safe levels.

Other concerns are more speculative at this stage, but never before have women been subjected to prolonged and virtually complete oestrogen deprivation, and the prevention studies have an obligation to examine very carefully what are the effects of this manoeuvre.

Losses in cognitive function have been suggested and this will be evaluated in a specific protocol, but careful long term follow-up of women in the trial will be essential.

References

Bonneterre J, Thurlimann B, Robertson J, Krzakowski M, Mauriac L, Koralewski P, Vergote I, Webster A, Steinberg M, von Euler M (2000) Anastrozole versus tamoxifen as first-line therapy for advanced breast cancer in 668 postmenopausal women – results of the target (tamoxifen or Arimidex randomized group efficacy and tolerability) study. J Clin Oncol 18:3748–3757

Bonneterre J, Buzdar A, Nabholtz JM, Robertson JF, Thurlimann B, von Euler M, Sahmoud T, Webster A, Steinberg M (2001) Anastrozole is superior to tamoxifen as first-line therapy in hormone receptor positive advanced breast carcinoma. Cancer 92:2247–2258

Cuzick J (2000) Future possibilities in the prevention of breast cancer. Breast cancer prevention trials. Breast Cancer Res 2:258–263

Fisher B, Constantino JP, Wickerham DL et al. (1998) Prevention of breast cancer with tamoxifen. Report of the National Surgical Adjuvant Breast and Bowel Project P-1 Study. J Nill Cancer Inst 96:1321–1387

IBIS Investigators (2002) First results from the International Breast Cancer Intervention Study (IBIS-I): a randomised prevent trial. Lancet 360:817–24

Mouridsen H, Gershanovich M, Sun Y, Perez-Carrion R, Boni C, Monnier A, Apffelstaedt J, Smith R, Sleeboom H (2001) Superior efficacy of letrozole versus tamoxifen as first-line therapy for postmenopausal women with advanced breast cancer: results of a phase III study of the International letrozole breast cancer group. J Clin Oncol 19:2596–2606

Nabholtz J, Buzdar A, Pollak M, Harwin W, Burton G, Mangalik A (2000) Anastrozole is superior to tamoxifen as first-line therapy for advanced breast cancer in postmenopausal women: results of a North American multicenter randomized trial. J Clin Oncol 18:3758–3776

Powles T, Eeles R, Ashley S, Easton D, Chang J, Dowsett M, Tidy A, Viggers J, Davey J (1998) Interim analysis of the incidence of breast cancer in the Royal Marsden Hospital tamoxifen randomised chemoprevention trial. Lancet 352:98–101

Veronesi U, Maisonneuve P, Costa A, Sacchini V, Maltoni C, Robertson C, Rotmensz N, Boyle P (1998) Prevention of breast cancer with tamoxifen: preliminary findings from the Italian randomised trial among hysterectomised women. Lancet 352:93–97

ATAC Trialists Group (2002) Anastrozole alone or in combination with tamoxifen versus tamoxifen alone for adjuvant treatment of postmenopausal women with early breast cancer: First results of the ATAC randomised trial. Lancet 359:2131–2139

HRT Opposed to Low-Dose Tamoxifen (HOT Study): Rationale and Design

Andrea Decensi, Arianna Galli, Umberto Veronesi

A. Decensi (✉)
European Institute of Oncology, Via Ripamonti 435, 20141 Milan, Italy

Abstract

The rationale for the HOT study is mainly based on the findings of the Italian Tamoxifen Prevention Study, where 5,408 healthy hysterectomized women aged 35–70 years were randomized to 20 mg/day of tamoxifen or placebo for 5 years. After 81.2 months median follow-up, 79 breast cancers occurred (34 on tamoxifen versus 45 on placebo, $p=0.215$). In the subgroup of 1,580 women who used estrogen replacement therapy (ERT) at some point during the study, 23 breast cancers were observed: 17 on placebo and 6 on tamoxifen (hazard ratio=0.35, 95% CI, 0.14–0.89). Pharmacokinetic and pharmacodynamic (surrogate endpoint biomarkers) studies showed that a lower dose of tamoxifen (such as 5 mg/day) does not affect the drug's activity on several biomarkers of both cardiovascular and breast cancer risk. We therefore propose a multicenter placebo-controlled phase III trial in postmenopausal healthy women on hormone replacement therapy (HRT) to assess whether the combination of HRT and low-dose tamoxifen retains the benefits while reducing the risks of either.
A number of different observations indicate that the combination of hormone replacement therapy (HRT) and a selective estrogen receptor modulator (SERM) such as tamoxifen may retain the benefits while reducing the risks of either agent. While epidemiological evidence suggests that HRT can substantially increase quality as well as length of life, a prolonged use of HRT can also increase the risk of developing breast cancer, particularly with the combination of estrogens and progestins. The increased risk has been associated with an increased expression of estrogen receptors in the healthy breast tissue, thus leading to an enhanced sensitivity to estrogen signal. Thus, the addition of a SERM which may be capable of reducing this growth promoting effect on the breast appears rationale for women's health maintenance. A post hoc analysis of the Italian study of Breast Cancer Chemoprevention with tamoxifen showed a borderline significant reduction of breast cancer among women who were

Recent Results in Cancer Research, Vol. 163
© Springer-Verlag Berlin Heidelberg 2003

on HRT continuously and tamoxifen as compared with continuous HRT users who received placebo.

Although the study was regarded as being affected by a high drop-out rate [1], a comparison of the three primary prevention trials of tamoxifen indicates that, in fact, the number of discontinuations for reasons other than major events was 20.7%, 28.8%, and 35.5%, in the Italian, American, and Marsden trials, respectively [2]. In the Italian trial, the drop-out rate was higher during the first year of recruitment and plateaued thereafter (2% per month in the first year versus 1% in years 2–5). Since most women who left the study voluntarily did so mainly because of menopausal symptoms, the combination of tamoxifen and estrogen replacement therapy (ERT) might reduce tamoxifen side effects. Indeed, the rate of voluntary withdrawals was different according to ERT use: compliance with treatment was 78% at 3 years and 75% at 5 years for women who never took ERT, while for women who were not on ERT at baseline but who took ERT at some time during the trial, the compliance was 92% at 3 years and 88% at 5 years. The figures for 3 years are based on 2,204, 385, and 433 women, respectively, while those at 5 years are based on 500, 111, and 151 for "never on ERT," "no ERT at baseline then on" and "always on ERT," respectively. These data suggest that compliance may be increased by concomitant use of ERT and tamoxifen.

The use of progestins in the HRT regimen might reduce the risk of endometrial cancer associated with tamoxifen treatment. Indeed, the NSABP P1 trial showed that women aged 50 years or younger had no increased incidence of adverse events, including endometrial cancer and venous thromboembolic events [3]. This might suggest that the concomitant presence of adequate circulating hormone levels prevent tamoxifen from acting as an estrogen agonist at these target tissues. In addition, previous studies have shown that the combination of HRT and tamoxifen does not adversely influence their biological effects, including bone density and clotting factors [4], and our group has recently shown that the beneficial effects of tamoxifen on cardiovascular risk factors are unchanged in current HRT users [5]. Altogether, these considerations provide a strong rationale for further investigations of the combination of tamoxifen and HRT in an attempt to reduce the risk while retaining the benefits of both agents.

As regards breast cancer risk associated with HRT use, the meta-analysis of 51 epidemiological studies, including 52,705 individuals with breast cancer and 108,411 control women accounting for 90% of the worldwide evidence, has shown that ever use of oral HRT is associated with an overall increased risk of breast cancer (RR=1.14, SE=0.03, p=0.00001) [6]. The risk increased with duration of HRT (RR=1.35, 95%CI =1.21–1.49 after an average of 11 years), and progressively decreased after HRT discontinuation with no excess risk after 5 years from cessation. Interestingly, the magnitude of the increased risk (2.3% per year, 95% CI, 1.1%–3.6%) is comparable to that associated with each year of delayed menopause (i.e., 2.8%, 95% CI, 2.1%–3.4%), strongly upholding the hypothesis that maintenance of a premenopausal hormonal milieu may account for the reported increased risk in HRT users. Importantly, the increased risk observed in current and recent HRT users was greater for women with lower body mass index (i.e., BMI <25 kg/m^2).

Although little information was available regarding hormonal type and dose and 80% of these women had used oral estrogen alone, the addition of progestins was associated with a higher RR of breast cancer than estrogen alone. The RR was 1.15 (SE, 0.19) and 1.53 (SE, 0.33) in current or recent users of estroprogestins for 5 years or less and for more than 5 years, respectively, compared with a RR of 0.99 (SE, 0.08) and 1.34 (SE, 0.09) for current or recent users of estrogens alone. Finally, cancers in women who had ever used HRT tended to be less advanced clinically than those in never users. In this regard, a prospective cohort study on 37,105 HRT users in the Iowa Women's Health Study has shown that exposure to HRT was associated with an increased risk of invasive breast cancer with a favorable histologic type, while there was little evidence of association with other invasive ductal or lobular cancers or ductal carcinoma in situ [7]. These findings have not been confirmed in other studies [8]. Also, a trend to longer survival in HRT users who developed breast cancer compared to never users has been observed in some studies [9]. A previous analysis from the Nurses' Health Study [10] showed a moderately elevated risk of breast cancer death among postmenopausal women who were taking oral estrogen or had previously used this therapy for 10 years or more. Notably, a recent update of the cohort shows that the addition of progestins was associated with a 9% (SE, 2.5) increased risk per year as compared to 3.3% (SE, 0.84) with estrogen alone [11]. Likewise, a recent analysis from the Breast Cancer Detection Demonstration Project (BCDDP) based on 2,082 incident breast cancer cases found that the estrogen-progestin regimens were associated with greater increases in breast cancer risk than estrogen alone (8% per year, 95% CI, 2%–16% compared to 1%, 95% CI, 0.2%–3% for each year of estrogen alone) [8]. Importantly, the increased risk is largely limited to current or recent users and is directly related to duration of use. An updated analysis in a Swedish cohort also found greater risks with combined therapy; for 6 or more years of current or recent use, the risk of breast cancer was increased by 70% for combined therapy but no increase was seen for estrogen alone [12]. A case-control study recently performed in California among 1,897 postmenopausal case subjects and 1,637 postmenopausal control subjects also showed that combined estroprogestin therapy was associated with a higher risk of breast cancer compared to unopposed estrogen replacement therapy [13]. The OR for 5 years of HRT use was 1.10 (95% CI, 1.02–1.18). Risk was higher for continuous HRT (estro-progestin) users (OR, 1.24, 95% CI, 1.07–1.45) than for ERT users (OR, 1.06, 95% CI, 0.97–1.15). There was a trend for sequential HRT (i.e., with progestins given for 10 or more days per month) being associated with a higher risk (OR, 1.38, 95% CI, 1.13–1.68) than combined continuous HRT (i.e., with progestins given continuously), where the OR was 1.09 (95% CI, 0.88–1.35), but this was not statistically significant. These results were not confirmed in the Swedish cohort, where continuous combined HRT was associated with a higher risk than sequential HRT (14). Differences between progesterone-derived and testosterone-derived progestin use may partly account for these discrepancies. Overall, these studies provide firm evidence that addition of progestin to estrogen does not reduce the risk of breast cancer and suggest that the risk is actually increased [15].

It must be emphasized that all the above data are based solely on studies making use of orally administered estrogens. Since the extensive use of transdermal HRT is relatively recent, no epidemiological data is available yet on its association with breast cancer risk. However, the parenteral route of administration, in contrast to the oral route, is associated with the following endocrine effects: a trend to an increase in circulating insulin-like growth factor-I (IGF-I) levels, one of the most potent breast mitogens [16, 17], a lower conversion to the weak estrogen estrone [18, 19], and a higher availability of free estrogen levels due to unchanged sex-hormone binding globulin (SHBG) levels [16, 18, 20]. These effects might be associated with an increased risk of breast cancer. While further studies are needed to clarify this issue, new strategies to minimize the risk of breast cancer in HRT users are demanded.

From the biological point of view, the increased risk of breast cancer associated with HRT use is linked to an increased expression of estrogen receptors in the breast tissue [21], thus leading to an enhanced sensitivity to the mitogenic effect of estrogen. The addition of a SERM, such as tamoxifen, capable of reducing this growth-promoting effect on the breast could therefore be useful for women's health maintenance. On the other hand, one of the major concerns about this drug is the increased risk of endometrial cancer. In the NSABP P1 prevention study, the rate of endometrial cancer was increased in the tamoxifen group (risk ratio=2.53; 95% CI=1.35–4.97), the increased risk occurring predominantly in women aged 50 years or older. In women aged 49 or younger, the RR was 1.21, 95% CI, 0.41–3.60; in women aged 50 years or more, the RR was 4.01, 95% CI, 1.70–10.90. This suggests that the woman's endocrine milieu can influence the pharmacodynamics of tamoxifen at the endometrial level. Specifically, progesterone could neutralize tamoxifen's agonistic activity on the endometrium in much the same manner as progesterone countered the proliferative effect of estrogen in this organ. Moreover, all endometrial cancers observed in the NSABP P1 trial were stage I and no endometrial cancer deaths were reported in the tamoxifen group [3].

There is also indirect evidence that the risk of endometrial cancer induced by tamoxifen is both time and dose dependent, the higher relative risk being observed with daily doses of 40 or 30 mg/day of adjuvant tamoxifen [22]. Thus, one plausible way to lower this risk is a reduction of the dose [23]. We therefore studied the biological activity of tamoxifen with a view to establishing a dosing schedule with a better risk–benefit ratio [24, 25]. The blood concentrations of tamoxifen and its main metabolites were measured in a dose titration study in 105 healthy women (placebo, tamoxifen 10 mg on alternate days, 10 mg/day, and 20 mg/day). Drug levels measured after 2 months of treatment were correlated with the changes in several biomarkers such as total cholesterol, HDL cholesterol, LDL cholesterol, triglycerides, lipoprotein (a), blood cell count, fibrinogen, antithrombin III, osteocalcin, and IGF-I. Mean (±SD) tamoxifen and N-desmethyltamoxifen (metabolite X) concentrations were dose-related, being, respectively, 0 and 0 ng/ml with placebo, 26.8±15.1 and 43.7±22.5 ng/ml with 10 mg every other day, 51.2±24.1 and 90.7±48 ng/ml with 10 mg/day, and 136±52.7 and 230.6±75.0 ng/ml with 20 mg/day of tamoxifen. In contrast, the biomarker changes were of comparable magnitudes at all drug concentrations, with the exception of platelet counts and triglyceride levels, both of which showed a trend toward increasing with increasing tamoxifen concentrations. Therefore, a 75% reduction of the conventional dose, which resulted in an 80% decrease in serum drug concentration, did not affect tamoxifen activity on several biomarkers of cardiovascular and breast cancer risk and may in fact have a more favorable safety profile [25].

We have subsequently set up an experiment that is reciprocal and complementary to our previous trial, namely, a study of the correlation of tamoxifen elimination with biomarker recovery in healthy subjects completing the 5-year intervention period [26]. Tamoxifen, N-desmethyltamoxifen and biomarker levels were measured at 0 (baseline), 2, 4, and 6 weeks after completion of treatment in 23 healthy postmenopausal women allocated to tamoxifen 20 mg/day and in six women allocated to placebo. Mean (±SD) serum tamoxifen and N-desmethyltamoxifen concentrations were, respectively, 141±50 and 226±77 ng/ml at baseline, 36±19 and 99±46 ng/ml at 2 weeks, 20±15 and 61±37 ng/ml at 4 weeks and 12±9 and 36±26 ng/ml at 6 weeks. Compared to baseline values, the percent increase in total cholesterol, LDL cholesterol and IGF-I four weeks after treatment completion was 5%, 9%, and 14%, respectively. No change during the 6-week period was observed in the placebo arm. After one month of treatment discontinuation, the biomarkers' recovery was far from complete despite tamoxifen concentrations in the range of 10 ng/ml, i.e., approximately 15 times lower than the steady-state concentrations attained with 20 mg/day [26]. Consistent with observations in breast cancer patients treated for a short term [27] or for longer periods [28], tamoxifen and N-desmethyltamoxifen serum concentrations were halved after 9 and 13 days, respectively. These findings underscore the importance of assessing the most appropriate schedule for preventive agents based on their pharmacokinetic characteristics. Although the limited observation time and the specific drug pharmacokinetics prevented us from inferring the minimal active concentration, our data suggest that biomarker recovery is slower than tamoxifen elimination from blood. This is in agreement with the observation that tamoxifen is retained in tissues for a long time [29], and indicates that tamoxifen may exert biological effects for several weeks after treatment interruption.

Since tamoxifen has a very high tissue/serum concentration ratio [29,30], the tissue level attainable with 10 mg every other day exceeds the growth inhibitory concentration of tamoxifen and N-desmethyltamoxifen in breast cancer cell lines, which is approximately 35 ng/ml [31–33]. In addition, the concomitant activity of metabolite X, which has a significant growth inhibitory activity in breast cancer cell lines, may further contribute to the total drug inhibitory activity. Moreover, in vivo studies in a spontaneous rat mammary tumor model showed that a dose equivalent to 1 mg/day in humans leads to a 94% inhibition of mammary tumor formation compared to control animals

Table 1. Potential benefit of the combination of tamoxifen and HRT

Breast cancer risk associated with HRT
Drop-out rate in tamoxifen studies[a]
Endometrial cancer associated with tamoxifen
Tamoxifen side effects? (vasomotor and urogenital symptoms)[a]

[a] Reduction in tamoxifen side effects is a major contributor to decreased drop-out rates in tamoxifen studies.

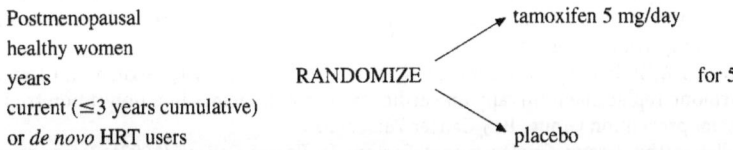

Postmenopausal
healthy women
years   RANDOMIZE   for 5
current (≤3 years cumulative)
or *de novo* HRT users

tamoxifen 5 mg/day

placebo

Fig. 1. HOT (hormone replacement therapy opposed to tamoxifen) study: design and endpoints. The study is a randomized, double-blind, placebo-controlled phase III trial with the following design: It will be a multicenter trial, and a total of 8,500 subjects are required, 4,250 per arm. *Primary endpoint*: Incidence of invasive and intraductal breast cancer. *Sample size*: 4,250 subjects per arm. Hazard ratio, 0.6; annual rate of events, 4/1,000; compliance, 80%. recruitment, 5 years; follow-up, 5 years; power, 80%

[34]. Interestingly, a recent cross-sectional study conducted in older nursing home residents in New York State long-term facilities has shown a significant reduction of bone fracture rate among women with breast cancer taking 10 mg/day of tamoxifen. During the first 1.5-year period for which bone fractures were documented, the fracture rates were 7.6% in 5,196 untreated control women, 3.2% in the 125 women receiving 10 mg/day of tamoxifen, and 6.7% in the 1,248 women receiving 20 mg/day of tamoxifen. The OR for 20 mg/day compared to controls is 0.92 (0.72–1.16), while for 10 mg/day versus controls is 0.31 (0.11–0.87, p=.025) [35]. Altogether, these findings provide a strong rationale to assess a lower dose of tamoxifen in a preventive context.

Taking into account all the above-mentioned considerations, it seems reasonable to test whether the combination of HRT and low doses of tamoxifen may retain the benefits while reducing the risks of either agent. A summary of the potential benefits of the combination of these two agents is reported in Table 1. We are therefore setting up a multicenter placebo-controlled phase III trial in postmenopausal healthy women currently on HRT (no more than 3 years are allowed) or in de novo users. Women will be randomized to tamoxifen 5 mg/day or placebo for 5 years. The study design is shown in Fig. 1. The study is powered to detect a 40% reduction in the incidence of invasive breast cancer and ductal carcinoma in situ in the tamoxifen arm. Secondary endpoints will be the incidence of other noninvasive breast disorders, endometrial cancer, bone fractures, cardiovascular events, venous thromboembolic events, cataracts, all other cancers (in particular, colorectal and ovary), and overall mortality.

References

1. Pritchard KI (1998) Is tamoxifen effective in prevention of breast cancer? Lancet 352:80–81
2. Veronesi U, Maisonneuve P, Costa A, et al (1999) Drop-outs in tamoxifen prevention trials. Lancet 353:244
3. Fisher B, Costantino JP, Wickerham DL, et al (1998) Tamoxifen for prevention of breast cancer: report of the National Surgical Adjuvant Breast and Bowel Project P-1 Study. J Natl Cancer Inst 90:1371–1388
4. Chang J, Powles TJ, Ashley SE, et al (1996) The effect of tamoxifen and hormone replacement therapy on serum cholesterol, bone mineral density and coagulation factors in healthy postmenopausal women participating in a randomised, controlled tamoxifen prevention study. Ann Oncol 7:671–675
5. Decensi A, Robertson C, Rotmensz N, et al (1998) Effect of tamoxifen and transdermal hormone replacement therapy on cardiovascular risk factors in a prevention trial. Italian Chemoprevention Group. Br J Cancer 78:572–578
6. Collaborative Group On Hormonal Factors In Breast Cancer (1997) Breast cancer and hormone replacement therapy: collaborative reanalysis of data from 51 epidemiological studies of 52 705 women with breast cancer and 108,411 women without breast cancer. Lancet 350:1047–1059
7. Gapstur SM, Morrow M, Sellers A (1999) Hormone replacement therapy and risk of breast cancer with a favorable histology: results of the Iowa Women's Health Study. JAMA 281:2091–2097
8. Schairer C, Lubin J, Troisi R, et al (2000) Menopausal estrogen and estrogen-progestin replacement therapy and breast cancer risk. JAMA 283:485–491
9. Schairer C, Gail M, Byrne C, et al (1999) Estrogen replacement therapy and breast cancer survival in a large screening study. J Natl Cancer Inst 91:264–270
10. Colditz GA, et al (1995) The use of estrogens and progestins and the risk of breast cancer in postmenopausal women. N Engl J Med 332:1589–1593
11. Colditz GA, Rosner B (1998) Use of estrogen plus progestin is associated with greater increase in breast cancer risk than estrogen alone. Am J Epidemiol 147:64S
12. Persson I, Weiderpass E, Bergkvist L, et al (1999) Risks of breast and endometrial cancer after estrogen and estrogen-progestin replacement. Cancer Causes Control 10:253–260
13. Ross RK, Paganini-Hill A, Wan PC, et al (2000) Effect of hormone replacement therapy on breast cancer risk: estrogen versus estrogen plus progestin. J Natl Cancer Inst 92:328–332
14. Magnusson C, Perssonh I, Adami O (2000) More about: effect of hormone replacement therapy on breast cancer risk: estrogen versus estrogen plus progestin. J Natl Cancer Inst 92:1183–1184
15. Willett W, Colditz CG, Stampfer M (2000) Postmenopausal estrogens–opposed, unopposed, or none of the above. JAMA 283:534–535
16. Slowinska-Srzednicka J, Zgliczynski S, Jeske W, et al (1992) Transdermal 17 beta-estradiol combined with oral progestogen increases plasma levels of insulin-like growth factor-I in postmenopausal women. J Endocrinol Invest 15:533–538
17. Weissberger AJ, Hol KK, Lazarus L (1991) Contrasting effects of oral and transdermal routes of estrogen replacement therapy on 24-hour growth hormone (GH) secretion, insulin-like growth factor I, and GH-binding protein in postmenopausal women. J Clin Endocrinol Metab 72:374–381
18. Van Erpecum KJ, Van Berge Henegouwen GP, Verschoor L, et al (1991) Different hepatobiliary effects of oral and transdermal estradiol in postmenopausal women. Gastroenterol. 100:482–488
19. Walsh BW, Li H, Sacks FM (1994) Effects of postmenopausal hormone replacement with oral and transdermal estrogen on high density lipoprotein metabolism. J Lipid Res 35:2083–2093

20. Chetkowski RJ, Meldrum DR, Steingold KA, et al (1986) Biologic effects of transdermal estradiol. N Engl J Med 314:1615–1620
21. Khan SA, Rogers MA, Khurana KK, et al (1998) Estrogen receptor expression in benign breast epithelium and breast cancer risk. J Natl Cancer Inst 90:37–42
22. Rutqvist E, Johansson H, Signomklao T, et al (1995) Adjuvant tamoxifen therapy for early stage breast cancer and second primary malignancies. Stockholm Breast Cancer Study Group. J Natl Cancer Inst 87:645–651
23. Jordan VC (1999) Tamoxifen: too much for a good thing? J Clin Oncol 17:2629–2630
24. Decensi A, Bonanni B, Guerrieri-Gonzaga A, et al (1998) Biologic activity of tamoxifen at low doses in healthy women. J Natl Cancer Inst 90:1461–1467
25. Decensi A, Gandini S, Guerrieri-Gonzaga A, et al (1999) Effect of blood tamoxifen concentrations on surrogate biomarkers in a trial of dose reduction. J Clin Oncol 17:2633–2638
26. Guerrieri-Gonzaga A, et al (2000) Correlation between tamoxifen wash-out and biomarkers recovery in a primary prevention trial (abstract). Proc Am Assoc Cancer Res 41:1419
27. Fabian C, Sternson L, El-Serafi M, et al (1981) Clinical pharmacology of tamoxifen in patients with breast cancer: correlation with clinical data. Cancer 48:876–882
28. Langan-Fahey SM, Tormey DC, Jordan VC (1990) Tamoxifen metabolites in patients on long-term adjuvant therapy for breast cancer. Eur J Cancer 26:883–888
29. Lien EA, Solheim E, Ueland PM (1991) Distribution of tamoxifen and its metabolites in rat and human tissues during steady-state treatment. Cancer Res 51:4837–4844
30. Robinson SP, Langan-Fahey SM, Johnson DA, et al (1991) Metabolites, pharmacodynamics, and pharmacokinetics of tamoxifen in rats and mice compared to the breast cancer patient. Drug Metab Dispos 19:36–43
31. Sutherland RL, et al (1987) Mechanisms of growth inhibition by nonsteroidal antioestrogens in human breast cancer cells. J Steroid Biochem 27:891–897
32. Lippman M, Bolan G, Huff K (1976) The effects of estrogens and antiestrogens on hormone-responsive human breast cancer in long-term tissue culture. Cancer Res 36:4595–4601
33. Wakeling AE (1989) Comparative studies on the effects of steroidal and nonsteroidal oestrogen antagonists on the proliferation of human breast cancer cells. J Steroid Biochem 34:183–188
34. Maltoni C, et al (1996) Experimental results on the chemopreventive and side effects of tamoxifen using a human-equivalent animal model. In: Maltoni C, Soffritti M, Davis W (eds) The scientific bases of cancer chemoprevention. pp 197–217
35. Breuer B, Wallenstein S, Anderson R (1998) Effect of tamoxifen on bone fractures in older nursing home residents. J Am Geriatr Soc 46:968–972

Secondary Prevention of Breast Cancer: 4
The Mammography Controversy

Is Mammography Screening for Breast Cancer Really Not Justifiable?

Anthony B. Miller

A.B. Miller (✉)
Division of Clinical Epidemiology,
Deutsches Krebsforschungszentrum (DKFZ),
Im Neuenheimer Feld 280, 69120 Heidelberg, Germany

Abstract

The consensus that breast screening is effective for women aged 50–59 years was shattered when Gotzsche and Olsen suggested that there are no reliable data to support screening by mammography. In practice, their concerns have been difficult to address because for many studies purporting to show effectiveness, adequate data have not been published to confirm that they were valid. Further, the trials in Canada for which such data are available did not show effectiveness of screening mammography. Since the 1990s, there has been an unprecedented reduction in breast cancer mortality in many countries. However, the reductions have no clear link to screening, but are probably due to the implementation of adjuvant treatment with chemotherapy and tamoxifen. Whether screening will have an additional impact in the future is unclear. After reviewing the published evidence, I conclude that the additional contribution of mammography over screening by good breast physical examinations and breast self examination is to detect good prognosis breast cancers, as the benefit of screening derives from the earlier detection of relatively advanced breast cancers, providing good therapy is given. If women choose mammography screening, they should understand that their risk of dying in the next few years may not be reduced.

Introduction

Mammography screening has become the mainstay of nearly all screening programmes for breast cancer. This is largely because a succession of expert groups have agreed that there is a significant benefit from such screening, especially among women age 50–69 (Day et al. 1986; Fletcher et al. 1993; Miller et al. 1990; US Preventive Services Task Force 1996).

However, periodically, doubts have surfaced. This has been particularly true for mammography screening among women age 40–49 (National Institutes of Health Consensus Development Panel1997). The consensus for women age 50–59 was shattered when Gotzsche and Olsen (2000) suggested that there are no reliable data to support screening by mammography, and the controversy was exacerbated by Olsen and Gotzsche (2001a), and the support they received from the editor of the *Lancet* (Horton 2001). In this manuscript, I shall first consider the Cochrane review of Olsen and Gotzsche (2001b), and then review the data that suggest that expert physical examinations of the breasts may be a viable alternative to mammography screening.

The Cochrane Review of Olsen and Gotzsche

Olsen and Gotzsche (2001b) suggested that randomisation was inadequate in achieving baseline comparability between the groups in at least two of the Swedish mammography screening trials, the Two-County and Stockholm trials, and possibly in the Göteborg trial as well. They were also concerned about the Edinburgh and HIP trials. Olsen and Gotzsche (2001b) were also concerned with what they called "early contamination" in the Two-County, Stockholm and Göteborg trials (the early screening of the control groups) and what they perceive as not reliable mortality data in most of the trials. I believe the concern over "early contamination" to be an error. This they define not in the usual way contamination is considered, but as introducing screening early in the control group. This may reduce the power of a trial, but it does not invalidate it, as what is being assessed is the effect of the numbers of screens given when there was no screening in the controls (ranging from 2 in the Stockholm trial to 8 in the Edinburgh trial).

However, the conclusion of Olsen and Olsen and Gotzsche (2001a,b) that because of the faults they identified, there are no reliable data to support screening by mammography, must be considered seriously. Although many have disputed their findings and analyses, it is notable that none of the investigators associated with the Swedish trials have refuted their suggestions with data on baseline comparability, presumably because these data were not collected. The problem is particularly acute for the Two-County trial, as that was the largest, had the greatest degree of benefit overall, and has been influential in establishing policy in many countries. Therefore I shall consider the criticisms made by Olsen and Gotzsche (2001b) in some detail, considering each of the trials they review in turn, but will first consider an issue they raised on the appropriate endpoint for screening trials.

The Issue of Endpoints of Screening Trials

All breast screening trials have so far reported their results in terms of the outcome cause-specific death (death due to breast cancer as the underlying cause). This approach has been criticised by Olsen and Gotzsche (2001b), who propose all cause mortality as the preferable endpoint, though they admit that such an endpoint would require very large trials. Using all cause mortality as an endpoint avoids problems with ascertaining cause of death precisely, and the concern that some deaths not apparently due to the cancer of interest may be a consequence of treatment for the cancer, but it causes major problems with trial power as death from the cancer, even one as common as breast cancer, is only a small component of all cause mortality. Olsen and Gotzsche (2001b) argue, for example, that radiotherapy, given after lumpectomy for screen-detected cancers, may cause unrecognised mortality from heart disease, which should have been regarded as a consequence of screening. However, this can not have been a problem in the HIP trial (see below), while in the Canadian trials we showed that there was an excess of mastectomies in the mammography screening arm, largely because of treatment of ductal carcinomas in situ (Miller 1994), and the major excess of lumpectomies expected by many did not appear to occur. Expert death review should solve these problems (Miller et al. 2000a; Miller 2001), though Gotzsche (2001) does not agree.

Nevertheless, Black et al. (2002) largely supported Olsen and Gotzsche (2001b), pointing out that in many screening trials the differential in all cause mortality is in the opposite direction to the differential in cause-specific mortality. They suggested that only when the differential for cause-specific and all cause mortality are both in the same direction in favour of the screened group, is it reasonable to conclude that screening is beneficial. This only occurred in the HIP trial. If the differential is in opposite directions in terms of sign, and all cause mortality is higher in the screened group, this suggests that screening may have been harmful, as in the Swedish Two-County trial and the Canadian 2 trial. Nevertheless, except for the Edinburgh breast screening trial, the differential in all cause mortality was very small and nonsignificant, supporting the contrary view that death review can usually be relied upon to reduce bias.

Lenner (1990) had earlier proposed the use of what he termed excess mortality rate, which is based upon the rate of death from all causes in the women with breast cancer less the similar rate of death in the women without breast cancer in the screened population expressed as the excess death rate in the total population offered screening. This rate can then be compared with the similar excess death rate in the women not offered screening. The method avoids the necessity to determine the cause of death, and it is believed in screening trials to be unbiased with regard to lead time and overdiagnosis. It should capture any deaths caused by the treatment for breast cancer and unrecognised as such, but will not capture deaths caused directly or indirectly by the screening procedure and associated diagnostic interventions if the woman was not diagnosed with breast cancer. Nyström et al. (1993) used this approach in the Swedish overview analysis as well as the conventional approach, and obtained very similar results. The method has so far not been used in analysing individual breast screening trials.

The HIP Trial

Olsen and Gotzsche (2001b) agreed the randomisation in HIP was adequate, but were concerned about the use of radiotherapy, and felt that post-randomisation exclusions may have led to lack of comparability in the HIP trial. Therefore they concluded that the published data are flawed.

I disagreed with that conclusion (Miller 2001). I pointed out that the HIP trial was performed in an era when the size of breast cancers was much larger than became usual in the subsequent two decades in North America. Lumpectomy was not practised in the HIP era, though radiotherapy was used frequently, especially for locally advanced disease. However, if an unrecognised consequence of radiotherapy was the cause of death, and was labelled as cardiovascular disease, such labelling would have been applied without bias as to treatment assignment. The major difficulty for the death reviewers was not whether the patient died of cancer, nor whether breast cancer had been diagnosed, but whether breast cancer was the cause of death when the patient had been diagnosed with another malignant disease. The decisions made were entirely masked, even after consultation between the reviewers for initial disagreement.

Olsen and Gotzsche (2001b) comment that equal numbers of patients, by allocation, were reviewed, but that the numbers assigned to breast cancer as a cause of death were fewer in the screening group, and this they cite as evidence of bias. An alternative explanation is more plausible. If screening was truly effective, then the numbers of deaths from breast cancer in a reviewed series would be less in the screened arm. The equal numbers reviewed could have resulted from a deliberate attempt to ensure that equivalent numbers of subjects in the two arms were reviewed at the same time to avoid bias. Further, the difference in numbers of women with breast cancer excluded from the two arms arose because when women in the screened group attended for screening, previously diagnosed breast cancers were identified, but this was not possible for the controls. The 18-year follow-up, however, enabled all deaths from breast cancer to be identified in the two groups; identification of the date of diagnosis was then possible from hospital records. Patients diagnosed before randomisation were excluded. Although this process did not eliminate the inequality in the numbers of patients with previously diagnosed breast cancers still living at 18 years who were not excluded, the small difference in person-years of observation is unlikely to have biased the results.

Therefore, I conclude that the HIP trial results are valid, and the trial should not be dismissed as flawed.

The Malmö Trial

The Malmö trial was the only Swedish trial that Olsen and Gotzsche (2001b) regarded as of sufficiently high quality to permit using its results. They noted some imbalance in numbers of missing women, and felt that the published data may not be fully reliable, but for the main trial (MMST I) classified the data as of medium quality. They noted that recently an additional cohort had been added (MMST II) which was not conducted with a formal protocol. This group of women age 45-49 were combined by Andersson and Janzen (1997) with women age 45-49 in MMST I in their report to the NIH breast cancer consensus conference, being one of two trials in this age group to show a significant reduction in breast cancer mortality. They have also been included in the updated Swedish overview analysis (Nyström et al. 2002). However, Olsen and Gotzsche (2001b) point out that randomisation was faulty, in that because of an administrative error, one total birth year cohort (1934) was invited to screening, and none to be controls. They also comment that no baseline data are available. They classified the data in this MMST II trial as of poor quality. I agree with that conclusion.

The Two-County Trial

Olsen and Gotzsche (2001b) describe many difficulties of the randomisation of this cluster randomised trial. They could not find adequate details of the randomisation process in Kopparberg with 18 clusters [6 passive study population (PSP), the controls, and 12 active study population (ASP) invited to the screen group]. They noted that in the other county – Östergötlund – with 24 clusters, randomisation was by tossing a coin in the presence of a witness. They also comment that baseline data relating to comparability have not been published, and conclude that the randomisation procedure may have been seriously flawed. They note that the breast cancer mortality in the control group in Kopparberg is higher than in Östergötlund, and that there are more pre-trial breast cancers in the control group areas in Kopparberg than in the intervention areas. They note an age difference in both areas between the ASP and PSP, and found contradictory information as to when control group screening started. They noted lack of information from Tabar, and it is notable that Tabar did not permit data from Kopparberg to be included in the updated Swedish Overview analysis (Nyström et al. 2002). They classified the published data as of poor quality and very likely flawed. This conclusion was disputed by Duffy et al. (2001), but they provide no data to document their rebuttal, other than that related to treatment that I consider below.

A special analysis by Nixon et al. (2000) contributes to the debate, however, as when they analysed the data by clusters, using appropriate techniques, they found that fixed effects, and a variety of random effects models, show a strong degree of agreement and yield a significant 29% or 30% reduction in breast cancer mortality. Further, the heterogeneity among clusters and strata was relatively small, supporting the claim that the investigators make that there is no evidence of lack in baseline comparability in the randomised groups, other than a small age imbalance, which it is easy to adjust.

This does not solve all problems with this trial, however. Comparison of survival at 13 years of breast cancers in the Two-County and Canadian trials in women age 50–59 show that outcome was similar in the screened groups in the Canadian and Swedish trials, but far worse in the controls in the Two-County trial (Miller 2000a). Although such comparisons are confounded by lead time, there is evidence that adjuvant chemotherapy or hormone therapy was not used in the Swedish trial (Holmberg et al. 1986; Tabar et al. 1997), but was used in the Canadian (Kerr 1991; Miller et al. 2000b, 2002), raising the possibility that this difference in the use of effective therapy was the main reason for the poorer outcome in the Swedish controls. Further, this must mean that the survival experienced by the women with breast cancer in the Swedish controls, and used as a basis for a number of analyses of the benefit expected from breast screening, is not the current expectation. This must have some impact, perhaps a major impact, on the estimated benefits that are likely to be derived from breast screening.

The Edinburgh Trial

Olsen and Gotzsche (2001b) comment extensively on the cluster randomisation process in this trial. They note that for various reasons, seven practices changed allocation status after the randomisation was complete. They also note the major difference in socioeconomic level of the participants, with 26% of the women in the control group and 53% in the screening group belonging to the highest socioeconomic level (Alexander et al. 1989). They noted differences in the recruitment procedures for screening and control practices, and that 338 women in the screened group and 177 in the control were excluded because of a previous diagnosis of breast cancer. They conclude that the trial is flawed. However, they do not consider whether the adjustment made by Alexander et al. (1999) for social class differences between the randomised clusters (general practices) took care of the admitted social class imbalance, and neither did Black et al. (2002). This may not take care of all the problems with the trial however, and therefore I conclude that the results of this trial, which also included breast physical examinations, must remain suspect.

The CNBSS

Olsen and Gotzsche (2001b) felt that the trial "appears to have been adequately randomised". They were not concerned with the excess of 4+ nodes in the MP group in CNBSS 1 as they agreed with our explanations, noting that differences that arise post-randomisation after intervention, can not be used to impute differences pre-randomisation. They concluded that the trial provides medium-quality data. I discuss the older age group in this trial (CNBSS 2) in more detail later.

The Stockholm Trial

Olsen and Gotzsche (2001b) indicate that this trial is technically two trials with partly overlapping control groups, randomised by birth date. The first trial comprised women age 40–64 born 1917–1941, and the second women of the same age born 1918–1942. The control women born in 1918–1941 were used twice, explaining the double counting in the reports of this trial (Frisell et al. 1997), and Olsen and Gotzsche (2001b) suggest they should have had two entry dates, approximately 1 year apart. They also found an imbalance of numbers in the second subtrial, with 508 more women belonging to the screened group than the control. Although they found no age imbalances, there were inconsistencies in the numbers excluded, and they classified the data published by the trialists and in the Swedish meta-analyses as of poor quality.

This trial has always been somewhat problematic, with the double counting of the controls and with invitation to screening of the controls after only two screens in the screened group. The randomisation process would not normally pass muster in a therapy trial, and it is unclear why it has simply been regarded as a form of cluster randomisation. However, the trial and its design have never been satisfactorily defended, and I have no reason to differ with Olsen and Gotzshe's conclusion.

The Göteborg Trial

This trial has only been reported for women age 39–49 (Bjurstam et al. 1997), even though it included women up to age 59. Olsen and Gotzsche (2001b) comment on uneven randomisation ratios, apparently dictated by the capacity of the mammography unit and staff. Randomisation in the younger ages was individual, and performed by the city's computer department, in the older age group (included in the Swedish overview analyses) it was by cluster. Olsen and Gotzsche (2001b) comment that the trial may have been well randomised, but further information is needed to check this. They suggest that the selective reporting of findings for the younger age group may be an example of publication bias, though it was probably predicated on the desire to include the trial results in the 1997 NIH consensus conference. They classified the available data as of poor quality.

I concur with that evaluation. When the Bjurstam et al. (1997) report was published, I expressed doubt over whether the randomisation process had resulted in comparable groups, citing the lack of excess of breast cancers in the screened group compared to the control as evidence that the controls had a higher incidence, and thus too high breast cancer mortality (Miller et al. 1998). In response, Bjurstam et al. (1998) indicated that they believed the excess in cancers was due to delayed screening of the controls, and provided additional data on incidence in the trial. I do not accept their explanation; screening the controls will bring the case numbers together, but not result in an excess, even if the control screen is delayed by 3 months. There has to be bias in the trial. Further, it seems clear from what little has been published about this trial on women age 50–59 in the Swedish overview analyses (Nyström et al. 1993, 2002) that the effect in this age group is not significant, which brings us back to the selective publication of the data that were.

Conclusion on the Gotzsche and Olsen Reviews

It is not clear whether it will ever be possible to completely resolve the controversies, even if original data are eventually submitted from all trials for a pooled analysis. Only the Edinburgh investigators have faced up to their problems, and attempted a resolution. The resolution attempted for the Two-County trial by Nixon et al. (2000) could not take care of all concerns, given the lack of published information. I conclude that Gotzsche and Olsen are not as far off base as many would like us to believe. The implication is that the overall estimates of effect derived from meta-analysis incorporating the trials with unresolved difficulties may be overestimating the likely public health benefit to be derived from mammography screening. This particularly affects those derived from the overview of the Swedish trials (Nyström et al. 1993, 2002).

The Miettinen et al. (2002) Analysis of the Malmö Trial

As indicated above, the Malmö trial was the only Swedish trial that Olsen and Gotzsche (2001a,b) regarded as of sufficiently high quality to permit using its results. However, they concluded that it did not show a benefit from mammography screening. Miettinen et al. (2002) disputed this. Their suggestion was that it is important to analyse trials according to the time benefit is to be expected. They evaluated the published Malmö data (Andersson et al. 1988) according to year of death from breast cancer from time of entry, and computed what they called rate ratios, though they are really ratios of numbers of breast cancer deaths. On this basis, for the women age 55–69 a statistically significant difference in favour of mammography screening arises from about 8 years from entry. However, this analysis ignores the nonsignificant excess earlier, and the women age 45–54 who had a much greater excess of deaths in the screened group than the control (Fig. 1). If both groups are combined, the early excess is more striking (Fig. 2), but the delayed apparent benefit persists. However, one has also to look at the overall effect, because that is what is important for public health purposes. In that respect, Olsen and Gotzsche (2001b) are correct in that the trial shows no overall benefit from mammography.
    The curve for the younger age group in Fig. 1 is very different from that published by Andersson and Janzon (1997) for women age 45–49 on entry. This must mean that the adverse effect was largely in the women age 50–54. This may explain the fact that Nyström et al. (2002) in the latest Swedish over-

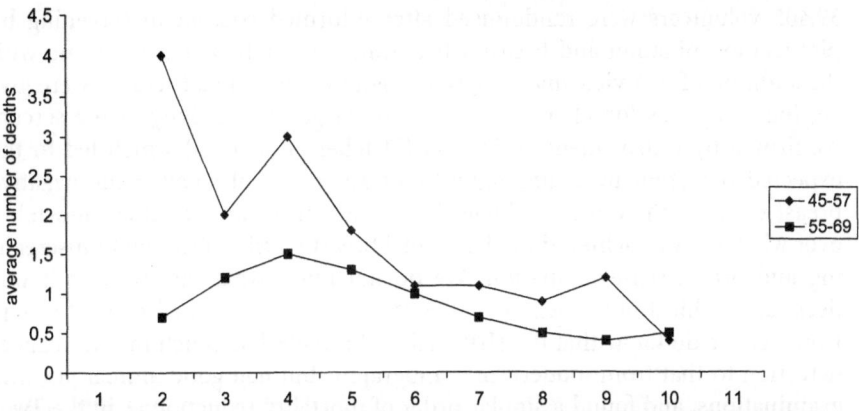

Fig. 1. Malmö trial, 3-year moving averages of breast cancer deaths for women age 45–57 and 55–64 years on entry to the trial. (Adapted from Miettinen et al. 2002 and Andersson et al. 1988)

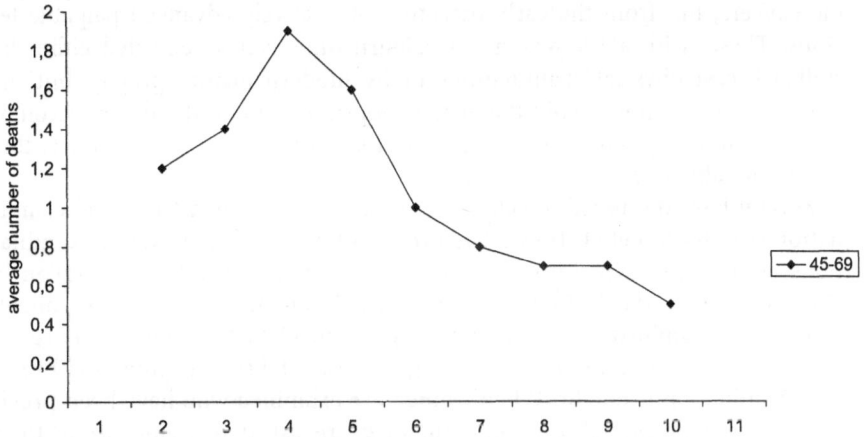

Fig. 2. Malmö trial, 3-year moving averages of breast cancer deaths for women age 45–64 years on entry to the trial. (Adapted from Miettinen et al. 2002 and Andersson et al. 1988)

view found a much lesser effect of mammography screening in women at this age, something noted before in other studies. This of course points to the fragility of the data, and the fact that you really should not analyse a trial in subsegments of age, if you did not plan it that way. The Malmö trial was planned for women age 45–64; the subdivision by age was data driven, and conventional statistical significance does not apply.

The Canadian National Breast Screening Study – 2

This trial among women age 50–59 was designed to evaluate how much mammography adds to good breast physical examinations, and the teaching and re-enforcement of breast self-examination (Miller et al. 2000b). A total of

39,405 volunteers were randomised after informed consent to screening by physical examination and breast self-examination only versus the same with the addition of two-view mammography. Four or five annual screens were given, follow-up was for 11–16 years. In spite of good sensitivity of the screen, confirmed by independent evaluation (Fletcher et al. 1993) which led to the expected detection by mammography of an excess of small, node-negative breast cancers, there was no benefit in reduction in breast cancer mortality over whatever was achieved by the annual breast physical examination screening and breast self-examination. We do not know what that was, as it was deemed unethical in women age 50–59 to have an unscreened control group. However, we do know that the HIP trial in the 1960s had much inferior cancer detection to that from modern mammography, but had good annual physical examinations, and found a similar order of mortality reduction as in the Two-County trial, suggesting, as does CNBSS 2, that much if not all of the benefit is achieved by good breast physical examinations. This must mean that the benefit from breast screening derives not from the early detection of impalpable cancers, but from the early detection of relatively advanced palpable lesions. These, with a 1.5 year mean sojourn time, can be detected either by skilled breast physical examinations or by modern mammography, but the physical examinations avoid the excess biopsies, many of the ductal carcinomas in situ, and possible overdiagnosis of small invasive breast cancers, that are inseparable from mammography.

Several have discussed the characteristics of a good breast physical examination (e.g. Barton et al. 1999). The protocol for the breast physical examinations used in the CNBSS was developed by an experienced breast surgeon in Toronto (Basset 1985). In brief, the examination has a visual component; women are examined sitting up and lying down; all parts of the breast are examined by firm pressure using the finger pads; it takes 7–10 min, and breast self-examination is taught. When women are examined who have been previously taught breast self-examination, they are asked to demonstrate their technique to the examiner, and any errors are corrected. In the CNBSS these examinations were largely given by specially trained nurses, who became very expert in the technique, and who performed many other functions in the screening centres (Miller et al. 1991)

Trends in Breast Cancer Mortality

Since the 1990s, there has been an unprecedented reduction in breast cancer mortality in many countries. This is depicted for women age 50–74, the age group expected to show an impact of screening mammography, for countries that have introduced breast screening in Fig. 3. Although percentage-wise the reduction is similar in the UK, the United States and Canada, it is less in Sweden, Finland, and the Netherlands and negligible in Denmark. Thus, the reductions seen in breast cancer mortality have no clear link to screening, but are probably due to the extensive implementation of adjuvant treatment with

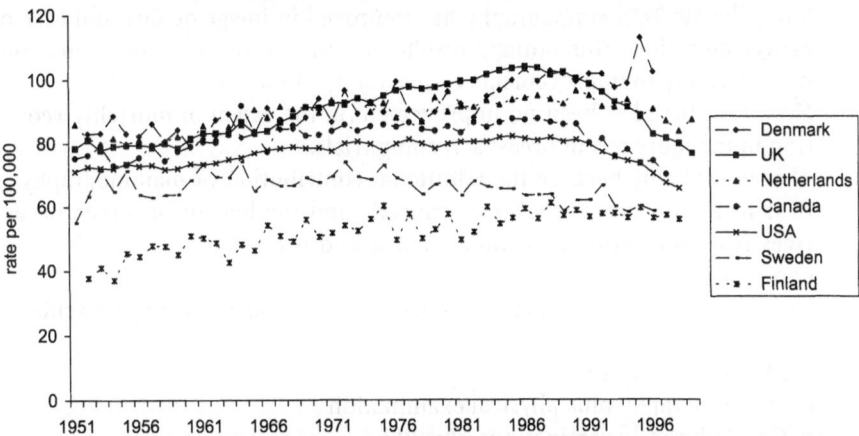

Fig. 3. Trends in mortality from breast cancer, in countries with breast screening programmes, for women age 50–74 years

chemotherapy and tamoxifen in North America. The timing of that introduction (the 1980s) is much more compatible with the fall than the later introduction of screening, especially in Canada (Pacquette et al. 2000; Miller 2000a). In the UK, there had been a major increase in breast cancer mortality, so far unexplained, and much of the reduction is to bring the rates down towards those in North America. Some of this could be due to the increase in standards of treatment, associated with their national breast screening programme. Blanks et al. (2000) with a model-based analysis, have calculated that perhaps two thirds of the reduction in the UK from 1990 to 1998 was due to improved treatment, and less than a third from screening. However, this analysis does not explain what caused the rise in breast cancer mortality in the UK prior to 1990, and also probably overestimates the contribution of screening (Miller 2000b). It remains to be seen whether the falls continue, and whether it is possible to determine the contribution of mammography more precisely over the next 5 years, when the major effect could be anticipated. However, with treatment for breast cancer continuing to improve, and the possibility raised by CNBSS 2 that screening is not additive to good treatment, the relative contribution of screening may remain small.

Conclusions

1. It is likely that the meta-analyses of screening effectiveness to date have over-estimated the benefit likely to be achieved by mammography screening in the era of adjuvant chemotherapy and hormone therapy.
2. In many countries, mortality from breast cancer is falling, but the contribution of screening is probably small.

3. Since the 1960s, mammography has improved in image quality and ease of cancer detection. This initially resulted in improvement in sensitivity, and more recently in improvements of specificity of the test.
4. However, there has been no improvement in the extent of mortality reduction in the more recent breast screening trials.
5. This is probably because the additional contribution of mammography is to detect good prognosis breast cancers, and the benefit of screening derives from the earlier detection of advanced breast cancers, coupled with good therapy.
6. In women age 50–69, reduction in breast cancer mortality may be achieved by:
   ● Mammography alone
   ● Mammography plus physical examination
   ● Good physical examinations plus BSE

However, as treatment improves, the contribution of screening will fall.

So my answer to the question posed in the title of this paper is "No, but only providing that women have access to skilled breast physical examinations. If women choose mammography screening, they should understand that their overall risk of dying in the next few years may not be reduced at all".

References

Alexander FE, Anderson TJ, Brown HK, Forrest APM, Hepburn W, Kirkpatrick AE, et al (1999) 14 years of follow-up from the Edinburgh randomised trial of breast-cancer screening. Lancet 353:1903–1908

Alexander F, Roberts MM, Lutz W, Hepburn W (1989) Randomisation by cluster and the problem of social class bias. J Epidemiol Community Health 43:29–36

Andersson I, Aspergren K, Janzon L, Lindholm K, Linell F, et al (1988) Mammographic screening and mortality from breast cancer: the Malmö mammographic screening trial. Br Med J 297:943–948

Andersson I, Janzon L (1997) Reduced breast cancer mortality in women under age 50: updated results from the Malmö mammographic screening program. NCI Monogr 22:63–67

Barton MB, Harris R, Fletcher SW (1999) Does this patient have breast cancer? The screening clinical examination: Should it be done? How? J A M A 282:1270–1280

Bassett AA (1985) Physical examination of the breast and breast self-examination. In: Miller AB (ed) Screening for cancer. Academic Press Inc. Orlando, pp 271–291

Black WC, Haggstrom DA, Welch HG (2002) All-cause mortality in randomised trials of cancer screening. J Natl Cancer Inst 94:167–173

Blanks RG, Moss SM, McGahan CE, Quinn MJ, Babb PJ (2000) Effect of NHS breast screening programme on mortality from breast cancer in England and Wales, 1990–8: comparison of observed with expected mortality. Br Med J 321:665–669

Bjurstam N, Björneld L, Duffy SW, Prevost TC (1998) Author reply. Cancer 83:188–190

Bjurstam N, Björneld L, Duffy SW, Smith TC, Cahlin E, Eriksson O, et al (1997) The Gothenberg breast screening trial. First results on mortality, incidence, and mode of detection for women ages 39–49 years at randomization. Cancer 80:2091–2099

Day NE, Baines CJ, Chamberlain J, et al (1986) UICC project on screening for cancer: Report of the workshop on screening for breast cancer. Int J Cancer 38:303–308

Duffy SW, Tabar L, Smith RA (2001) Screening for breast cancer with mammography. Lancet 358:2166

Fletcher SW, Black W, Harris R, Rimer BK, Shapiro S (1993) Report on the International Workshop on Screening for breast cancer. J Natl Cancer Inst 85:1644-1656

Frisell J, Glas U, Hellstrom L, Rutqvist LE (1997) Follow-up after 11 years - update of mortality results in the Stockholm mammographic screening trial. Breast Cancer Res Treat 45:263-270

Gotzsche PC (2001) Author's reply. Lancet 358:2167-2168

Gotzsche PC, Olsen O (2000) Is screening for breast cancer with mammography justifiable? Lancet 355:129-34

Holmberg LH, Tabar L, Adami HO, Bergstrom R (1986) Survival in breast cancer diagnosed between mammographic screening examinations. Lancet 2: 27-30

Horton R (2001) Screening mammography-an overview revisited. Lancet 358:1284-1285

Lenner P (1990) The excess mortality rate. A useful concept in cancer epidemiology. Acta Oncol 29: 573-576

Kerr M (1991) A case-control study of treatment adequacy and mortality from breast cancer for women age 40-49 years at entry into the National Breast Screening Study. Masters Thesis, University of Toronto, Toronto

Miettinen OS, Henschke CI, Pasmantier MW, Smith JP, Libby DM, Yankelevitz DF (2002) Mammography screening: no supporting evidence? Lancet 359:404-405

Miller AB (1994) May we agree to disagree, or how do we develop guidelines for breast cancer screening in women? J Natl Cancer Inst 86:1729-1731

Miller AB (2000a) Organized breast cancer screening programs in Canada. Can Med Ass J 163:1150-1151

Miller AB (2000b) Effect of screening programme on mortality from breast cancer. Benefit of 30% may be substantial overestimate. Br Med J 321:1527

Miller AB (2001) Screening for breast cancer with mammography. Lancet 358:2164

Miller AB, Baines CJ, To T (1998) The Gothenburg Breast Screening Trial. First results on mortality, incidence and mode of detection for women ages 39-49 years at randomization. Cancer 83:186-188

Miller AB, Baines CJ, Turnbull C (1991) The role of the nurse-examiner in the National Breast Screening Study. Can J Pub Health 82:162-167

Miller AB, Chamberlain J, Day NE, Hakama M, Prorok PC (1990) Report on a workshop of the UICC project on evaluation of screening for cancer. Int J Cancer 46:761-769

Miller AB, To T, Baines CJ, Wall C (2000b) Canadian National Breast Screening Study-2: 13-year results of a randomized trial in women age 50-59 years. J Natl Cancer Inst 92:1490-1499

Miller AB, To T, Baines CJ, Wall C (2002) The Canadian National Breast Screening Study - 1. A randomized screening trial of mammography in women age 40-49: Breast cancer mortality after 11-16 years of follow-up. Ann Int Med 137:305-320

Miller AB, Yurgalevitch S, Weissfeld JL (2000a) Death review process in the Prostate, Lung, Colorectal and Ovarian (PLCO) cancer screening trials. Control Clin Trials 21:400S-406S

National Institutes of Health Consensus Development Panel (1997) Consensus statement. NCI Monogr 22:vii-xii

Nixon RM, Prevost TC, Duffy SW, Tabar L, Vitak B, Chen HH (2000) Some random-effects models for the analysis of matched-cluster randomised trials: application to the Swedish Two-County trial of breast-cancer screening. J Epidemiol Biostat 5:349-358

Nyström L, Andersson I, Bjurstam N, Frisell J, Nordenskjold B, Rutqvist L-E (2002) Long-term effects of mammography screening: updated overview of the Swedish randomized trials. Lancet 359:909-919

Nyström L, Rutqvist LE, Wall S, Lindgren A, Lindqvist M, Ryden S, et al (1993) Breast cancer screening with mammography: overview of Swedish randomized trials. Lancet 341:973-978

Olsen O, Gotzsche P (2001a) Cochrane review on screening for breast cancer with mammography. Lancet 358:1340-1342

Olsen O, Gotzsche PC (2001b) Screening for breast cancer with mammography (Cochrane Review). In: The Cochrane Library, Issue 4, Oxford: Update software

Paquette D, Snider J, Bouchard F, Olivotto I, Bryant H, Decker K, et al (2000) Performance of screening mammography in organized programs in Canada in 1996. Can Med Ass J 163:1133–1138

Tabar L, Chen H-H T, Duffy SW, Kruesmo UB (1999) Primary and adjuvant therapy, prognostic factors and survival in 1,053 breast cancers diagnosed in a trial of mammography screening. Jpn J Clin Oncol 29:608–616

US Preventive Services Task Force (1996) Guide to clinical preventive services, 2nd edn. Washington DC. US Department of Health and Human Services

How Reliable Is the Evidence for Screening Mammography?

Stephen A. Feig

S.A. Feig (✉)
Department of Radiology, The Mount Sinai Hospital,
One Gustave L. Levy Place, New York, NY 10029-6574, USA

Abstract

Substantial reduction in breast cancer mortality has been proven in randomized trials of screening mammography. These trials have found a statistically significant benefit both for women ages 40–49 years and for women age 50 years and older at onset of screening. In fact, it is likely that the trials actually underestimate the benefit for an individual woman who is screened. Service screening programs have shown a 63% reduction in deaths from breast cancer among women who are screened. Virtually all major medical organizations now advise screening mammography for women ages 40 and older. Two recent studies that questioned the validity of results from screening mammography trials are themselves fatally flawed.

Results from Randomized Clinical Trials

Proof of benefit from screening women ages 40–74 years has been obtained by means of randomized clinical trials (RCTs). An RCT is a prospective comparison of breast cancer death rates among study group women offered screening and control group women not offered screening. These two groups should have no other significant differences. There have been seven randomized trials of populations, each comprised of several age decades. Screening was performed by mammography alone or in combination with physical examination. Three of these RCTs, the Health Insurance Plan of Greater New York (HIP) trial, the Swedish Two-County trial, and the Edinburgh, Scotland trial have reported statistically significant reduction in breast cancer mortality of 23%, 32%, and 29%, respectively (Shapiro et al. 1998; Tabar et al. 2000; Alexander et al. 1999). The other three trials, Malmö (1976–1986), Stockholm (1981–1985), and Gothenburg, Sweden (1982–1988) have found nonsignificant reductions in breast cancer deaths of 19%, 10%, and 22% (Nystrom et al.

Recent Results in Cancer Research, Vol. 163
© Springer-Verlag Berlin Heidelberg 2003

2002). A recent meta-analysis of five Swedish trials found a statistically significant 21% reduction in breast cancer deaths (Nystrom et al. 2002).

How Well Do Randomized Trials Estimate Benefit from Screening?

There are several reasons why results from RCTs underestimate the benefit to an individual woman undergoing screening with modern mammography. First, there have been many improvements in mammographic technique and quality control since the early 1980s when nearly all trials were conducted (Haus 1999; Conway et al. 1994). Better image quality facilitates detection of early breast cancer (Feig 2002a; Taplin 2002; Young 1994). Second, women in the RCTs were mostly screened with one view per breast rather than the current standard of two views per breast, a protocol that would have increased the detection rate by 7%–14% (Feig 1995). Third, screening intervals in all except the HIP trial ranged from 18 to 33 months. These are longer than the annual interval now recommended by the American College of Radiology and the American Cancer Society (Feig et al. 1997; Leitch et al. 1997). There is compelling evidence that annual screening should result in substantially greater mortality reduction (Feig et al. 1997; Leitch et al. 1997).

Finally, RCTs compare breast cancer deaths among study group women offered screening versus control group women not offered screening. However, some study group women refuse to be screened while many control group women obtain screening on their own, outside the trial. Comparative tabulation of deaths from breast cancer was not restricted to study group women who accepted the invitation to screening versus those control group women who were not screened. Thus, both "noncompliance" of some study women and "contamination" of control group women reduce the calculated benefit from RCTs.

Several investigators have used mathematical models of RCT data to calculate the benefit to an "average" women who is screened every year and where results are not affected by "noncompliance" and "contamination" (Falun Meeting Committee 1996; Feig 1994, 1997; Tabar et al. 1995). For example, based on an observed 45% reduction in breast cancer mortality among women age 39–49 offered screening every 18 months at the Gothenburg trial, Feig calculated that the mortality reduction could have been as high as 65% with annual screening at the observed 80% compliance rate and as high as 75% at a 100% compliance rate (Feig 1997). In addition, Michaelson et al. using a computer simulation based on biological data from cancer growth rates and metastatic spread, calculated that annual mammography for all age groups combined could affect a 51% reduction in breast cancer deaths (Michaelson et al. 1999).

Benefit from Screening Women Ages 40–49

Initial reports from the HIP trial, the first RCT ever conducted, found a difference in breast cancer death rates between study and control groups for women age 50 and over at entry that was apparent by year 4. However, a difference for women ages 40–49 did not emerge until 7–8 years of follow-up. By 18 years of follow-up, the reduction in breast cancer deaths among study women ages 40–49 at entry was 23%, the same as ages 50–64 at entry. However, even by that time, benefit for younger women was still not statistically significant according to Shapiro et al. (1998). This lack of statistical significance was a consequence of the relatively smaller number of younger women enrolled and their lower breast cancer incidence. Nevertheless, it led to controversy regarding screening women in their forties (Smith 2000).

The HIP study, however, was not designed to determine the efficacy of screening separate age groups, but rather a single age group of all women ages 40–65. Attempts to subdivide the study group reduced statistical power. The observation that results for younger women lacked statistical significance was often cited in the screening debate. The fact that the data for women ages 50–59 and for those age 60 and older at entry, when analyzed separately also lacked statistical significance was largely ignored (Hurley and Kaldor 1992). Some commentators failed to recognize that Chu et al. (1988), using a different method of analysis, found statistically significant mortality reductions of 24% for women ages 40–49 and 21% for those ages 50–64 at entry into the HIP trial.

Despite the analysis of Chu et al. (1988), some observers were still not convinced that screening would benefit women in their forties. There were several reasons for their opinion. First, in all trials, the reduction in the breast cancer death rates for younger women did not appear until several years after it was seen for women over age 50 (Smith 2000). Second, results for younger women were not statistically significant for any other individual trial until 1997.

The controversy intensified in 1992 with publication of the 7 year follow-up report from the National Breast Screening Study of Canada (NBSS) trial (Miller et al. 1992). This study found no evidence of benefit among women age 40–49 who were offered five annual screenings by mammography and physical examination. There was still no evidence of benefit for longer term 11–16-year follow-up (Miller et al. 2002b) There are several explanations for these disappointing results. First, the technical quality of mammography was poor (Baines et al. 1990; Boyd et al. 1993; Warren-Burhenne and Burhenne 1993). During most of the trial, more than 50% of the mammograms were poor or completely unacceptable, even as assessed by the standards of the day (Kopans 1990; Kopans and Feig 1993). Second, there is reason to believe that the randomization process through which women were assigned into study and control groups may have been flawed (Bailar and MacMahon 1997; Boyd 1997; Mettlin and Smart 1993). All women were given a physical examination prior to their randomization. This protocol may have allowed preferential allocation of women with breast masses, and thereby late-stage breast cancers into the study group. As a likely consequence, an excess of late-stage breast cancers and breast cancer deaths was found in the study group compared with the control group throughout the trial (Kopans and Feig 1993; Tarone 1995).

Beginning in 1993, several successive meta-analyses of combined data for multiple RCTs were performed in order to accrue a greater number of women-years of follow-up than possible from any one RCT alone. However, the earliest meta-analyses, published in 1993 and 1995, suggested that there is little if any benefit from screening women under 50 years of age (Kerlikowske et al. 1995).

Subsequent meta-analyses published by Smart et al. (1995) and the Falun Meeting Committee (1996) included more recent follow-up. These studies showed statistically significant mortality reductions of 24% for women ages 40–49 at entry into the seven population-based RCTs. These and other meta-analyses found a 15%–16% mortality reduction when a nonpopulation-based RCT, the National Breast Screening Study of Canada (NBSS), was also included (Humphrey et al. 2002). A recent meta-analysis, by Hendrick et al. (1997), found a statistically significant mortality reduction for women invited to screening in their forties of 18% for all eight RCTs and 29% for the five Swedish RCTs. Thus, with increasing length of follow-up, successive meta-analyses have shown progressively greater and statistically significant mortality reductions for women ages 40–49. Regardless of whether NBSS results are included or excluded, meta-analyses for screening women ages 40–49 now show statistically significant benefit.

Moreover, meta-analyses are no longer necessary to prove benefit for screening younger women. Two other RCTs besides the HIP study have now shown statistically significant benefit for women ages 40–49. Bjurstam et al. (1997) reported a statistically significant 45% mortality reduction for women ages 39 to 49 at randomization in the Gothenburg, Sweden trial. Andersson and Janzon (1997) reported a statistically significant 35% breast cancer mortality reduction for women at the Malmo Trial who began screening mammography at age 45–49.

As a result of data from the RCTs and other studies, screening beginning at age 40 years is now recommended by the American Cancer Society, the American College of Obstetrics and Gynecology, the American College of Radiology, and the American Medical Association. Screening every 1–2 years between ages 40–49 and annual screening from age 50 years is recommended by the National Cancer Institute and the U.S. Preventive Services Task Force.

The Most Recent Screening Controversy

Based on results from randomized trials conducted over the past quarter of a century and involving over 500,000 women, there has been consensus in the medical community in favor of screening mammography. In the face of such near unanimous agreement, two recent articles made the seemingly incredible claim that none of the trials provided convincing evidence that screening prevents breast cancer deaths (Gotzsche and Olsen 2000; Olsen and Gotzsche 2001). The authors asserted that only two of the eight screening trials – Malmo, Sweden and the National Breast Screening Study of Canada (NBSS) – were valid, and that neither of these trials found evidence of benefit. The Gotzsche and Olsen papers received enormous publicity because of the sensational nature of their claim, which questioned the widely held belief in the efficacy of early detection.

The only points on which Gotzsche and Olsen and all other observers agree was that the NBSS: (1) failed to find benefit for screening women 50–70 years old with mammography and clinical examination versus clinical examination alone (Miller et al. 2002a); and (2) found no benefit for mammographic screening of women aged 40–49 years (Miller et al. 1992b, 2002b). However, at that point screening advocates part ways with Gotzsche and Olsen because their explanations for the negative NBSS results are vastly different.

Because serious deficiencies at the NBSS have been well documented, it is astonishing that Gotzsche and Olsen view the NBSS as the paradigm of a well-conducted study. First, independent reviews found that the technical quality of mammography at NBSS was poor even when measured by the standards of the 1980s when the trial was conducted (Kopans 1990; Kopans and Feig 1993). Second, performance of clinical breast examination prior to randomization may have allowed channeling of symptomatic women into the study group. The finding of excess advanced cancers in the 40–49-year study group suggests that randomization was not blindly performed (Tarone 1995).

Third, NBSS was not population-based. Rather, participants were self-selected volunteers. Because self-selected women are more likely to be symptomatic, adequate randomization will be more problematic, especially when clinical examination has already been performed. Because self-selected asymptomatic women may have higher survival rates than randomly selected asymptomatic women, benefit may be harder to demonstrate than in a population-based trial. Contrary to the sentiments of Gotzsche and Olsen, almost any of these fatal flaws in trial design and implementation render the NBSS incapable of providing meaningful results.

The statement by Gotzsche and Olsen that the Malmo trial showed no evidence of benefit is even more inconceivable. For some inexplicable reason, Gotzsche and Olsen only considered an early report by Andersson et al. (1988) of a small, insignificant 5% mortality reduction among women aged 45–70. They totally ignored later reports of breast cancer mortality reductions of 19% among women age 45–70, 26% among women 55–70 (Andersson and Nystrom 1995), and 36% among women age 45–50 at entry into the Malmo trial (Anderson and Janzon 1997). Moreover, several months after publication of the latest Gotzsche and Olsen (2001) paper, Miettinen and Henschke (2002) used 3-year moving averages of relative risk estimates to estimate that the true mortality reduction from the Malmo trial was 55% for women age 55–69, and 60% for those age 45–57 at entry into screening.

The next point made by Gotzsche and Olsen was that apart from the Malmo and NBSS trials they claimed to have identified major age differences between study and control groups that rendered results from the HIP, Edinburgh, and remaining Swedish trials invalid. The authors suggested that the observed reductions in breast cancer death rates were due to these age differences rather than the screening process itself. To support their hypothesis, Gotzsche and Olsen cited the age differences of 1–5 months between study and control groups in those other trials. However, in presuming to have discovered a fatal flaw in the randomized trials, Gotzsche and Olsen were unaware that when screening trials use cluster randomization rather than individual randomization such relatively small age differences are not only expected but acceptable (de Koning 2000, Duffy 2001).

Screening trials and therapeutic trials are different in nature, and may be different in design. In therapeutic trials, all participants have disease. The main variables are treatment versus no treatment, and dose regimen. Study and control groups are small. Individual randomization is required and small age differences are study significant. In screening mammography trials there is a low disease prevalence so that extremely large study and control groups are necessary. For this reason, individual randomization may not be practical and cluster randomization is usually necessary.

The age difference between the two groups which Gotzsche and Olsen purported to have discovered in the Swedish Two-County Trials had been previously acknowledged by Tabar et al. (1989). In fact, after adjustment for age, mortality rates were only minimally different: 31% versus 30% for women aged 40–70 in the Swedish Two-County Trial (Duffy 2001), and 45% instead of 46% for women aged 39–49 years in the Gothenburg, Sweden trial (Bjurstam et al. 1998).

In another criticism, Gotzsche and Olsen suggested that assignment of the cause of death among women in the Swedish screening trials may have been inaccurate. Accurate assignment of cause of death is of course critical to proper assessment of trial results. Death in a woman with breast cancer may be causally related or unrelated to a malignancy. Because screening trials compare deaths due to breast cancer in study group women versus control group women, attribution of the cause of death must be performed in a consistent and unbiased manner. However, the criticism by Gotzsche and Olsen was baseless. The methods for cause of death assignment in the Swedish trials had been previously described in detail by Nystrom et al. (1995). The process consisted of independent blind evaluation by four physicians and resulted in a remarkable unanimous agreement in 93.1% of cases (Nystrom et al. 1993, 1995, 2002).

Gotzsche and Olsen also jumped on the fact that no statistically significant decrease in death rates from all causes combined had yet been shown in any of the Swedish trials. This observation was interpreted by Gotzsche and Olsen to mean that any benefit from reduction in breast cancer deaths would be countered by increased deaths from other causes. This incorrect conclusion disregarded the fact that breast cancer accounts for only about 5% of total mortality. Thus, even the largest individual trial would be unlikely to demonstrate any statistically significant decrease in all-cause mortality. Much to their chagrin, Gotzsche and Olsen were again proven wrong. Subsequent to publication of the second Gotzsche and Olsen (2001) paper, Nystrom et al. (2002) were in fact able to find a 2% decrease in all-cause mortality among study group women in five Swedish trials combined. Thus, the Gotzsche and Olsen conjecture regarding all-cause mortality was incorrect.

To further their thesis that data from the Swedish Two-County trial was unreliable, Gotzsche and Olsen asserted that the reported study group size had changed between different articles by Tabar et al. In response to this criticism, Duffy and Tabar (2000) acknowledged that the study population size did in fact differ among their published reports. In fact, Tabar et al. (1989) had previously noted that these differences were due to progressive identification and exclusion of women diagnosed with breast cancer before the trial began. This is an acceptable and in fact a commendable practice. This observation had escaped Gotzsche and Olsen, who obviously did not read the articles thoroughly and did not appreciate the rationale for such fastidious data collection. The irony of this unjustified criticism is that Tabar et al. were faulted for practicing good science.

In their papers, Gotzsche and Olsen also reiterated the conclusion of a study by Sjonell and Stahle (1999), which claimed that widespread screening in Sweden had not affected population breast cancer mortality. The basic mistake by Sjonell and Stahle was that they had measured death rates too early. Decreased mortality should not be expected until 5–8 years after the start of screening. Sjonell and Stahle had mistakenly begun to tally breast cancer deaths before the beginning of the service screening programs that they were attempting to assess (Rosen and Rehnquist 1999; Nystrom 2000). Additionally, their calculations did not consider the increase in breast cancer incidence over time.

When properly measured, service-screening in Sweden has been shown to reduce breast cancer deaths in the entire population by as much as 50% (Feig 2002b). Seven published studies have shown a reduction in population breast cancer death rates ranging from 19%–50% in different regions of Sweden and Finland (Duffy and Tabar 2002; Garne et al. 1997; Hakama et al. 1997; Jonsson et al. 2001; Lerner and Jonsson 1997; Tornberg et al. 1994; Tabar et al. 2001). Most of this benefit has been attributed to screening mammography.

A recent study by Tabar et al. (2001) employs a unique method to measure the effect of mammography in a population where service screening is offered to all women age 40 and over. This method is not affected by study group noncompliance nor control group contamination. Their paper compares breast cancer death rates in two Swedish counties over 3 periods of time: 1968–1977, when virtually no women were screened, 1978–1987, when half the population was offered screening in the RCT, and 1988–1996, after completion of the trial when screening was offered to all women and 85% of the population were being screened.

Table 1. Reduction in breast cancer death rates[a] (from Tabar et al. 2001)

	Time of diagnosis	
	1978–1987	1988–1996
Screening status of women	Randomized trial	Service screening
Screened	57%	63%
Invited to screening	43%	48%
Screened plus nonscreened	21%	50%

[a] Women aged 40–69 years in two Swedish counties. Compared with the period 1969–1977 before screening began. All results were statistically significant at 95% confidence level.

When compared with breast cancer death rates among women ages 40–69 in the prescreening year, breast cancer death rates in 1988–1996 were reduced 63% for screened women and 50% for the entire population (85% screened + 15% nonscreened; Table 1). During this time, reduction in death rates from breast cancer for screened women were similar to those for women screened during the trial, i.e., 63% versus 57%. However, during the trial (1978–1987) only half the population was offered screening. For that era, breast cancer death rate reduction in the entire population was only 21%.

Tabar et al. believed that screening rather than advances in treatment was responsible for nearly all the benefit. The relative risk of breast cancer death among nonscreened women aged 40–69 was similar (1.0, 1.17, and 1.19) during the three consecutive periods. Moreover, the breast cancer death rate for women ages 20–39, virtually none of whom were screened, showed no significant difference, i.e., 1.0, 1.10, and 0.81, respectively, during these three consecutive periods.

Possibly, women who agree to be screened have selection bias factors which apart from the screening process improve their survival rates. However, even assuming the maximum effect of selection bias, screening was shown to reduce breast cancer deaths by at least 50%. In this study, all results for breast cancer mortality reduction were statistically significant.

Even more recently, Duffy and Tabar (2002) have expanded their service-screening study to include a total of seven Swedish counties. They have found an overall reduction in breasts cancer deaths of 32% in counties screening for 10 years or more. They also provided evidence that the majority of this benefit was due to screening rather than changes in treatment.

Conclusion

Benefit from screening women age 40–74 has been proven in randomized trials. Subset analysis of women who began screening between ages 40–49 has found significant benefit for them as well. Recent questions regarding the validity of randomized trial data have been thoroughly answered by trial investigators and other experts. After careful review of the data, the validity of screening mammography has been reaffirmed by major medical organizations in the United States, including the National Cancer Institute, U.S. Preventive Services Task Force, American Cancer Society, American College of Physicians, American Society of Internal Medicine, American Medical Association, American College of Obstetrics and Gynecology, and American Academy of Family Practice.

References

Alexander FE, Anderson TJ, Brown HK, et al. (1999) 14 years of follow-up from Edinburgh randomized trial of breast cancer screening. Lancet 3353:1903–1909

Andersson I, Aspegren K, Janzon L, et al. (1988) Mammographic screening and mortality from breast cancer: the Malmo Mammographic Screening Trial. BMJ, Brit Med J 297:943–948

Andersson I, Janzon L (1997) Reduced breast cancer mortality in women under 50: updated results from the Malmo Mammographic Screening Program. NCI Monogr 22:63–68

Andersson I, Nystrom L (1995) Mammography screening. J Natl Cancer Inst 87:1263

Bailar JC III, MacMahon B (1997) Randomization in the Canadian National Breast Screening Study: a review of evidence for subversion. Can Med Assoc J 156:193–199

Baines CJ, Miller AB, Kopans DB, et al (1990) Canadian National Breast Screening Study: assessment of technical quality by external review. AJR Am J Roentgenol 155:743–747

Bjurstam N, Bjorneld L, Duffy SW (1997) The Gothenburg Breast Screening Trial: first results on mortality, incidence, and mode of detection for women ages 39–49 years of randomization. Cancer 80:2091–2099

Bjurstam N, Bjorneld L, Duffy SW, Prevost TC (1998) The Gothenburg Breast Screening Trial (authors' reply). Cancer 83:188–190

Boyd NF (1997) The review of randomization in the Canadian National Breast Screening Study: Is the debate over? Can Med Assoc J 156:207–209

Boyd NF, Jong RA, Yaffe MJ, et al (1993) A critical appraisal of the Canadian National Breast Screening Study. Radiology 189:681–663

Chu KC, Smart CR, Tarone RE (1988) Analysis of breast cancer mortality and stage distribution by age for the Health Insurance Plan Trial. J Natl Cancer Inst 80:1125–1132

Conway BJ, Suleiman OH, Reuter FG, Antonsen RG, Slayton RJ (1994) National survey of mammographic facilities in 1985, 1988, and 1992. Radiology 191:323–330

de Koning HJ (2000) Assessment of nationwide cancer-screening programmes. Lancet 355:80–81

Duffy SW (2001) Interpretation of the breast screening trials: a commentary on the recent paper by Gotzsche and Olsen. The Breast 10:209–212

Duffy SW, Tabar L (2000) Screening mammography re-evaluated (letter to the editor) Lancet 355:747–748

Duffy SW, Tabar L, Chen H-H, et al. (2002) The impact of organized mammography service screening on breast cancer mortality in seven Swedish counties: a collaborative evaluation. Cancer 95:458–469

Falun Meeting Committee and Collaborators (1996) Falun meeting on breast cancer screening with mammography in women aged 40–49 years: report of the organizing committee and collaborators. Int J Cancer 68:693–699

Feig SA (1994) Determination of mammographic screening intervals with surrogate measures for women aged 40–49 years. Radiology 193:311–314

Feig SA (1995) Estimation of currently attainable benefit from mammographic screening of women aged 40–49 years. Cancer 75:2412–2419

Feig SA (1997) Increased benefit from shorter screening mammography intervals for women ages 40–49 years. Cancer 80:2035–2039

Feig SA, D'Orsi CJ, Hendrick RE, et al (1997b) American College of Radiology Guidelines for Breast Cancer Screening. AJR Am J Roentgenol 171:29-33

Feig SA (2002a) Screening mammography: effect of image quality on clinical outcome. AJR, Am J Roentgenol 178:805-807

Feig SA (2000b) Effect of service screening mammography on population mortality from breast carcinoma. Cancer 95:451-457

Garne JP, Aspegren K, Balldin G, Ranstam J (1997) Increasing incidence of and declining mortality from breast carcinoma: trends in Malmo, Sweden, 1961-1992. Cancer 79:69-74

Gotzsche PC, Olsen O (2000) Is screening for breast cancer with mammography justifiable? Lancet 355:129-1134

Hakama M, Pukkala E, Heikkila M, Kallio M (1997) Effectiveness of the public health policy for breast cancer screening in Finland: a population based cohort study. Brit Med J 314:864-867

Haus AG (1999) Dedicated mammographic x-ray equipment, screen-film processing systems, and viewing conditions for mammography. Seminars in Breast Disease 2:30-54

Hendrick RE, Smith RA, Rutledge JH III, et al. (1997) Benefit of screening mammography in women aged 40-49: a new meta-analysis of randomized controlled trials. NCI Monogr 33:87-92

Humphrey LL, Helfant M, Chan BKS, Woolf SH (2002) Breast cancer screening: a summary of the evidence for the U.S. Preventive Services Task Force. Ann Intern Med 137:347-360

Hurley SF, Kaldor JM (1992) The benefits and risks of mammographic screening for breast cancer. Epidemiol Rev 14:101-130

Jonsson H, Nystrom L, Tornberg S, Lenner P (2001) Service screening with mammography of women aged 50-69 years in Sweden: effects on mortality from breast cancer. J Med Screen 8:152-160

Kerlikowske K, Grady D, Rubin SM, et al (1995) Efficacy of screening mammography: a meta-analysis. JAMA 273:149-154

Kopans DB (1990) The Canadian Screening Program: a different perspective. AJR Am J Roentgenol 155:748-749

Kopans DB, Feig SA (1993) The Canadian National Breast Screening Study: a critical review. AJR Am J Roentgenol 161:755-760

Leitch AM, Dodd GD, Costanza M, et al (1997) American Cancer Society Guidelines for the Early Detection of Breast Cancer. CA Cancer J Clin 47:150-153

Lerner P, Jonsson H (1997) Excess mortality from breast cancer in relation to mammography screening in northern Sweden. J Med Screen 4:6-9

Mettlin CJ, Smart CR (1993) The Canadian National Breast Screening Study: an appraisal and implications for early detection policy. Cancer 72:1461-1465

Michaelson JS, Halpern E, Kopans DB (1999) Breast cancer computer simulation method for estimation of optimal intervals for screening. Radiology 212:551-560

Miettinen OS, Henschke CI, Pasmantier MW, et al. (2002) Mammographic screening: no reliable supporting evidence? Lancet 359:404-406

Miller AB, Baines CJ, To T, Wall C (1992) Canadian National Breast Screening Study: 1. Breast cancer detection and death rates among women aged 40 to 49 years. Can Med Assoc J 147:1459-1476

Miller A, To T, Baines CJ, Wall C (2002a) Canadian National Breast Screening Study: 2. 13-year results of a randomized trial in women aged 50-59 years. J Natl Cancer Inst 92:1490-1499

Miller AB, To T, Baines CJ, Wall C (2002b) The Canadian National Breast Screening Study-1: breast cancer mortality after 11 to 16 years of follow-up. A randomized trial of mammography in women age 40 to 49 years. Ann Intern Med 137:305-312

Nystrom L (2000) Screening mammography re-evaluated (letter to the editor). Lancet 355:748-749

Nystrom L, Andersson I, Bjurstam N, Frisell J, Nordenskjold B, Rutqvist LE (2002) Long-term effects of mammography screening: updated overview of the Swedish randomized trials. Lancet 359:909-919

Nystrom L, Rutqvist L-E, Wall S, et al (1993) Breast cancer screening with mammography: overview of Swedish randomized trials [published erratum appears in Lancet 1993; 342:1372]. Lancet 341:973–978

Nystrom L, Larsson L-G, Rutqvist L-E, et al (1995) Determination of cause of death among breast cancer cases in the Swedish randomized mammography screening trials. A comparison between official statistics and validation by an end point committee. Acta Oncol 34:145–152

Olsen O, Gotzsche PC (2001) Cochrane review on screening for breast cancer with mammography. Lancet 358:1340–1342

Rosen M, Rehnqvist N (1999) No need to reconsider breast screening programme on basis of results from defective study (letter to the editor). Br Med J 318:809–810

Shapiro S, Venet W, Strax P, Venet L (1988) Periodic screening for breast cancer. The Health Insurance Plan Project and its sequelae, 1963–1986. Johns Hopkins University Press, Baltimore

Sjonell G, Stahle L (1999) Mammography screening does not reduce breast cancer mortality [Swedish]. Lakartidningen 96:904–913

Smart CR, Hendrick RE, Rutledge JH III, et al (1995) Benefit of mammography screening in women ages 40–49 years: current evidence from randomized trials. Cancer 75:1619–1626 [errratum appears in Cancer 75: 2788, 1995]

Smith RA (2000) Breast cancer screening among women younger than 50: a current assessment of the issues. CA Cancer J Clin 50:312–336

Tabar L, Fagerberg G, Chen H-H, et al (1995) Efficacy of breast cancer screening by age: new results from the Swedish Two-County Trial. Cancer 75:2507–2517

Tabar L, Fagerberg G, Duffy SW, Day NE (1989) The Swedish Two-County Trial of mammographic screening for breast cancer: recent results and calculation of benefit. J Epidemiol Comm Hlth 43:107–114

Tabar L, Vitak B, Chen H-H, et al (2000) The Swedish Two-County Trial twenty years later. Updated mortality results and new insights from long-term follow-up. Radiol Clin North Am 38:625–651

Tabar L, Vitak B, Chen H-H, Yen M-F, Duffy SW, Smith RA (2001) Beyond randomized controlled trials: organized mammographic screening substantially reduces breast carcinoma mortality. Cancer 91:1724–1731

Taplin SH, Rutter CM, Finder C, Mandelson MT, Houn F, White E (2002) Screening mammography: clinical image quality and the risk of interval breast cancer. AJR Am J Roentgenol 178:797–804

Tarone RE (1995) The excess of patients with advanced breast cancer in young women screened with mammography in the Canadian National Breast Screening Study. Cancer 75:997–1003

Tornberg S, Carstensen J, Hakulinen T, Lenner P, Hatschek T, Lundgren B (1994) Evaluation of the effect on breast cancer mortality of population based mammography screening programmes. J Med Screen 1:184–187

Warren-Burhenne LJ, Burhenne HJ (1993) The Canadian National Breast Screening Study: a Canadian critique. AJR Am J Roentgenol 161:761–763

Young KC, Wallis MG, Ramsdale ML (1994) Mammographic film density and detection of small breast cancers. Clin Radiol 49:461–465

Political Interpretation of Scientific Evidence – Case Study of Breast Cancer Screening Policies Around the World

Gad Rennert

G. Rennert (✉)
Department of Community Medicine and Epidemiology,
Carmel Medical Center and Technion Faculty of Medicine,
and Clalit Health Services (CHS) National Cancer Control Center,
National Israeli Breast Cancer Detection Program, 7 Michal St.,
Haifa 34362, Israel

Abstract

Early detection of breast cancer has been studied for effectiveness in reducing mortality for more than four decades. During this period numerous studies took place, with more than half a million participating women. In spite of large amounts of nonconflicting data, different countries took varying lengths of time to establish a policy, and came up with a variety of policies, quite different from one another. Inherent differences between the countries in structure of the health system, in the commitment to public health activities, and in opinions and health habits of the relevant populations may explain these different outcomes.

The Scientific Process

Data Acquisition

The scientific process of acquiring information about the efficacy of breast cancer screening was initiated by Sam Shapiro in 1963. Shapiro introduced the HIP study [1] in New York, the first randomized controlled trial studying the effect of mammography and clinical breast examination on mortality reduction from breast cancer.

This study opened the era of randomized controlled trials for evaluation of screening technologies. Cancer screening technologies invented beforehand such as the Pap Smear never underwent proper randomized evaluation prior to their introduction as a population screening means. Randomized controlled trials have since been criticized many times for being expensive and slow to provide results. The BCDDP [2], a "demonstration project" in the United States, was initiated to provide short-cut data on the efficacy of breast cancer screening and provided its first results in 1979, 3 years before the publication of the HIP study results.

Three more studies: Malmö [3], Edinburgh [4], and the Swedish Two-County study [5], were initiated 13–14 years after the launching of the HIP study, followed by another three studies initiated in 1980–1982: Canadian CNBSS [6], Stockholm [7], and Gothenburg [8]. Thus, a total of seven randomized controlled trials, initiated in five different countries over a 20-year period, set the base for the evidence in the field of mammography screening. Several more case-control studies (DOM [9], Nijmegen [10], United Kingdom [11], Florence[12]) had also been running during the same period.

Study Results

The first trial results became available in 1981. Results of the HIP study demonstrated the benefits of breast cancer screening and equally valued clinical breast examination and mammography [1]. The results of the Swedish Two-County study, employing a single intervention with a more advanced mammography technology than in the HIP study, were published in 1985 [5]. In total, 456,349 women participated in the seven randomized controlled studies (248,192 as cases and 208,157 as controls). This is possibly the largest trial effort ever taken to prove the effectiveness of any technology. All studies, with the exception of the Canadian trial [6, 13] demonstrated a reduction in mortality from breast cancer (Fig. 1). The total cumulative effect was of a magnitude of 30% in women ages 50 and over [8]. A less clear, and smaller mortality reduction, taking more years of follow-up to appear, was noticed among women under the age of 50 years [14].

These results, together with the results of the various case-control studies, set grounds to the beginning of the policy making process on breast cancer screening.

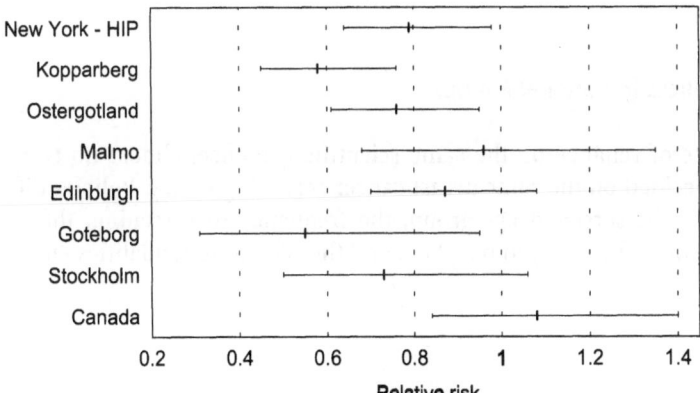

Fig. 1. Relative risk of death from breast cancer in screening mammography trials

The Political Process

National Screening Programs Start Evolving

Mammography was first officially introduced in Iceland and in several districts in Sweden in 1987. This was followed in 1988 by The Netherlands and several regions in Canada, and in 1989 in Finland. In 1988, the American Cancer Society and the US Preventive Services Task Force established policy in favor of screening for breast cancer in the United States [15]. In contrast to policies in other countries, the United States policy emphasized the need for a triple approach of breast self-examination, clinical breast examination, and mammography. The Europe Against Cancer program initiated simultaneously a series of pilot screening programs in a variety of countries in Europe [16, 17]. The rationale behind the pilot programs was the need to develop expertise in planning and running a high-quality population-based screening program before incorporating it into a country-wide policy. The early 1990s saw the initiation of national screening programs in Australia and the United Kingdom, followed by organized programs in a variety of states in the United States, in Israel, and later in France.

Experience acquired by the mid-1990s with large-scale screening mammography, as well as the influx of more follow-up data from the trials, led to newer discussions on the value of mammography in women younger than 50. While an NCI expert committee, in a consensus conference in 1997, recommended against inclusion of young women in screening mammography programs [18], the United States Congress, under pressure from a variety of medical and public interest groups, ruled against this decision and decided to change the formal screening policy to include these younger women [19, 20]. This is an interesting example of the involvement of lay, nonexpert, political powers in determining a professional policy.

Germany and Switzerland were among the last Western countries to join the international trend with plans to introduce national screening in the beginning of the twenty-first century (Fig. 2).

Differences in National Policies

In spite of reliance on the same scientific evidence, almost no two countries have decided on the same breast cancer screening policy. Policies differ by the target to-be-screened age-group, the frequency of screening, the number of mammography views to be taken, and the screening modalities employed.

Age

While there was no debate on the 50–69-year age group, pressures have mounted leading to discussions on the value of mammography in ages young-

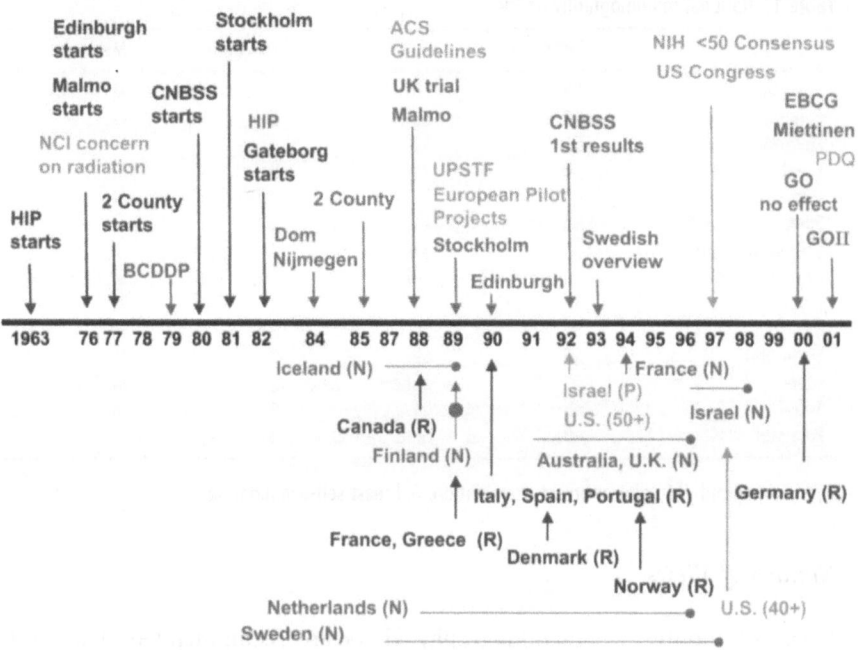

Fig. 2. Mammography screening – timeline of science and policy

er than 50 and in women ages 70 and over. The United Kingdom program stuck out as the most restrictive program, including only women up to the age of 64, while the United States policy included the widest age group, starting at 40 and not stating an upper age limit. The United States policy to screen women younger than 50 was set in contrast with the recommendation of an expert committee of the NCI on this issue. Most countries in the world offer mammography to postmenopausal women only. A trend towards increasing the upper limit of screening resulted in a change in the Dutch policy, which currently offers mammography to women up to the age of 74, as does Israel.

Frequency

Screening every 2 years in postmenopausal women is the most common policy in the world. Yet the American policy recommends annual screening, while the United Kingdom program recommends mammography once every 3 years. Other policies based their screening frequencies on breast tissue characteristics found in the prevalence round.

Table 1. National mammography policies

	From age	To age	Frequency	Methods
Australia	50	69	2	M
Canada	50	69	2	M, C, B
Finland	50	59	2	M
Israel	50	74	2	M
Netherlands	50	74	2	M
Sweden	50	74	2	M
United Kingdom	50	64	3	M
United States	50	none	1–2	M, C, B
France	50	69	2–3	M
Italy	50	69	2	M
Denmark	50	69	2	M
Greece	40	none	2	M, C, B
Spain	45	64	2	M
Portugal	40	none	2	M

M, mammography; C, clinical breast examination, B, breast self-examination.

Number of Views

Most commonly, two mammography views are recommended. The United Kingdom program offers only one medio-lateral oblique view, although most screening centers in the United Kingdom were found not to comply with this regulation. Policies of several countries recommend a two-view approach in the prevalence round followed by a single view in subsequent rounds.

Screening Modalities

Mammography is the exclusive recommended screening modality in most countries. Japan's policy originally relied on clinical breast examination until recent years, when it decided to add mammography. North American policies traditionally include clinical breast examination and breast self examination in spite of lack of any evidence of effectiveness of these modalities [13, 21–24], again pointing to the political angles of the medical decision-making process (Table 1).

Why Differences in Mammography Policies?

A question of major interest is why, in the face of what seems to be solid scientific evidence, have different countries developed different policies and followed different timelines in reaching a decision regarding breast cancer screening and its contents.

Difference in the policy setting process can be clearly attributed to the types of health systems in the involved countries. Countries with a National

Health Service (NHS) type of service such as the United Kingdom, Sweden and other Scandinavian countries, and Canada were the first to include active screening, to use a cost-effectiveness approach to decide on the contents of such screening and to provide nationwide financial coverage. In the United Kingdom, this approach led to a very restrictive program. Most of these programs reached very high uptake levels. Countries with a social health insurance which provides service through organized providers or health maintenance organizations express three different models:

1. Holland, Israel – A health system where the GPs are the gatekeepers and specialists are usually based in hospitals. This system is usually characterized by highly centralized, public health-oriented authorities, therefore usually leading to early action in public health issues. These countries were among the early initiators of national screening programs.
2. French-speaking countries model – The health system motto is liberal medicine. The freedom of the expert physicians is such that it precludes regulation and central control. These countries took part in the European pilot activities, but were late to establish a national program with national regulation.
3. German-speaking countries – A health system granting a very high degree of freedom to health care providers. Specialists are often based in the community. The high degree of freedom inhibits regulatory activity and lowers the probability of public health-oriented policy. These countries were the last to discuss national screening activity, the last to decide on implementation and were first to withdraw when negative reports started showing up in the literature.
4. The United States model – A model of a mixed health system. Private providers, HMOs, and Federal agencies such as the VA system and the Medicare/Medicaid systems operate and influence the system. The American medical organizations, the American Cancer Society and the US Preventive Services Task Force are usually the first to recommend activities relating to preventive oncology. Yet, with the exclusion of the last body (USPSTF), which is a professional authority with no vested interest, the others usually produce policy statements long before there is solid evidence of an effect. Their policy is usually broader than any other policy statement and usually ignores central issues in public health, such as acceptability to the population and cost-effectiveness. This policy is many times driven by other, non-medical bodies. Because of the relative lack of central public health action, organized screening programs are few and late to form. Due to issues of health insurance coverage, uptake of screening is many times low, especially in underserved regions or populations. On the other hand, the personal awareness of preventive medicine in the United States is probably higher than in most other countries.

New Threats to Mammography Screening

Claims of Ineffectiveness

In spite of the vast amount of information available from a large number of randomized controlled trials pointing at a significant reduction in mortality, various scientific groups have in recent years cast doubts on the value of this technology. The first doubts were introduced by the research team behind the Canadian CNBSS study, which found no protective effect [6, 13]. Second came a Cochrane Group review which published two different reports in the *Lancet* in 2001 rejecting most existing results based on poor study design and claiming no overall effect of mammography [25, 26]. This claim came under debate, between the Cochrane report authors and the Cochrane Advisory Board [27]. A rare situation has developed in which two reports have been issued, on the same day by the same authors, carrying different and conflicting messages [26, 28]. An editorial of the *Lancet* editor [29] added to the feeling that it is politics and not science which is the driving force of the events. Since this ordeal, the PDQ scientists of the NCI have also raised doubts as to the cost-effectiveness of mammography screening in the United States in an as yet unpublished report [30].

An even newer analysis of the data of the Malmö study, deemed to be a valid study, showed significant mortality benefits using different analytic approaches by a nonrelated scientific group [31].

Summary

From this case study it is obvious that the existence of a large database of trial results is not the sole requirement for a timely setting of a policy. In spite of large amounts of nonconflicting data, different countries took varying lengths of time to establish a policy, and came up with a variety of policies, quite different from one another. Inherent differences between the countries in structure of the health system, in the commitment to public health activities, and in opinions and health habits of the relevant populations may explain these different outcomes.

Future policy setting in the field of breast cancer screening will need to take into account not only the currently available data, and the re-evaluation of these data, but also other issues such as the expected reduction in the sensitivity of screening programs due to the increased use of hormone replacement therapy in peri- and postmenopausal women [32–36], as well as the introduction of new imaging modalities such as the breast MRI [37–39].

References

1. Shapiro S, Venet W, Strax, Venet L (1988) Periodic screening for breast cancer: The Health Insurance Plan Project and its Sequelae, 1963–1986. Baltimore, The Johns Hopkins University Press
2. Baker LH (1982) Breast Cancer Detection Demonstration Project: five year summary report. Ca Cancer J Clin 32:194–225s
3. Andersson L, Aspegren K, Janzon L, et al (1988) Mammographic screening and mortality from breast cancer: the Malmö mammographic screening trial. BMJ 297:943–948
4. Roberts MM, Alexander FE, Anderson TJ, et al (1990) Edinburgh trial of screening for breast cancer. Mortality at seven years. Lancet 335:241–246
5. Tabar L, Fagerberg G, Duffy SW, et al (1992) Update of the Swedish two-county program of mammographic screening for breast cancer. Radiol Clin North Am 30:187–210
6. Miller AB, Baines C, To T, Wall C (1992) Canadian National Breast Screening Study: 2. Breast cancer detection and death rates among women aged 50 to 59 years. CMAJ 147:1477–1488
7. Frisell J, Eklund G, Hellstrom, et al (1991) Randomized study of mammography screening-preliminary report on mortality in the Stockholm trial. Breast Cancer Res Treat 18:49–56
8. Nystrom L, Rutqvist LE, Wall S, et al (1993) Breast cancer screening with mammography: an overview of the Swedish randomized trials. Lancet 341:973–978
9. de-Waard F, Collette HJ, Rombach JJ, Baanders van Halewijn EA, Honing C (1984) The DOM project for the early detection of breast cancer, Utrecht, The Netherlands. J Chronic Dis 37:1–44
10. Verbeek AL, Hendriks JH, Holland R, Mravunac M, Sturmans F, Day NE (1984) Reduction of breast cancer mortality through mass screening with modern mammography. First results of the Nijmegen project, 1975–1981. Lancet 1:1222–1224
11. United Kingdom trial of Early Detection of breast cancer group (1988) 16-year mortality from breast cancer in the United Kingdom Trial of early detection of breast cancer. Lancet 2:411–416
12. Palli D, Del Turco MR, Buiatti E, Carli S, Ciatto S, Toscani L, Maltoni G (1986) A case-control study of the efficacy of a nonrandomized breast cancer screening program in Florence (Italy). Int J Cancer 38:501–504
13. Miller AB, To T, Baines C, Wall C 2000 Canadian National Breast Screening Study-2: 13 Year results of a randomized trial in women aged 50–59 Years. JNCI 92:1490–1499
14. Ringash J (2001) Canadian Task Force on Preventive Health Care. Screening mammography among women aged 40–49 years at average risk of breast cancer. CMAJ 164:469–476
15. Guide to Clinical Preventive Services (1996) Report of the US Preventive Services Task Force, 2nd edn. Williams & Wilkins, Baltimore, pp 73–88.
16. Recommendations of the Committee of Cancer Experts on Breast Cancer Screening (1992) 6 April. European Commission
17. Shapiro S, Coleman EA, Broeders M, Codd M, de-Koning H, Fracheboud J, Moss S, Paci E, Stachenko S, Ballard-Barbash R (1998) Breast cancer screening programmes in 22 countries: current policies, administration and guidelines. International Breast Cancer Screening Network (IBSN) and the European Network of Pilot Projects for Breast Cancer Screening. Int J Epidemiol 27:735–42
18. National Institutes of Health. National Cancer Institute (1997) Consensus development conference on screening mammography in women under age 50. L. Gordis, Chairman
19. United States Congress decision, 105th Congress, 1st Session, February 4, 1997, 4:59 pm, Page S-936 Temp. Record, Vote No. 5
20. NCI-PDQ (1997) Cancer Facts. Research studies on screening mammography
21. Thomas DB, Gao DL, Self SG, Allison CJ, Tao Y, Mahloch J, et al (1997) Randomized trial of breast self-examination in Shanghai: methodology and preliminary results. JNCI 9:355–365

22. Semiglazov VF, Sagaidak VN, Moiseyenko VM, Mikhailov EA (1993) Study of the role of breast self-examination in the reduction of mortality from breast cancer. The Russian Federation/World Health Organization Study. Eur J Cancer 29A:2039-2046

23. Holmberg L, Ekbom A, Calle E, Mokdad A, Byers T (1997) Breast cancer mortality in relation to self-reported use of breast self examination. A cohort study of 450,000 women. Breast Cancer Res Treat 43:137-140

24. Baxter N, CTFPHC (2001) Should women be routinely taught breast self-examination to screen for breast cancer? CMAJ 164:1837-1846

25. Gotzsche PC, Olsen O (2000) Is screening for breast cancer with mammography justifiable? Lancet 355:129-134

26. Olsen O, Gotzsche PC (2001) Cochrane review on screening for breast cancer with mammography. Lancet 358:1340-1342

27. EBCG editors, Cochrane Collaboration (2002) Screening mammography: setting the record straight. Lancet 359:439-440

28. Olsen O, Gotzsche PC (2001) Screening for breast cancer with mammography (Cochrane Review). In: The Cochrane Library. Issue 4. Oxford: Update software

29. Horton R (2001) Screening mammography-an overview revisited. Lancet 358:1284-1285

30. P.D.Q. Screening and Prevention Editorial Board. January 24, 2002 Expert Panel Cites Doubts on Mammogram1s Worth By GINA KOLATA, New York Times, 2002, US

31. Miettinen OS, Henschke C, Pasmantier MW, Smith JP, Libby DM Yankelevitz DF (2002) Mammographic screening: no reliable supporting evidence? Lancet 359:404-406

32. Roubidoux MA, Wilson TE, Orange RJ, Fitzgerald JT, Helvie MA, Packer S-A (1998) Breast cancer in women who undergo screening mammography: relationship of hormone replacement therapy to stage and detection method. Radiology 208:725-8

33. Banks E (2001) Hormone replacement therapy and the sensitivity and specificity of breast cancer screening: a review. J Med Screen 8:29-34

34. Rutter CM, Mandelson MT, Laya MB, Seger DJ, Taplin S (2001) Changes in breast density associated with initiation, discontinuation, and continuing use of hormone replacement therapy. JAMA 285:171-176

35. Kavanagh AM, Mitchell H, Giles GG (2000) Hormone replacement therapy and accuracy of mammographic screening. Lancet 355:270-274

36. Seradour B, Esteve J, Heid P, Jacquemier J (1999) Hormone replacement therapy and screening mammography: analysis of the results in the Bouches du Rhone programme. J Med Screen 6:99-102

37. Stoutjesdijk MJ, Boetes C, Jager GJ, Beex I, Bult P, Herndriks JH, Laheij R, Massuger L, van Die LE, Wobbes T, Barentsz JO (2001) Magnetic resonance imaging and mammography in women with a hereditary risk of breast cancer. JNCI 18:1095-102

38. Tilanus-Linthorst MM, Obdeijn IM, Bartels KC, de Koning HJ, Oudkerk M (2000) First experience in screening women at high risk for breast cancer with MR imaging. Breast Cancer Res Treat 63:53-60

39. Warner E, Plewes DB, Shumak RS, Catzavelos GC, Di Prospero LS, Yaffe MJ, Goel V, Ramsay E, Chart PI, Cole DE, Taylor GA, Cutrara M, Samuels TH, Murphy JP, Narod SA (2001) Comparison of breast magnetic resonance imaging, mammography and ultrasound for surveillance of women at high risk for hereditary breast cancer. J Clin Oncol 19:3524-31

Chemoprevention of Skin and Lung Cancer 5

Skin Cancer Chemoprevention: Strategies to Save Our Skin

Janine G. Einspahr, G. Timothy Bowden, David S. Alberts

J.G. Einspahr (✉)
Arizona Cancer Center, University of Arizona, P.O. Box 245024, Tucson,
AZ 85724, USA

Abstract

There are over 1 million cases of skin cancer diagnosed yearly in the United
States. The majority of these are nonmelanoma (NMSCs) and are associated
with chronic exposure to ultraviolet light (UV). Actinic keratosis (AK) has
been identified as a precursor for SCC, but not for BCC. AKs are far more
common than SCC, making them excellent targets for chemoprevention. Cancer chemoprevention can prevent or delay the occurrence of cancer in high-
risk populations using dietary or chemical interventions. We have developed
strategies that have rational mechanisms of action and demonstrate activity
in preclinical models of skin cancer. Promising agents proceed to phase I-III
trials in subjects at high risk of skin cancer. UV light induces molecular signaling pathways and results in specific genetic alterations (i.e., mutation of
p53) that are likely critical to skin cancer development. UVB-induced changes
serve as a basis for the development of novel agents. Targets include inhibition
of polyamine or prostaglandin synthesis, specific retinoid receptors, and components of the Ras and MAP kinase signaling pathways. Agents under study
include: epigallocatechin gallate (EGCG), a green tea catechin with antioxidant
and sunscreen activity, as well as UVB signal transduction blocking activity;
perillyl alcohol, a monoterpene derived from citrus peel that inhibits Ras farnesylation; difluoromethylornithine (DFMO), an inhibitor of ornithine decarboxylase and polyamines; retinoids that target retinoid X receptors and AP-1
activity; and nonsteroidal anti-inflammatory agents that inhibit cyclooxygenase and prostaglandin synthesis. We performed a series of Phase I-II trials in
subjects with multiple AK. For example, a phase II randomized trial of topical
DFMO reduced AK number, suppressed polyamines, and reduced p53 protein.
Our goal is to develop agents for use in combination and/or incorporation
into sunscreens to improve chemoprevention efficacy and reduce skin cancer
incidence.

Recent Results in Cancer Research, Vol. 163
© Springer-Verlag Berlin Heidelberg 2003

Skin Cancer, a Worldwide Problem

Over 1 million new skin cancers are diagnosed yearly in the United States, accounting for approximately 40% of all new cancer diagnoses. The incidence of skin cancer is increasing due to many factors, including aging of the population and larger amounts of ultraviolet radiation reaching the earth's surface due to depletion of the ozone layer (Johnson et al. 1998). Approximately 80% of skin cancers are basal cell carcinomas (BCC), 16% are squamous cell carcinomas (SCC), and 4% are melanomas.

In 2002 there will be approximately 53,600 cases with 7,400 deaths (National Cancer Institute 2001). Melanoma, while associated with exposure to sunlight, appears to be related to severe sunburns or intermittent exposure, rather than chronic sun exposure (Gilchrest et al. 1999). While vitally important to the reduction of skin cancer mortality, melanoma chemoprevention has been limited (Halpern et al. 1994; Meyskens et al. 1986; Stam-Posthuma et al. 1998).

BCC is a slow growing tumor that rarely metastasizes, but can cause tremendous morbidity. In contrast, SCCs can metastasize, accounting for approximately 1,200 deaths in 1998 (a number equivalent to the yearly mortality attributed to Hodgkin's lymphoma) (Greenlee et al. 2000; Marks 1995; Moller et al. 1979). Furthermore, a high percentage of patients with SCC develop a second primary skin cancer within 5 years (Frankel et al. 1992; Karagas et al. 1992; Preston and Stern 1992). NMSCs occur primarily on sun-exposed areas of the body and have been strongly associated with chronic sun exposure (Kwa et al. 1992). A premalignant lesion or actinic (or solar) keratosis has been identified for SCC, but not for BCC.

Actinic Keratoses, Intraepithelial Neoplasia

There is strong evidence that AKs are precursors of SCC with shared risk factors, a histologic continuum, and the presence of common molecular/genetic alterations (Salasche 2000). Although the exact incidence of AK is unknown, 40%–50% of Australians 40 years of age or older harbor AK and the incidence increases with advancing age (Fritzgerald 1998; Marks et al. 1988; Salasche 2000). The rate of SCC in the population is much lower than the rate of AK, demonstrating that not all AK progress to SCC (Marks et al. 1988). Approximately 60% of SCCs arise from pre-existing AKs and the rate of malignant transformation to SCC is 6%–10% or 1 per 1,000 per year in individual lesions (Dodson et al. 1991). While most AKs do not progress to SCC, AK represents SCC in situ at its earliest stages (Cockerell 2000).

Clinically, AKs appear as red/brown, scaly, nonsubstantive patches on chronically sun-exposed areas such as the face, ears, and dorsal surface of hands (Kuflik and Schwartz 1994). Histologically, AKs are characterized by dysplasia of the keratinocytes with changes in cellular polarity and nuclear atypia. The diagnosis of SCC is made when atypical cells invade underlying dermis.

Skin adjacent to AKs often harbor similar histologic changes, suggesting that AKs develop on a background of sun-damaged skin. These findings support the concept that there is a field of cancerization due to chronic exposure to UV light (Marks 1990).

Multistep Model of UVB-Induced SCC

UV-induced human skin cancer progresses in stages from sun-damaged epidermis, to AK, to SCC and metastasis, as demonstrated in Fig. 1. UV is a complete carcinogen in UVB-induced animal models, capable of initiation, promotion, and progression of SCCs (Matsui and DeLeo 1995). This sequence of lesions provides an excellent opportunity to study the progression of genetic and epigenetic alterations that take place during UV-induced carcinogenesis. AKs and sun-damaged skin may serve as surrogate endpoint biomarkers (SEBs) in chemoprevention studies.

Mutations in the p53 gene have been identified in chronically sun-damaged skin, AK, and SCC (Brash et al. 1991; Campbell et al. 1993; Kubo et al. 1994; Moles et al. 1993; Nelson et al. 1994; Pierceall et al. 1991; Taguchi et al. 1994;

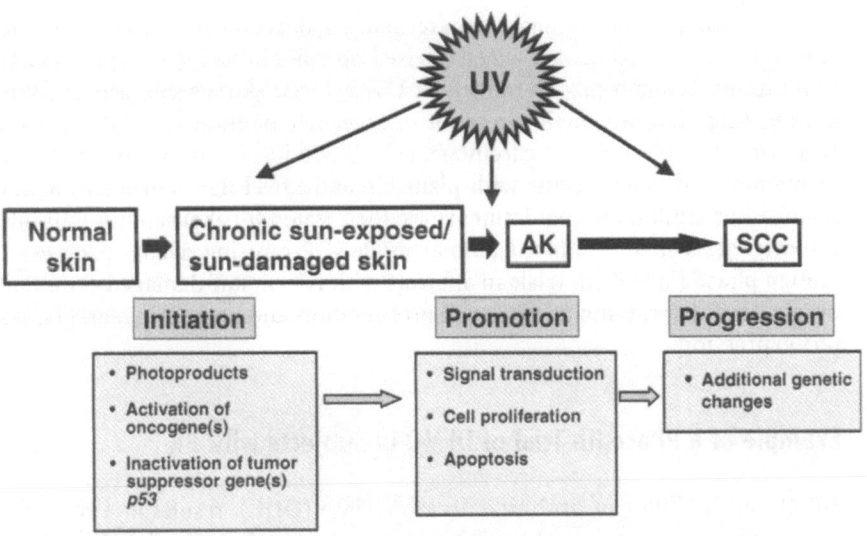

Fig. 1. Multistep UV-induced skin carcinogenesis. Human UV-induced SCC is a multistep process where premalignant AKs develop on a background of chronically sun-damaged skin. AKs can than progress to SCC. The ultraviolet or UV portion of sunlight is a complete carcinogen capable of initiation with formation of UV-induced photoproducts and genetic alterations in oncogenes and tumor suppressor genes (mutation and overexpression the p53 gene). Promotion involves activation of signal transduction pathways, as well as alterations in cell proliferation and apoptosis while progression requires additional genetic alterations

Ziegler et al. 1994). This high incidence of p53 mutations early in UV-induced carcinogenesis strongly supports an important role for the p53. Furthermore, these p53 mutations are consistent with UV as the causative agent (i.e., CC to TT and C to T substitutions at dipyrimidine sites) (Brash et al. 1991; Campbell et al. 1993; Kubo et al. 1994; Moles et al. 1993; Nelson et al. 1994; Pierceall et al. 1991; Taguchi et al. 1994; Ziegler et al. 1994). Mutation of p53 often leads to a stabilization of the protein, which can than be measured by immunohisto-chemistry (Jonason et al. 1996; McNutt et al. 1991; Nagano et al. 1993; Nelson et al. 1994; Ren et al. 1996; Ro et al. 1993; Shea et al. 1992; Sim et al. 1991, 1992; Taguchi et al. 1994; Urano et al. 1992, 1995).

The p53 gene is essential in maintaining genomic integrity by blocking DNA replication in response to DNA damage from exposure to agents like UV light. Cells with extensive damage are blocked from entering the cell cycle and instead undergo apoptosis (Leffell 2000; Nataraj et al. 1995). p53 is present at low levels in normal cells but in response to DNA damage, the half-life of p53 increases posttranslationally from minutes to hours. Exposure of normal epidermal keratinocytes to UV light results in a transient increase in p53 protein levels and resultant arrest in the G1 phase of the cell cycle (Campbell et al. 1993; Gujuluva et al. 1994; Hall et al. 1993; Healy et al. 1994).

Decision Tree for Selection of Chemoprevention Agents

At the Arizona Cancer Center we are using a decision tree where leads for chemoprevention agents are selected based on epidemiologic evidence and activity in in vitro and in vivo models of UV-induced skin carcinogenesis. With the identification of genetic alterations, molecular pathways, and cellular targets critical to UV-induced carcinogenesis, it will be important to use this information to develop agents with plausible and novel mechanisms of action. Agents that fulfill these requirements are then tested for their ability to inhibit tumorigenesis in UV-induced animal models. Promising agents progress to human phase IIa and IIb trials in subjects with AK or sun-damaged skin. Endpoints, or SEBs, can include AK, cell proliferation and apoptotic markers, and p53 expression.

Example of a Phase IIb Trial of DFMO in Subjects with AK

DFMO, an inhibitor of ornithine decarboxylase (ODC), results in a reduction of polyamine synthesis and inhibition of both chemically and UVB-induced skin tumorigenesis in rodent models. Upregulation of polyamines occurs in the promotion phase of chemically and UVB-induced skin carcinogenesis models and is likely to be a critical factor in skin cancer development (Boone et al. 1990; Pegg et al. 1988; Fischer et al. 1999, 2001; Weeks et al. 1982; Gilmour et al. 1987; Meyskens and Gerner 1999; Gensler 1991; Takigawa et al. 1983). Polyamines are ubiquitous polycations that are essential for normal cell growth (Smith et al. 2000). Both oral and topical administration of DFMO inhibits the development of UVB-induced mouse skin tumors. Topical administration of 3 mg DFMO in acetone three times a week reduced tumor formation by 40% (p=0.05) (Gensler 1991).

This led to the topical formulation of 10% DFMO in a hydrophilic ointment (Alberts et al. 2000). Males and females, at least 30 years of age, with ten or more clinical AKs on forearms were eligible for the study. Details of the study population and design are described in Alberts et al. (Alberts et al. 2000).

Briefly, a 1-month placebo run-in was performed prior to randomization to placebo or DFMO to the right or left arm so that one arm served as a control for the contralateral arm. Participants were randomized to ensure that males and females were equally distributed between the two groups (right arm treated versus left arm treated) and that the distributions of initial AKs were the same in both groups.

During the placebo run-in and at the end of 6 months of placebo or DFMO topical treatment there was a clinical evaluation of AK number. Skin punch biopsy specimens were obtained for polyamine levels and shave biopsy specimens were obtained for PCNA, p53 protein expression, p53 mutations, and apoptosis. All biopsy specimens were obtained from AKs on the dorsal surface of forearms.

Data were available for 42 subjects. Topical DFMO reduced the number of AKs (23.5% reduction) and the skin level of spermidine (21% reduction), a polyamine known to be involved in cell proliferation. Additionally, p53 protein expression was significantly reduced (26% reduction) by DFMO, while cell proliferation and apoptosis were not affected (Alberts et al. 2000; Einspahr et al. 2002).

UVB-Induced Signal Transduction

UV radiation can initiate carcinogenesis through DNA mutations and chromosomal alterations. However, at least some of the promoting effects of UV involve activation of signal transduction pathways. One of these UVB-induced pathways is the mitogen-activated protein kinase (MAPK) cascade which affects the regulation of transcription factors, and consequently the control of genes involved in biological processes like cell proliferation, apoptosis, and tumorigenesis.

Activator Protein-1 (AP-1) transcription factor plays a critical role in skin tumor promotion in both chemical and UVB-induced skin carcinogenesis models. Induction of AP-1 occurs through stimulation of MAPK pathways in UVB-irradiated mouse and human keratinocytes and epidermis (Dong et al. 1994; Huang et al. 1996, 1997; Young et al. 1999). UVB can induce the MAPK cascade through activation of acidic sphingomyelinases followed by ceramide activation of atypical PKCs as illustrated in Fig. 2. Atypical PKCs activate MAPK/extracellular signal-regulated kinase (ERK)-kinase or MEK (Huang et al. 2000). The pathway continues with activation of ERK by MEK, followed by

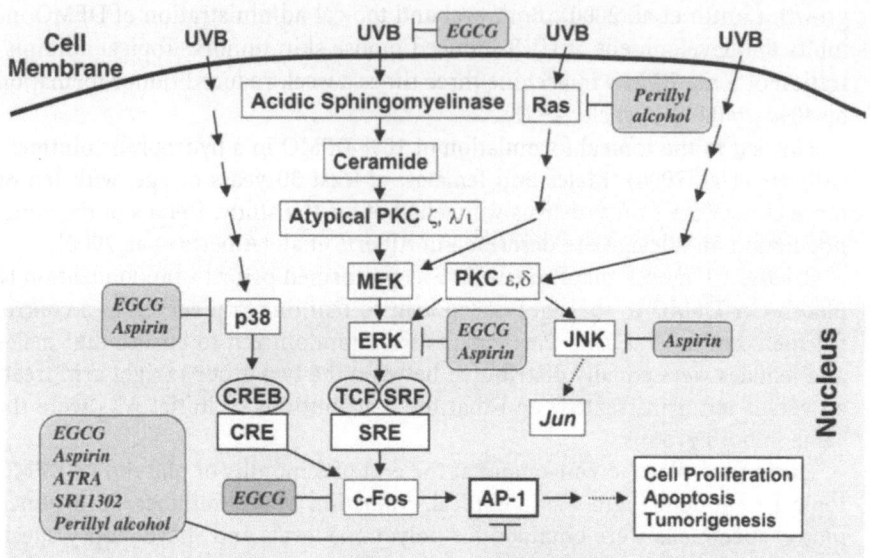

Fig. 2. UVB-induced MAPK signaling pathways. UVB signals through the MAPK cascade that includes ERK, JNK, and p38. In this simplified model, UVB activates sphingomyelinases which in turn activate ceramide followed by activation of atypical PKCs. Atypical PKCs phosphorylate and activate MEK, followed by ERK. ERK phosphorylates and activates TCF and binding of SRF to an SRE site within the promoter of specific genes. Activation of this pathway results in c-Fos expression followed by AP-1 activation. Another effect of UVB is activation of the p38 pathway. UVB can also induce signaling through the Ras pathway. These signal transduction cascades result in cellular responses that include proliferation, apoptosis or tumorigenesis. The postulated molecular targets of the chemoprevention agents EGCG (a green tea polyphenol), perillyl alcohol, aspirin, and retinoids (all trans-retinoic acid or ATRA and SR11302) are shown

activation of ternary complex factor (TCF). In mouse keratinocytes, UVB-induced translocation of the atypical PKC isoform PKCς (cytosol to membrane), activation of MAPK family members, and AP-1 transcriptional activation occur via activation of ERKs, but not JNKs or p38 (Huang et al. 2000).

This pathway through MEK and ERK ultimately results in transcription of c-Fos. UVB-induced c-Fos expression is an early epigenetic event and occurs through the binding of the transcription factors TCF and serum response factor (SRF) to specific sites within the DNA referred to as the serum response element (SRE). In human skin, UVB induces the activity of all three major MAPKs: JNK, ERK, and p38 (Fisher et al. 1998).

UVB-Induced Signal Transduction and Skin Cancer Chemopreventive

Illustrated in Fig. 2 are chemoprevention agents and points in the UVB-induced signal transduction pathway where these agents appear to be acting.

Elucidation of these and other pathways is key to determining the mechanism of action of UVB-induced skin cancer chemopreventive agents.

Green and black tea polyphenols and black tea theaflavins inhibit UVB-induced activation of AP-1, MAP kinase, and ERK; moreover, they inhibit enhanced expression of c-Fos in human keratinocytes (Barthelman et al. 1998; Chen et al. 1999; Chung et al. 1999; Nomura et al. 2000). Epigallocatechin-3-gallate (EGCG), the green tea polyphenol proposed to have the highest antioxidant activity (Mukhtar and Ahmad 1999), inhibits autophosphorylation of the epidermal growth factor receptor (EGFR) and suppresses cell proliferation (Liang et al. 1997). EGCG differentially induces apoptosis and cell cycle arrest in epidermoid carcinoma cells, with no affect on normal cells (Chen et al. 1998; Lin et al. 1999). Tea is one of the most widely consumed beverages worldwide (Lin et al. 1999; Mukhtar and Ahmad 1999; Yang and Wang 1993). Green and black tea have antitumor activity in both chemically and UVB-induced skin carcinogenesis models (Ahmad and Mukhtar 1999; Kuroda and Hara 1999). The antitumor activity of tea remains when administered after UVB exposure, indicating that activity goes beyond a simple antioxidant or sunscreen effect (Ahmad and Mukhtar 1999; Kuroda and Hara 1999; Mukhtar et al. 1994; Nomura et al. 2000).

Perillyl alcohol, a monoterpene derived from citrus peel, has antitumor activity in a number of tumor types that include UVB-induced skin carcinogenesis (Barthelman et al. 1998; Crowell 1999). As an inhibitor of Ras farnesylation, perillyl alcohol prevents attachment of Ras to the cell membrane thereby inhibiting Ras signaling pathways. This disruption of Ras can affect downstream signaling pathways that would likely include inhibition of AP-1 transcriptional activity (Barthelman et al. 1998; Crowell et al. 1994). Perillyl alcohol can induce apoptosis and/or inhibit proteins that require isoprenylation for activity, such as Ras (Bardon et al. 1998).

Nonsteroidal anti-inflammatory drugs (NSAIDs), like aspirin, inhibit COX activity rather than expression, producing a reduction of growth stimulatory eicosinoids (i.e., prostaglandins). Prostaglandins are involved in the promotion phase of both chemically and UVB-induced skin carcinogenesis animal models (Fischer et al. 1999; Pentland et al. 1999). Oral administration of celecoxib, a selective COX-2 inhibitor, decreases the incidence and number of UVB-induced mouse skin cancers and decreases COX-2 activity in skin tumors. This upregulation of COX-2 in tumors suggests that the COX-2 plays an important role in UVB-induced carcinogenesis (Fischer et al. 1999; Pentland et al. 1999). COX-2 inhibitors are effective in both the early and late stages of UVB-induced skin carcinogenesis (Pentland et al. 1999). Aspirin, a nonselective NSAID, inhibits UVB-induced AP-1 activation though inhibition of MAP kinase signaling that includes suppression of JNK, ERK, and p38 activity (Huang et al. 1997; Ma et al. 1998). NSAIDs can also have COX-2-independent mechanisms (Kubba 1999).

Retinoids have antitumor activity against skin cancer models (Evans and Kaye 1999; Lippman and Lotan 2000; Lotan 1996). Retinoids function through activation of the nuclear receptors; retinoic acid receptors (RAR), and retinoid x receptors (RXR). These receptors bind specific DNA sequences called retinoic acid response elements (RARE) and retinoid x response elements (RXRE) that are present in retinoid responsive genes. Regulation of retinoid receptors is highly complex with variation in tissue expression, ligand specificity, and the ability to regulate other signaling pathways (i.e., AP-1) (DiSepio et al. 1999; Levine 1998). Retinoids with selective receptor activity are currently under development (Evans and Kaye 1999; Lippman and Lotan 2000).

Potential mechanisms for the chemopreventive properties of retinoids include activation of nuclear retinoid receptors and transrepression of AP-1, growth arrest, and induction of apoptosis and differentiation (Niles 2000; Nicholson et al. 1990; Schule et al. 1991). Topical application of a synthetic AP-1 specific retinoid (SR11302) or trans-retinoic acid, a retinoid that has both AP-1 and RARE affects, suppresses TPA-induced papilloma formation in mice, inhibits AP-1 transactivation, and inhibits transformation of mouse epidermal cells in vitro (Li et al. 1996). In contrast, a retinoid with selective RARE transactivating activity (SR11235) did not reduce papilloma number or inhibit AP-1 transactivation. These experiments provide strong evidence that the antitumor activity of retinoids occurs via AP-1 transrepression (Li et al. 1996; Fanjul et al. 1994). Furthermore, an RXRα-selective retinoid (SR11235) inhibits RARE-dependent gene expression but did not significantly inhibit AP-1 transactivation or neoplastic transformation in vitro (Li et al. 1996; Huang et al. 1997; Fanjul et al. 1994). Additionally, retinoic acids suppress both TPA and EGR-mediated expression of COX-2 in squamous carcinoma cells (Mestre et al.). Inhibition of COX-2 may be mediated through AP-1 and/or cyclic AMP response element (CRE) dependent pathways (Xie and Herschman 1995).

Another chemopreventive target is the phosphatidylinositol-3 kinase (PI-3K) signaling pathway. TPA, EGF, and insulin induce PI-3K and AP-1 activation as well as malignant transformation in mouse epidermal cells, while inositol hexaphosphate blocks these effects (Dong et al. 1999). Recently, Dr. Bowden's group has shown a role for p38 MAP kinase (Chen et al. 2001) and PI-3 kinase (Tang et al. 2001) in UVB-induced transcriptional regulation (Tang et al. 2001) of the COX-2 gene in human keratinocytes. His group has demonstrated that activation of p38 is required for UVB-induced COX-2 gene expression. It appears that UVB-induced p38 activity mediates phosphorylation of CRE binding protein (CREB) at serine 133. He has shown that phospho-CREB binds to a critical CRE in the promoter region of the human COX-2 gene in response to UVB. His group also has demonstrated in human keratinocytes that UVB activation of PI-3 kinase leads to phosphorylation of AKT, which in turn leads to enhanced phosphorylation of GSK-3β on serine 9. Serine 9 phosphorylation of GSK-3β inactivates this enzyme. His group showed that inactivation of GSK-3β leads to increased transactivation of the COX-2 promoter and increased expression of COX-2 protein. Therefore, both p38 MAP kinase and the PI-3 kinase pathways play a role of UVB-induced COX-2 expression in keratinocytes. These two pathways may be potential targets for chemoprevention of skin cancer.

Conclusion

NMSC is a significant and increasing health problem worldwide. Epidemiologic evidence has determined that chronic exposure to sunlight is the etiologic agent responsible for most cases of skin cancer. Subsequent studies in animal models and in vitro have identified UV radiation, particularly UVB, as a complete carcinogen (Brash et al. 1996). UV-induced human skin carcinogenesis is a multistep process having discreet steps that include chronically sun-damaged skin, AK, and SCC. This multistep process provides an excellent model for testing chemopreventive strategies to reduce the incidence of SCC and its precursor lesion, AK. A sensible approach would be to combine primary prevention and secondary chemoprevention to maximize their effectiveness (Harvey et al. 1996; Naylor et al. 1995).

Useful strategies for development of chemopreventive agents would be to identify agents that inhibit components of UV signal transduction pathways. Promising agents would then be tested for activity in UVB-induced animal models and finally advanced to clinical trials in high-risk subjects. The ideal chemoprevention agent, in addition to inhibiting skin cancer, must have minimal toxicity for use in healthy populations and would differentially affect premalignant or malignant cells leaving normal cells unaffected (Lippman et al. 1998).

Chemoprevention studies also include biological measures of the carcinogenesis process, markers of cancer risk, and/or surrogate endpoint biomarkers of the affect of an intervention. Biological markers can include genetic alterations (e.g., mutation of the tumor suppressor gene p53) as well as biological processes (e.g., cell proliferation or apoptosis). It will be important to validate these SEBs as surrogates for the carcinogenesis process and/or as measures of an intervention effect.

Acknowledgements. This publication was supported in part by Public Health Service grant CA27502 from the National Cancer Institute. Its contents are solely the responsibility of the authors and do not necessarily represent the official views of the National Cancer Institute.

References

Ahmad N, Mukhtar H (1999) Green tea polyphenols and cancer: biologic mechanisms and practical implications. Nutr Rev 57:78–83

Alberts DS, Dorr RT, Einspahr JG, Aickin M, Saboda K, Xu MJ, Peng YM, Goldman R, Foote JA, Warneke JA, Salasche S, Roe DJ, Bowden GT (2000) Chemoprevention of human actinic kerotoses by topical 2-(difluoromethyl)-dl-ornithine. Cancer Epidemiol Biomarkers Prev 9:1281–1286

Bardon S, Picard K, Martel P (1998) Monoterpenes inhibit cell growth, cell cycle progression, and cyclin D1 gene expression in human breast cancer cell lines. Nutr Cancer 32:1–7

Barthelman M, Bair WB 3rd, Stickland KK, Chen W, Timmermann BN, Valcic S, Dong Z, Bowden GT (1998) (-)-Epigallocatechin-3-gallate inhibition of ultraviolet B-induced AP-1 activity. Carcinogenesis 19:2201–2204

Barthelman M, Chen W, Gensler HL, Huang C, Dong Z, Bowden GT (1998) Inhibitory effects of perillyl alcohol on UVB-induced murine skin cancer and AP-1 transactivation. Cancer Res 58:711–716

Boone CW, Kelloff GJ, Malone WE (1990) Identification of candidate cancer chemopreventive agents and their evaluation in animal models and human clinical trials: a review. Cancer Res 50:2–9

Brash DE, Rudolph JA, Simon JA, Lin A, McKenna GJ, Baden HP, Halperin AJ, Ponten J (1991) A role for sunlight in skin cancer: UV-induced p53 mutations in squamous cell carcinoma. Proc Natl Acad Sci U S A 88:10124–10128

Brash DE, Ziegler A, Jonason AS, Simon JA, Kunala S, Leffell DJ (1996) Sunlight and sunburn in human skin cancer: p53, apoptosis, and tumor promotion. J Investig Dermatol Symp Proc 1:136–42

Campbell C, Quinn AG, Angus B, Farr PM, Rees JL (1993) Wavelength specific patterns of p53 induction in human skin following exposure to UV radiation. Cancer Res 53:2697–2699

Chen W, Dong Z, Valcic S, Timmermann BN, Bowden GT (1999) Inhibition of ultraviolet B-induced c-fos gene expression and p38 mitogen-activated protein kinase activation by (-)-epigallocatechin gallate in a human keratinocyte cell line. Mol Carcinog 24:79–84

Chen W, Tang Q, Gonzales MS, Bowden GT (2001) Role of p38 MAP kinases and ERK in mediating ultraviolet-B induced cyclooxygenase-2 gene expression in human keratinocytes. Oncogene 20:3921–3926

Chen YR, Wang W, Kong AN, Tan TH (1998) Molecular mechanisms of c-Jun N-terminal kinase-mediated apoptosis induced by anticarcinogenic isothiocyanates. J Biol Chem 273:1769–1775

Chung JY, Huang C, Meng X, Dong Z, Yang CS (1999) Inhibition of activator protein 1 activity and cell growth by purified green tea and black tea polyphenols in H-ras-transformed cells: structure-activity relationship and mechanisms involved. Cancer Res 59:4610–4617

Cockerell CJ (2000) Histopathology of incipient intraepidermal squamous cell carcinoma ("actinic keratosis"). J Am Acad Dermatol 42:11–17

Crowell PL (1999) Prevention and therapy of cancer by dietary monoterpenes. J Nutr 129:775S–778S

Crowell PL, Ren Z, Lin S, Vedejs E, Gould MN (1994) Structure-activity relationships among monoterpene inhibitors of protein isoprenylation and cell proliferation. Biochem Pharmacol 47:1405–1415

DiSepio D, Sutter M, Johnson AT, Chandraratna RA, Nagpal S (1999) Identification of the AP1-antagonism domain of retinoic acid receptors. Mol Cell Biol Res Commun 1:7–13

Dodson JM, DeSpain J, Hewett JE, Clark DP (1991) Malignant potential of actinic keratoses and the controversy over treatment. A patient-oriented perspective. Arch Dermatol 127:1029–1031

Dong Z, Birrer MJ, Watts RG, Matrisian LM, Colburn NH (1994) Blocking of tumor promoter-induced AP-1 activity inhibits induced transformation in JB6 mouse epidermal cells. Proc Natl Acad Sci USA 91:609–613

Dong Z, Huang C, Ma WY (1999) PI-3 kinase in signal transduction, cell transformation, and as a target for chemoprevention of cancer. Anticancer Res 19:3743–3748

Einspahr JG, Nelson MA, Saboda K, Warneke J, Bowden GT, Alberts DS (2002) Modulation of biologic endpoints by topical difluoromethylornithine (DFMO), in subjects at high-risk for nonmelanoma skin cancer. Clin Cancer Res 8:149–155

Evans TR, Kaye SB (1999) Retinoids: present role and future potential. Br J Cancer 80:1–8

Fanjul A, Dawson MI, Hobbs PD, Jong L, Cameron JF, Harlev E, Graupner G, Lu XP, Pfahl M (1994) A new class of retinoids with selective inhibition of AP-1 inhibits proliferation. Nature 372:107–111

Fischer SM, Lee M, Lubet RA (2001) Difluoromethylornithine is effective as both a preventive and therapeutic agent against the development of UV carcinogenesis in SKH hairless mice. Carcinogenesis 22:83–88

Fischer SM, Lo HH, Gordon GB, Seibert K, Kelloff G, Lubet RA, Conti CJ (1999) Chemopreventive activity of celecoxib, a specific cyclooxygenase-2 inhibitor, and indomethacin against ultraviolet light-induced skin carcinogenesis. Mol Carcinog 25:231-240

Fisher GJ, Talwar HS, Lin J, Lin P, McPhillips F, Wang Z, Li X, Wan Y, Kang S, Voorhees JJ (1998) Retinoic acid inhibits induction of c-Jun protein by ultraviolet radiation that occurs subsequent to activation of mitogen-activated protein kinase pathways in human skin in vivo. J Clin Invest 101:1432-1440

Frankel DH, Hanusa BH, Zitelli JA (1992) New primary nonmelanoma skin cancer in patients with a history of squamous cell carcinoma of the skin. Implications and recommendations for follow-up. J Am Acad Dermatol 26:720-726

Fritzgerald DA (1998) Cancer precursors. Semin Cut Med Surg 17:108-113

Gensler HL (1991) Prevention by alpha-difluoromethylornithine of skin carcinogenesis and immunosuppression induced by ultraviolet irradiation. J Cancer Res Clin Oncol 117:345-350

Gilchrest BA, Eller MS, Geller AC, Yaar M (1999) The pathogenesis of melanoma induced by ultraviolet radiation. N Engl J Med 340:1341-1348

Gilmour SK, Verma AK, Madara T, O'Brien TG (1987) Regulation of ornithine decarboxylase gene expression in mouse epidermis and epidermal tumors during two-stage tumorigenesis. Cancer Res 47:1221-1225

Greenlee RT, Murray T, Bolden S, Wingo PA (2000) Cancer statistics, 2000. CA Cancer J Clin 50:7-33

Gujuluva CN, Baek JH, Shin KH, Cherrick HM, Park NH (1994) Effect of UV-irradiation on cell cycle, viability and the expression of p53, gadd153 and gadd45 genes in normal and HPV-immortalized human oral keratinocytes. Oncogene 9:1819-1827

Hall PA, McKee PH, Menage HD, Dover R, Lane DP (1993) High levels of p53 protein in UV-irradiated normal human skin. Oncogene 8:203-207

Halpern AC, Schuchter LM, Elder DE, Guerry Dt, Elenitsas R, Trock B, Matozzo I (1994) Effects of topical tretinoin on dysplastic nevi. J Clin Oncol 12:1028-1035

Harvey I, Frankel S, Marks R, Shalom D, Nolan-Farrell M (1996) Nonmelanoma skin cancer and solar keratoses II analytical results of the South Wales Skin Cancer Study. Br J Cancer 74:1308-1312

Healy E, Reynolds NJ, Smith MD, Campbell C, Farr PM, Rees JL (1994) Dissociation of erythema and p53 protein expression in human skin following UVB irradiation, and induction of p53 protein and mRNA following application of skin irritants. J Invest Dermatol 103:493-499

Huang C, Li J, Chen N, Ma W, Bowden GT, Dong Z (2000) Inhibition of atypical PKC blocks ultraviolet-induced AP-1 activation by specifically inhibiting ERKs activation. Mol Carcinog 27:65-75

Huang C, Ma W, Bowden GT, Dong Z (1996) Ultraviolet B-induced activated protein-1 activation does not require epidermal growth factor receptor but is blocked by a dominant negative PKClambda/iota. J Biol Chem 271:31262-31268

Huang C, Ma W, Ding M, Bowden GT, Dong Z (1997) Direct evidence for an important role of sphingomyelinase in ultraviolet-induced activation of c-Jun N-terminal kinase. J Biol Chem 272:27753-27757

Huang C, Ma WY, Dawson MI, Rincon M, Flavell RA, Dong Z (1997) Blocking activator protein-1 activity, but not activating retinoic acid response element, is required for the antitumor promotion effect of retinoic acid. Proc Natl Acad Sci USA 94:5826-5830

Huang C, Ma WY, Hanenberger D, Cleary MP, Bowden GT, Dong Z (1997) Inhibition of ultraviolet B-induced activator protein-1 (AP-1) activity by aspirin in AP-1-luciferase transgenic mice. J Biol Chem 272:26325-26331

Johnson TM, Dolan OM, Hamilton TA, Lu MC, Swanson NA, Lowe L (1998) Clinical and histologic trends of melanoma. J Am Acad Dermatol 38:681-686

Jonason AS, Kunala S, Price GJ, Restifo RJ, Spinelli HM, Persing JA, Leffell DJ, Tarone RE, Brash DE (1996) Frequent clones of p53-mutated keratinocytes in normal human skin. Proc Natl Acad Sci USA 93:14025-14029

Karagas MR, Stukel TA, Greenberg ER, Baron JA, Mott LA, Stern RS (1992) Risk of subsequent basal cell carcinoma and squamous cell carcinoma of the skin among patients with prior skin cancer. Skin Cancer Prevention Study Group. JAMA 267:3305–3310

Kubba AK (1999) Non steroidal anti-inflammatory drugs and colorectal cancer: is there a way forward? Eur J Cancer 35:892–901

Kubo Y, Urano Y, Yoshimoto K, Iwahana H, Fukuhara K, Arase S, Itakura M (1994) p53 gene mutations in human skin cancers and precancerous lesions: comparison with immunohistochemical analysis. J Invest Dermatol 102:440–444

Kuflik AS, Schwartz RA (1994) Actinic keratosis and squamous cell carcinoma. Am Fam Physician 49:817–820

Kuroda Y, Hara Y (1999) Antimutagenic and anticarcinogenic activity of tea polyphenols. Mutat Res 436:69–97

Kwa RE, Campana K, Moy RL (1992) Biology of cutaneous squamous cell carcinoma. J Am Acad Dermatol 26:1–26

Leffell DJ (2000) The scientific basis of skin cancer. J Am Acad Dermatol 42:18–22

Levine N (1998) Role of retinoids in skin cancer treatment and prevention. J Am Acad Dermatol 39:S62–S66

Li JJ, Dong Z, Dawson MI, Colburn NH (1996) Inhibition of tumor promoter-induced transformation by retinoids that transrepress AP-1 without transactivating retinoic acid response element. Cancer Res 56:483–489

Liang YC, Lin-Shiau SY, Chen CF, Lin JK (1997) Suppression of extracellular signals and cell proliferation through EGF receptor binding by (-)-epigallocatechin gallate in human A431 epidermoid carcinoma cells. J Cell Biochem 67:55–65

Lin JK, Liang YC, Lin-Shiau SY (1999) Cancer chemoprevention by tea polyphenols through mitotic signal transduction blockade. Biochem Pharmacol 58:911–915

Lippman SM, Lee JJ, Sabichi AL (1998) Cancer chemoprevention: progress and promise. J Natl Cancer Inst 90:1514–1528

Lippman SM, Lotan R (2000) Advances in the development of retinoids as chemopreventive agents. J Nutr 130:479S–482S

Lotan R (1996) Retinoids in cancer chemoprevention. FASEB J 10:1031–1039

Ma WY, Huang C, Dong Z (1998) Inhibition of ultraviolet C irradiation-induced AP-1 activity by aspirin is through inhibition of JNKs but not erks or P38 MAP kinase. Int J Oncol 12:565–568

Marks R (1990) Solar keratosis. Br J Dermatol 122[Suppl 35]:49–60

Marks R (1995) An overview of skin cancers. Incidence and causation. Cancer 75:607–612

Marks R, Rennie G, Selwood TS (1988) Malignant transformation of solar keratoses to squamous cell carcinoma. Lancet 1:795–797

Matsui MS, DeLeo VA (1995) Photocarcinogenesis by ultraviolet A and B. In: Mukhtar H (ed) Skin cancer: mechanisms and human relevance. CRC Press, Boca Raton, pp 21–30

McNutt NS, Saenz-Santamaria C, Volkenandt M, Shea CR, Albino AP (1991) Abnormalities of p53 protein expression in cutaneous disorders. Arch Dermatol 130:225–232

Mestre JR, Subbaramaiah K, Sacks PG, Schantz SP, Tanabe T, Inoue H, Dannenberg AJ (1997) Retinoids suppress epidermal growth factor-induced transcription of cyclooxygenase-2 in human oral squamous carcinoma cells. Cancer Res 57:2890–2895

Mestre JR, Subbaramaiah K, Sacks PG, Schantz SP, Tanabe T, Inoue H, Dannenberg AJ (1997) Retinoids suppress phorbol ester-mediated induction of cyclooxygenase-2. Cancer Res 57:1081–1085

Meyskens FL Jr, Edwards L, Levine NS (1986) Role of topical tretinoin in melanoma and dysplastic nevi. J Am Acad Dermatol 15:822–825

Meyskens FL Jr, Gerner EW (1999) Development of difluoromethylornithine (DFMO) as a chemoprevention agent. Clin Cancer Res 5:945–951

Moles JP, Moyret C, Guillot B, Jeanteur P, Guilhou JJ, Theillet C, Basset-Seguin N (1993) p53 gene mutations in human epithelial skin cancers. Oncogene 8:583–588

Moller R, Reymann F, Hou-Jensen K (1979) Metastases in dermatological patients with squamous cell carcinoma. Arch Dermatol 115:703–705

Mukhtar H, Ahmad N (1999) Green tea in chemoprevention of cancer. Toxicol Sci 52:111–117

Mukhtar H, Katiyar SK, Agarwal R (1994) Green tea and skin – anticarcinogenic effects. J Invest Dermatol 102:3-7

Nagano T, Ueda M, Ichihashi M (1993) Expression of p53 protein is an early event in ultraviolet light-induced cutaneous squamous cell carcinogenesis. Arch Dermatol 129:1157-1161

Nataraj AJ, Trent JC 2nd, Ananthaswamy HN (1995) p53 gene mutations and photocarcinogenesis. Photochem Photobiol 62:218-230

National Cancer Institute, National Institutes of Health, Public Health Service, U.S. Department of Health and Human Services (2001) Cancer Progress Report 2001 (http://progress-report.cancer.gov)

Naylor MF, Boyd A, Smith DW, Cameron GS, Hubbard D, Neldner KH (1995) High sun protection factor sunscreens in the suppression of actinic neoplasia. Arch Dermatol 131:170-175

Nelson MA, Einspahr JG, Alberts DS, Balfour CA, Wymer JA, Welch KL, Salasche SJ, Bangert JL, Grogan TM, Bozzo PO (1994) Analysis of the p53 gene in human precancerous actinic keratosis lesions and squamous cell cancers. Cancer Lett 85:23-29

Nicholson RC, Mader S, Nagpal S, Leid M, Rochette-Egly C, Chambon P (1990) Negative regulation of the rat stromelysin gene promoter by retinoic acid is mediated by an AP1 binding site. EMBO J 9:4443-4454

Niles RM (2000) Recent advances in the use of vitamin A (retinoids) in the prevention and treatment of cancer. Nutrition 16:1084-1089

Nomura M, Ma WY, Huang C, Yang CS, Bowden GT, Miyamoto K, Dong Z (2000) Inhibition of ultraviolet B-induced AP-1 activation by theaflavins from black tea. Mol Carcinog 28:148-155

Pegg AE, Madhubala R, Kameji T, Bergeron RJ (1988) Control of ornithine decarboxylase activity in alpha-difluoromethylornithine-resistant L1210 cells by polyamines and synthetic analogues. J Biol Chem 263:11008-11014

Pentland AP, Schoggins JW, Scott GA, Khan KN, Han R (1999) Reduction of UV-induced skin tumors in hairless mice by selective COX-2 inhibition. Carcinogenesis 20:1939-1944

Pierceall WE, Mukhopadhyay T, Goldberg LH, Ananthaswamy HN (1991) Mutations in the p53 tumor suppressor gene in human cutaneous squamous cell carcinomas. Mol Carcinog 4:445-449

Preston DS, Stern RS (1992) Nonmelanoma cancers of the skin. N Engl J Med 327:1649-1662

Ren ZP, Hedrum A, Ponten F, Nister M, Ahmadian A, Lundeberg J, Uhlen M, Ponten J (1996) Human epidermal cancer and accompanying precursors have identical p53 mutations different from p53 mutations in adjacent areas of clonally expanded non-neoplastic keratinocytes. Oncogene 12:765-773

Ro YS, Cooper PN, Lee JA, Quinn AG, Harrison D, Lane D, Horne CH, Rees JL, Angus B (1993) p53 protein expression in benign and malignant skin tumours. Br J Dermatol 128:237-241

Salasche SJ (2000) Epidemiology of actinic keratoses and squamous cell carcinoma. J Am Acad Dermatol 42:S4-S7

Schule R, Rangarajan P, Yang N, Kliewer S, Ransone LJ, Bolado J, Verma IM, Evans RM. (1991) Retinoic acid is a negative regulator of AP-1-responsive genes. Proc Natl Acad Sci USA 88:6092-6096

Shea CR, McNutt NS, Volkenandt M, Lugo J, Prioleau PG, Albino AP (1992) Overexpression of p53 protein in basal cell carcinomas of human skin. Am J Pathol 141:25-29

Sim CS, Slater SD, McKee PH (1991) Mutant p53 protein is expression in solar keratosis: an immunohistochemical study. J Cutan Pathol 19:302-308

Sim CS, Slater SD, McKee PH (1992) Mutant p53 protein is expressed in Bowen's disease. Am J Dermatopathol 14:195-199

Smith WL, DeWitt DL, Garavito RM (2000) Cyclooxygenases: structural, cellular, and molecular biology. Annu Rev Biochem 69:145-182

Stam-Posthuma JJ, Vink J, le Cessie S, Bruijn JA, Bergman W, Pavel S (1998) Effect of topical tretinoin under occlusion on atypical naevi. Melanoma Res 8:539-548

Taguchi M, Watanabe S, Yashima K, Murakami Y, Sekiya T, Ikeda S (1994) Aberrations of the tumor suppressor p53 gene and p53 protein in solar keratosis in human skin. J Invest Dermatol 103:500–503

Takigawa M, Verma AK, Simsiman RC, Boutwell RK (1983) Inhibition of mouse skin tumor promotion and of promoter-stimulated epidermal polyamine biosynthesis by alpha-difluoromethylornithine. Cancer Res 43:3732–3738

Tang Q, Chen W, Gonzales MS, Finch J, Inoue H, Bowden GT (2001) Role of cyclic AMP responsive element in the UVB induction of cyclooxygenase-2 transcription in human keratinocytes. Oncogene 20:5164–5172

Tang Q, Gonzales M, Inoue H, Bowden GT (2001) Roles of Akt and glycogen synthase kinase 3beta in the ultraviolet B induction of cyclooxygenase-2 transcription in human keratinocytes. Cancer Res 61:4329–4332

Urano Y, Asano T, Yoshimoto K, Iwahana H, Kubo Y, Kato S, Sasaki S, Takeuchi N, Uchida N, Nakanishi H (1995) Frequent p53 accumulation in the chronically sun-exposed epidermis and clonal expansion of p53 mutant cells in the epidermis adjacent to basal cell carcinoma. J Invest Dermatol 104:928–932

Urano Y, Oura H, Sakaki A, Nagae H, Matsumoto K, Fukuhara K, Nagae T, Arase S, Ninomiya Y, Nakanishi H (1992) Immunohistological analysis of p53 expression in human skin tumors. J Dermatol Sci 4:69–75

Weeks CE, Herrmann AL, Nelson FR, Slaga TJ (1982) alpha-Difluoromethylornithine, an irreversible inhibitor of ornithine decarboxylase, inhibits tumor promoter-induced polyamine accumulation and carcinogenesis in mouse skin. Proc Natl Acad Sci USA 79:6028–6032

Xie W, Herschman HR (1995) v-src induces prostaglandin synthase 2-gene expression by activation of the c-Jun N-terminal kinase and the c-Jun transcription factor. J Biol Chem 270:27622–27628

Yang CS, Wang ZY (1993) Tea and cancer. J Natl Cancer Inst 85:1038–1049

Young MR, Li JJ, Rincon M, Flavell RA, Sathyanarayana BK, Hunziker R, Colburn N (1999) Transgenic mice demonstrate AP-1 (activator protein-1) transactivation is required for tumor promotion. Proc Natl Acad Sci U S A 96:9827–9832

Ziegler A, Jonason AS, Leffell DJ, Simon JA, Sharma HW, Kimmelman J, Remington L, Jacks T, Brash DE (1994) Sunburn and p53 in the onset of skin cancer. Nature 372:773–776

Chemoprevention of Nonmelanoma Skin Cancer: Experience with a Polyphenol from Green Tea

Kenneth G. Linden, Philip M. Carpenter, Christine E. McLaren,
Ronald J. Barr, Pamela Hite, Joannie D. Sun, Kou-Tung Li, Jaye L. Viner,
Frank L. Meyskens

K.G. Linden (✉)
Department of Dermatology, University of California, Irvine,
101 The City Drive, Orange, CA 92868, USA

Abstract

Nonmelanoma skin cancer is extremely common and is increasing in incidence. It would be very useful to have forms of therapy that would prevent
precancerous changes from going on to form cancer, or to reverse the precancerous changes. Epidemiologic evidence in humans, in vitro studies on human
cells, and clinical experiments in animals have identified polyphenol compounds found in tea to be possibly useful in reducing the incidence of various
cancers, including skin cancer. To examine the potential for a polyphenol
from green tea, epigallocatechin gallate, to act as a chemopreventive agent for
nonmelanoma skin cancer, a randomized, double-blind, placebo-controlled
phase II clinical trial of topical epigallocatechin gallate in the prevention of
nonmelanoma skin cancer was performed.

Background

Nonmelanoma skin cancer is a significant and increasing medical problem. In
the United States, over one million new cases of nonmelanoma skin cancer are
diagnosed each year, probably exceeding the incidence of all other types of
cancer combined (Jemal et al. 2002). The two most common types of nonmelanoma skin cancer are basal cell carcinoma and squamous cell carcinoma.
The greatest risk factors for these types of cancers are a fair skin type and
high cumulative exposure to sunlight.

The most readily identifiable premalignant lesion for nonmelanoma skin
cancers is actinic keratosis (solar keratosis), which is considered to be a premalignant precursor to squamous cell carcinoma. There is some controversy
over this designation among dermatologists, some of whom consider actinic
keratoses to be a form of squamous cell carcinoma in situ of the skin (Heaphy
and Ackerman 2000). The risk factors for actinic keratoses are the same as

Recent Results in Cancer Research, Vol. 163
© Springer-Verlag Berlin Heidelberg 2003

those for nonmelanoma skin cancer, as described above. Given these risk factors, it is not surprising that fair-skinned populations inhabiting sunny climates at latitudes closer to the equator such as Australia have the highest risk for, and incidence of, actinic keratoses (Marks 1990).

Actinic keratoses are readily identifiable precursors to nonmelanoma skin cancer; as a result they are useful clinical markers for cancer prevention research. Interventions that lead to the regression or decrease in the rate of formation of actinic keratoses would be expected to lead to a decrease in the formation of nonmelanoma skin cancers, particularly squamous cell carcinoma of the skin. It is for this reason that actinic keratoses are being extensively studied as modulable clinical endpoints in trials testing the chemopreventive potential of promising agents against the development of nonmelanoma skin cancer.

The purpose of this chapter is to discuss important aspects of study design for clinical trials of potential chemopreventive agents administered to prevent, regress, or retard the development of actinic keratoses and nonmelanoma skin cancer. Our experiences with a polyphenol from green tea will be used as an example.

Choice of Potential Chemopreventive Agents for Actinic Keratoses and Nonmelanoma Skin Cancer

In choosing a candidate chemopreventive agent for nonmelanoma skin cancer, several factors must be considered. The factors include epidemiologic evidence indicating that the chemopreventive agent may be useful in the prevention of the cancer of interest and observational data on drugs developed for other applications (e.g., oncologic agents such as topical 5-fluorouracil). Activity of the potential chemopreventive agent in animal model systems is an important form of preliminary evidence. Additionally, in vitro activity against precancerous and cancerous cells may be of use. If there is a potential molecular mode of action postulated for the agent, various forms of biochemical and molecular studies may be used to evaluate a potential chemopreventive agent as well. In our study of the chemoprevention of actinic keratoses and squamous cell carcinoma, epigallocatechin gallate satisfied many of the above-mentioned criteria for advancement into clinical testing.

Epidemiologic evidence suggests that green tea may have anticancer activity against a number of cancers. However, the evidence is equivocal and various studies in different populations show that green tea may be associated with a preventive effect, no effect, or even an increased risk of cancer in nearly every epithelial cancer studied (see Bushman 1998 for review). In addition to differences in study design, plant variety, growth conditions, horticultural practices, processing, and variable tea consumption may contribute to the mixed data arising from epidemiologic studies (Katiyar and Mukhtar 1997). The bulk of the epidemiologic evidence probably does favor some chemopreventive effects for certain cancers. Animal model studies of epigallocatechin gallate, a tea constituent, have demonstrated inhibitory effects against carcinogenesis at a number of organ sites. Particularly convincing preliminary evidence is that the compound has been shown to reverse squamous papilloma formation in the mouse model of UV carcinogenesis that is most analogous to actinic keratoses in humans (Mukhtar et al. 1994; Gensler et al. 1996). There is also in vitro evidence using human skin cancer lines that epigallocatechin gallate may possess anticancer properties (Valcic et al. 1996). Numerous molecular mechanisms have been suggested to account for the possible chemopreventive activity of green tea against various cancers. The polyphenols, including epigallocatechin gallate, are powerful antioxidants that may act to quench free radicals produced during the carcinogenic process; also, they may act at many sites in the carcinogenic pathway (Dreosti 1997). Given the epidemiologic, animal model, in vitro, and molecular evidence, it was felt that epigallocatechin gallate was a good candidate agent for chemoprevention of human nonmelanoma skin cancer and a clinical trial was designed to test this hypothesis.

Another consideration is that any new chemopreventive agent will be judged against current therapies, which for actinic keratoses mainly consist of liquid nitrogen treatment, treatment with the topical chemopreventive agent 5-fluorouracil, photodynamic therapy (Jeffes et al. 2001), and more recently, treatment with the topical agent diclofenac (Rivers et al. 2002).

Clinical Trial Design for Chemoprevention of Nonmelanoma Skin Cancer

There are several important elements that must be included in a clinical trial of potential chemopreventive agents for actinic keratoses and nonmelanoma skin cancer. The trial must include a control arm. This is essential because actinic keratoses and visual signs of photodamage are usually graded and monitored clinically, which introduces a large element of subjectivity. For example, the application of emollient type vehicles can appear to regress actinic keratoses and photodamage simply by inducing immediate surface changes. For these reasons, it is necessary that the study be double-blinded, such that neither study participants nor investigators know whether the area under evaluation is being treated with the study agent or the placebo. Even for oral agents, the inherent subjectivity of clinical grading systems mandates inclusion of a control group and randomized, blinded studies.

Study Population Considerations

In regards to the population at risk and to be studied, the study cohort will primarily consist of fairer skinned individuals with a considerable amount of sun exposure. This translates into the need to recruit subjects mainly in their 60s or older, though rarely people even as young as those in their late 20s may have enough sun damage and actinic keratoses to qualify as study subjects.

Study subjects can be referred from associated dermatology clinics or recruited directly from the community through directed advertising. For our study of a topical green tea polyphenol, study participants were recruited from associated university and private dermatology clinics, and by various forms of print and radio advertising, which targeted the age demographics of the eligible study participants.

Design of Treatment Methodologies in Skin Cancer Chemoprevention Studies

Treatment methodology will depend on whether the agent is topical or oral. For topical formulations, study subjects can often serve as their own controls, with one body part designated as a target area to be treated with the active agent and the mirror area on the opposite side of the body receiving the placebo control. Again, the sides to receive the treatment and the control should be assigned in a random and double-blinded fashion. For clinical trials with oral agents, each participant must be randomized to active treatment or control, though there does not need to be an equal number of treatment and control subjects – the control arm can consist of a smaller number of study subjects. Statistical analysis will determine the proportion of subjects that should be allotted to the control group so that the study achieves an acceptable balance between statistical power and the desire of subjects to receive potentially active treatment rather than placebo.

For our trial, epigallocatechin gallate was compounded in a topical vehicle to a final assayed concentration of 5.5–8.5%, 0.5 ml was applied by the subject nightly for 12 weeks to target actinic keratoses on one of the forearms. A matched placebo ointment was applied to target actinic keratoses on the opposite forearm. Prior to treatment, at least two actinic keratoses were identified on each forearm target area, and these target actinic keratoses were mapped, followed, and clinically graded at 2-week intervals during the 12-week treatment period.

Statistical Considerations in Treatment Methodology Design

It is necessary to design the study such that it will have adequate power to detect the hypothesized differences between the agent and the control group for the parameters under study.

For our study with epigallocatechin gallate, 51 participants were randomized to either active agent or placebo, which provided more than adequate power to detect a 50% difference between active and placebo groups. It was felt that this level of activity would be necessary for the agent to be promising for future studies and possible development.

Surrogate Endpoint Biomarker Analyses

If possible, in addition to monitoring the clinical status of actinic keratoses during the trial of chemopreventive agents, it is desirable to include analyses of surrogate endpoint biomarkers for the actinic keratoses and the squamous cell carcinomas into which they may evolve. The elucidation of useful surrogate endpoint biomarkers is at an early stage for nonmelanoma skin cancer. The most likely candidate surrogate endpoint biomarker for actinic keratoses and squamous cell carcinoma is p53 (Brash et al. 1991; Einspahr et al. 1997). Good candidate surrogate endpoint biomarkers have yet to be identified for basal cell carcinoma.

For our study, we tried to choose a variety of potential surrogate endpoint biomarkers, with a goal being the evaluation of the usefulness of these biomarkers in chemoprevention studies for actinic keratoses and non-melanoma skin cancer. The biomarkers selected were: (1) p53, a cell cycle regulatory protein; (2) Ki-67, a marker of proliferation; (3) CD1A, a Langerhans cell marker – Langerhans cells being the main immune surveillance cells of the skin; (4) nucleolar number; and (5) various measures of nuclear morphometry, including nuclear size and shape and variability in size and shape.

We chose these markers because we felt that they have good potential to be useful surrogate endpoint biomarkers for actinic keratoses and nonmelanoma skin cancer. They represent a wide variety of categories of possible biomarkers including cell cycle regulation, cell proliferation, and cellular morphology, and because all of these biomarkers can be measured quantitatively in an objective manner with computer-assisted image analysis.

Skin biopsies were performed on actinic keratoses, sun-damaged skin, and nonsun-damaged skin pretreatment. Also, skin biopsies were performed on actinic keratoses and sun-damaged skin in the areas that agent or placebo was applied to posttreatment as well. This was done for histopathologic analysis of the changes and surrogate endpoint biomarker analysis between the different groups represented by the biopsies.

Results of Our Study Using Topical Epigallocatechin Gallate as a Chemopreventive Agent for Actinic Keratoses and Nonmelanoma Skin Cancer

A total of 51 study subjects completed the 12-week study, wherein the agent was applied to one forearm with actinic keratoses and placebo ointment to the other forearm nightly. Analysis of the clinical monitoring of the target actinic keratoses at 2-week intervals revealed a slight, progressive decrease in grade of severity of the actinic keratoses over the course of the study in both the treatment and control groups. There were no statistically significant differences between the treatment and control groups. This illustrates the necessity of including a control group, without which we might have concluded that the agent showed efficacy in the treatment of actinic keratoses.

Analysis of the surrogate endpoint biomarkers is ongoing; however, analyses have been completed on the majority of the biomarkers. For those completed, there was no significant difference between the treatment and control groups. However, for all biomarkers analyzed to date except CD1A, there are statistically significant differences between biomarkers between actinic keratoses and sun-damaged skin and actinic keratoses and nonsun-damaged skin. There were nonstatistically significant differences for the surrogate endpoint biomarkers so far analyzed between sun-damaged and nonsun-damaged skin.

Discussion of Results of Topical Epigallocatechin Gallate as a Chemopreventive Agent in Nonmelanoma Skin Cancer

Preliminary analysis of the clinical and surrogate endpoint biomarker data indicates that topical epigallocatechin gallate is not active in the formulation used in our study. There are several possible explanations for this. Epigallocatechin gallate may simply not be an effective clinical agent for actinic keratoses/nonmelanoma skin cancer. This is certainly a possibility, but one that is not easy to reconcile with the impressive animal model data (Mukhtar et al. 1994; Gensler et al. 1996). Another possibility is that the particular formulation used was not effective. Reasons for this could be that the active compound, epigallocatechin gallate, is not stable in the current formulation, or that the compound is stable, but is not being delivered in an effective manner to the target site in the skin tissue. The epigallocatechin gallate formulation used in this study has undergone repeated stability testing throughout the course of the study and shows minimal degradation over the time frame in question. As a result, compound instability is not likely to account for the inactivity of this formulation. Questions about the bioavailability of the specific formulation used and possible design of a more effective formulation are areas that merit further study.

Although the current study did not demonstrate agent efficacy, surrogate endpoint biomarker analysis is yielding useful data that tentatively support the biomarkers chosen (with the exception of CD1A) as having potential in differentiating sun-damaged from precancerous and cancerous states.

Further conclusions await complete analysis of the data.

Summary

Nonmelanoma skin cancer constitutes a significant human disease burden and new methods of prevention need to be developed. Given the limited success of primary behavioral prevention, there is a strong need for chemopreventive agents against nonmelanoma skin cancer. Our study of epigallocatechin gallate for the treatment of actinic keratoses has shown minimal to no clinical activity; however, this might be attributable to the particular formulation used. Further data analysis and experiments are underway to better understand these findings. The surrogate endpoint biomarker analysis, which showed differences between actinic keratoses and sun-damaged skin, has yielded promising information that will provide insights into biomarkers for skin carcinogenesis and potentially help identify surrogate endpoints that may prove useful in the design and interpretation of future clinical trials.

Acknowledgments. This research and publication were made possible by United States National Cancer Institute Contract N01-CN-85182. The authors would like to thank Carol Sekeris and Susan Sperling (Research Coordinators) from the Department of Dermatology, Sharon Maxwell, Janis DeJohn, and Lorene Kong, Pharm. D. from the Chao Family Comprehensive Cancer Center, and Shehla Arain, M.D. from the Department of Pathology, University of California, Irvine, for all their work on this research study.

References

Brash DE, Rudolph JA, Simon JA, et al (1991) A role for sunlight in skin cancer: UV-induced p53 mutations in squamous cell carcinoma. Proc Natl Acad Sci USA 88:10124–10128

Bushman JL (1998) Green tea and cancer in humans: a review of the literature. Nutr Cancer 31:151–159

Dreosti IE (1997) Cancer biomarkers in the field of tea. Cancer Lett 114:319–321

Einspahr J, Alberts DS, Aickin M, et al (1997) Expression of p53 protein in actinic keratosis, adjacent, normal-appearing, and nonsun-exposed human skin. Cancer Epidemiol Biomarkers Prev 6:583–587

Gensler HL, Timmermann BN, Vlacic S, et al (1996) Prevention of photocarcinogenesis by topical administration of pure epigallocatechin gallate isolated from green tea. Nutr Cancer 26:325–335

Heaphy MR Jr, Ackerman AB (2000) The nature of solar keratosis: a critical review in historical perspective. J Am Acad Dermatol 43:138–50

Jeffes EW, McCullough JL, Weinstein GD, et al (2001) Photodynamic therapy of actinic keratoses with topical aminolevulinic acid hydrochloride and fluorescent blue light. J Am Acad Dermatol 45:96–104

Jemal A, Thomas A, Murray T, et al (2002) Cancer statistics, 2002. CA Cancer J Clin 52:23–47

Katiyar SK, Mukhtar H (1997) Tea antioxidants in cancer chemoprevention. J Cell Biochem Suppl 27:59–67

Marks R (1990) Solar keratoses. Br J Dermatol 122:49–54

Mukhtar H, Katiyar SK, Agarwal R, et al (1994) Green tea and skin-anticarcinogenic effects. J Invest Dermatol 102:3–7

Rivers JK, Arlette J, Shear N, et al (2002) Topical treatment of actinic keratoses with 3.0% diclofenac in 2.5% hyaluronan gel. Br J Dermatol 146:94–100

Valcic S, Timmermann BN, Alberts DS, et al (1996) Inhibitory effect of six green tea catechins and caffeine on the growth of four selected human tumor cell lines. Anticancer Drugs 7:461–468

Chemoprevention of Lung Cancer: New Directions

Eva Szabo, Thea Kalebic

E. Szabo (✉)
Lung and Upper Aerodigestive Cancer Research Group,
Division of Cancer Prevention, National Cancer Institute,
6130 Executive Blvd., Room 2132, Bethesda, MD 20892, USA

Abstract

The refractoriness of advanced lung cancer to current treatment modalities requires new approaches to reduce the public health burden associated with this disease. One strategy that is currently being tested is chemoprevention, which aims to prevent the development of cancer in populations that are at high risk for cancer due to a variety of genetic or environmental factors. The key to the success of this approach, however, requires the identification of appropriately targeted efficacious, non-toxic agents as well as the methodologies to efficiently test them. Given the lack of success of previous phase III definitive lung cancer chemoprevention trials, there is a need for smaller scale phase II trials with molecular, imaging, or histologic endpoints to demonstrate preliminary safety and efficacy. The identification of molecular pathways critical to lung carcinogenesis offers the opportunity to develop targeted therapies for prevention. Means of optimizing the risk/benefit ratio associated with treatment include regional drug delivery that minimizes systemic toxicities and combination therapies. Identification of the most appropriate cohorts, such as former smokers without ongoing DNA damage due to carcinogen exposure, may uncover benefits that are hidden in a mixed population. Equally important is the identification of appropriate study endpoints that are predictive of patient outcomes such as cancer incidence. Further understanding of lung cancer biology will be critical to the success of future clinical trials.

Introduction

Despite major advances in our understanding of the molecular pathogenesis of lung cancer, survival after the diagnosis of lung cancer has not improved significantly over the past several decades (Greenlee et al. 2001). Lung cancer continues to be a leading cause of death worldwide, with an estimated 1.2 million new cases in 2000 (Parkin 2001). In the United States alone, there were an estimated 169,500 new cases and 157,400 deaths in 2001 (Greenlee et al. 2001). The 5-year survival rate of 14% has not improved appreciably since the 1970s, primarily due to the relatively late stage at diagnosis. The refractory nature of advanced disease to current treatment modalities mandates the development of alternate strategies to reduce its public health burden.

Targeting early phases of carcinogenesis that may be more amenable to treatment, thereby preventing the development of invasive and metastatic disease, offers one such attractive option. However, progress in prevention science depends on simultaneous advances in the identification of targeted, nontoxic agents and in the development of methodologies to evaluate promising new agents efficiently and appropriately. Definitive phase III cancer prevention trials with cancer incidence endpoints require thousands of patients, substantial resources, and many years for completion. Therefore, phase II studies examining the effect of interventional agents on molecular, imaging, and histologic endpoints are needed to demonstrate preliminary safety and efficacy prior to embarking on large-scale trials. This review will focus on new strategies for lung chemoprevention trials.

A Historical Perspective

The underlying principles of lung cancer chemoprevention are based on the notions that lung carcinogenesis evolves through various stages over a lengthy period of time in individuals exposed to carcinogens, and that the entire exposed epithelial surface is subject to damage from carcinogens (Saccomanno et al. 1974; Lippman et al. 1994). Chemopreventive agents theoretically block, reverse, or delay these changes. An effective chemopreventive agent should therefore inhibit the progression of histopathologic changes resulting from a stepwise accumulation of molecular alterations leading to cancer. In particular, chemopreventive intervention aimed at reducing lung cancer mortality should reverse bronchial precancerous lesions, such as dysplasia, or prevent formation of second primary tumors.

Chemoprevention combines investigation of basic biological mechanisms regulating the carcinogenic process with clinical approaches aimed at decreasing cancer-associated mortality. Primary prevention is aimed at inhibiting the development of lung cancer in ostensibly healthy, but high-risk, populations. Approaches designed to induce the reversal of premalignant lesions are considered secondary prevention. Tertiary preventive measures focus on prevention of second primary tumors in previously treated individuals (Lippman and Spitz 2001).

A number of previous large lung chemoprevention studies have focused on β-carotene, vitamin A, and vitamin A derivatives. The results of these studies are summarized in Table 1. The rationale for this approach (summarized in Omenn 1998) was based on epidemiological studies that have demonstrated the association between the increased incidence of lung cancer and a diet defi-

Table 1. Phase III lung chemoprevention trials

Trial	Cohort	Intervention	Outcome
ATBC, 1994	29,133 smokers	β-Carotene, vitamin E, both, or placebo	18% increase in lung cancer
CARET, 1996	18,314 smokers or asbestos exposed	β-carotene + retinol vs. placebo	Increased lung cancer, RR=1.36
EUROSCAN, 2000	2,592 lung or head and neck cancer patients	Retinyl palmitate, NAC, both, or placebo	No benefit
Intergroup, 2001	1,166 stage I NSCLC patients	Isotretinoin	No benefit (increased recurrence current smokers)

cient in fruit and vegetables containing β-carotene, a provitamin A. Preclinical data demonstrated that a decrease in vitamin A induces neoplastic transformation of bronchial epithelium, while the addition of vitamin A restores the normal respiratory epithelium in experimental animals. Animal carcinogenesis studies provided evidence of reduced tumor burden and longer latency after treatment with various retinoids or vitamin A during and after carcinogen exposure.

The Alpha-Tocopherol Beta Carotene Cancer Prevention Study (ATBC) investigated the effectiveness of β-carotene (20 mg per day) and α-tocopherol (50 mg per day), alone or in combination, in reducing lung cancer incidence in 29,133 Finnish male smokers (ATBC Study Group 1994). With a follow-up period ranging from 5 to 8 years, the treatment did not reduce lung cancer incidence. Moreover, subjects receiving β-carotene, alone or in combination with α-tocopherol, showed an 18% higher incidence of lung cancer compared with the placebo group. This effect was confined to the active smoker subgroup, suggesting that high doses of β-carotene are not efficacious and can actually be harmful in current smoker cohorts.

The CARET study (Beta-Carotene and Retinol Efficacy Trial) was a randomized double-blinded placebo-controlled chemoprevention trial which recruited 18,314 participants to evaluate the efficacy of the β-carotene and retinol in a population at high risk for developing lung cancer (Ommen et al. 1996). Current smokers, former smokers, and individuals exposed to asbestos were treated with 30 mg β-carotene and 25, 000 IU retinyl palmitate (vitamin A) or placebo. The primary endpoint of the study was lung cancer incidence. After results of the Finnish ATBC study became available, the CARET trial was stopped 21 months early since no benefit was seen. In contrast, the data showed that study participants receiving the active combination had an adverse outcome compared with the placebo group, with a relative risk (RR) of 1.36 [95% confidence interval (CC)=1.07–1.73, P=0.01] for lung cancer incidence and an RR of 1.59 (95% CI=1.13–2.23, P=0.01) for lung cancer mortality.

In contrast to the primary prevention studies exemplified by the ATBC and CARET, the EUROSCAN study (European Study on Chemoprevention with Vi-

Table 2. Phase II lung chemoprevention trials

Investigator	Intervention	Primary endpoint	Outcome
Arnold 1992	Etretinate	Sputum atypia	Negative
Lee 1994	Isotretinoin	Metaplasia	Negative
McLarty 1995	β-carotene+retinol	Sputum atypia	Negative
Kurie 2000	4-HPR	Metaplasia	Negative

tamin A and N-Acetylcysteine) was a tertiary prevention study designed to assess whether a combination of retinyl palmitate and the anti-oxidant N-acetylcysteine could prevent second primary tumors in 2,592 patients with curatively treated head and neck or lung cancers (van Zandwijk 2000). Intervention consisted of daily administration of retinyl palmitate, 300,000 IU daily for 1 year, followed by 150,000 IU daily throughout the second year versus 600 mg of N-acetylcysteine versus both agents versus neither agent. No statistically significant improvement in overall survival or tumor-free survival was observed in treated individuals. These results failed to confirm a previous smaller study of 307 patients with stage I lung cancer who received high-dose vitamin A, 300,000 IU, or placebo daily for 12 months, which showed a statistically significant increase in time to second primary tumors in vitamin A-treated patients (Pastorino 1993).

Clinical trials with isotretinoin (13-cis-retinoic acid, 13cRA) have demonstrated efficacy in treating oral leukoplakia, a precursor to cancer of the oral cavity (Hong et al. 1986; Lippman et al. 1993) as well as prevention of second primary tumors in patients previously treated for head and neck cancers (Hong et al. 1990). However, trials of retinoids for lung chemoprevention have not been successful to date. A number of phase II trials examining the effects of retinoids, vitamin A, or β-carotene on intermediate endpoints such as sputum atypia or bronchial metaplasia have all failed to show any benefit to treatment (Table 2). Arnold et al. and McLarty et al. evaluated the effects of a synthetic retinoid, etretinate, or β-carotene/retinol, respectively, on sputum atypia, with negative results (Arnold et al. 1992; McLarty et al. 1995). Lee et al. and Kurie et al. examined the effects of isotretinoin or N-(4-hydroxyphenyl)retinamide (4-HPR), respectively, on bronchial metaplasia (Lee et al. 1994; Kurie et al. 2000). While the incidence of metaplasia decreased after isotretinoin treatment, a similar decrease was noted in the placebo treated group and was most closely correlated with smoking cessation. The synthetic retinoid 4-HPR had no effect on histology or molecular markers.

The Phase III Intergroup Trial randomized 1,166 patients with resected stage I non-small-cell lung cancer (NSCLC) to low dose isotretinoin (30 mg/day) or placebo for 3 years (Lippman et al. 2001). Treatment did not improve the rates of second primary tumors, recurrence, or mortality. Subset analysis suggested that isotretinoin was harmful in current smokers, with a higher recurrence rate in this population than in never-smokers or former smokers.

As discussed above, no agent has been shown to be efficacious for lung chemoprevention to date. However, a large double-blinded randomized trial involving 1,312 patients with a history of skin cancer demonstrated that supplementation with selenium (200 µg/day) correlated with a significant decrease in the incidence of lung, colon, and prostate cancers (Clark et al. 1996). While there was not a significant decrease in skin cancers, selenium supplementation resulted in 17 cases of lung cancer compared with 31 cases in the placebo group (RR=0.54, 95% CI=0.30–0.98, P=.04). As a result of this observation, ongoing now is a randomized phase III trial prospectively assessing whether selenium supplementation can prevent second primary tumors after curative resection of stage I NSCLC.

New Molecular Targets

Identification of new agents with chemopreventive potential is of paramount importance for progress in lung chemoprevention. Identification of new agents for the prevention or treatment of cancer typically occurs via three pathways:

1. Epidemiologic data can be very informative regarding possible chemopreventive strategies, as exemplified by the use of nonsteroidal anti-inflammatory agents (NSAIDs) for colorectal chemoprevention (Xu 2002)
2. Secondary endpoints from prior clinical trials, as with the observation of reduced contralateral breast cancers after adjuvant tamoxifen treatment (Fisher et al. 1998)
3. Identification of specific molecular abnormalities that are crucial to carcinogenesis, as exemplified by the recent development of STI 571 targeting the Bcr-Abl tyrosine kinase in chronic myelogenous leukemia (Druker et al. 2001).

As we understand the molecular biology of lung cancer more thoroughly, new molecular targets for chemoprevention are becoming evident.

Recent attention has begun to focus on the role of metabolites of arachidonic acid in cancer development. Conversion of arachidonic acid by cyclooxygenases (COXs) and lipoxygenases (LOXs) results in the formation of a variety of bioactive metabolites, including prostaglandins, thromboxanes, HETEs (hydroxyeicosatetraenoic acids), and leukotrienes. Whereas the constitutive COX-1 and the inducible COX-2 are the major cyclooxygenases, multiple LOX enzymes that catalyze the stereospecific oxygenation of different carbon atoms of arachidonic acid exist (Steele et al. 1999; Shureiqi and Lippman 2001; Xu 2002). Several of these products are implicated in carcinogenesis. Inhibitors of the key enzymes involved in arachidonic acid metabolism now exist and are entering chemoprevention trials in a variety of target organs.

COX-2 has emerged as an important molecular target for colon chemoprevention. This is based on epidemiologic data linking NSAID use to decreased colon cancer incidence, animal models demonstrating inhibition of tumorigenesis by NSAIDs and COX-2 selective agents after carcinogen exposure or in tumor-prone genetically abnormal mice, and clinical trial data demonstrating decreased colorectal adenoma number after treatment of patients with familial polyposis coli (FAP) with the COX-2 selective celecoxib (Xu 2002; Steinbach et al. 2000). In the case of lung chemoprevention, there is limited epidemiologic evidence of NSAID's impact on lung cancer incidence (Schreinemachers et al. 1994). COX-2, however, is frequently expressed in lung cancers and has been documented to be expressed in atypical alveolar lesions that may be precursors to adenocarcinomas (Hida et al. 1998; Wolff et al. 1998; Watkins et al. 1999). COX-2 overexpression also confers a worse clinical prognosis (Achiwa et al. 1999; Khuri et al. 2001). Animal studies indicate that various NSAIDs, including the COX-2 selective NS-398, significantly inhibit adenoma formation in carcinogen-exposed mice by as much as 60% (Castonguay et al. 1998; Rioux and Castonguay 1998a). For these reasons, COX-2 targeting strategies are being explored in ongoing lung chemoprevention trials.

There is also data implicating the 5-lipoxygenase (5-LO) pathway in lung chemoprevention. Moody et al. and Rioux and Castonguay showed that general LO inhibitors and specific 5-LO inhibitors significantly reduce adenoma multiplicity in carcinogen-exposed mice (Moody et al. 1998; Rioux and Castonguay 1998b). Combination of a 5-LO inhibitor and aspirin synergistically lowered tumor incidence and multiplicity. Other studies confirm that human lung tumors express 5-LO and that 5-LO products stimulate NSCLC cell growth, while 5-LO inhibitors interfere with growth factor-stimulated proliferation (Avis et al. 1996). Inhibitors of 5-LO and leukotriene receptor antagonists are currently in use for the treatment of asthma, and some of these agents are being used in lung chemoprevention studies.

Another example of molecularly targeted therapy with potential relevance to lung chemoprevention includes the use of selective inhibitors of the epidermal growth factor receptor (EGFR) tyrosine kinase. EGFR overexpression occurs frequently in NSCLC, including in potentially preneoplastic bronchial metaplasias (Raben et al. 2002; Kurie et al. 1996). Inhibitors of EGFR-mediated signaling are currently in clinical trials for the treatment of advanced lung cancer, as well as other cancers, and lung chemoprevention studies are in development (Raben et al. 2002). Future efforts will focus on identifying additional molecular targets and their appropriate effector agents to study in the chemoprevention context.

Intermediate Endpoints

Identification of appropriate study endpoints is a critical aspect of chemoprevention trials. While phase III cancer prevention trials aim to demonstrate changes in cancer incidence, phase II preliminary efficacy cancer prevention trials rely on short term, or intermediate, endpoints that are theoretically predictive of patient outcomes such as cancer incidence. To be useful, intermediate markers should meet three major criteria (Lippman et al. 1990; Szabo and Shaw 1997). First, there must be a predictable relationship between the intermediate endpoint and cancer risk. Specifically, there must be a high association with the development of cancer, a low spontaneous reversion rate, differential expression between normal and premalignant or high-risk tissues, and the reduction in the marker should correlate with disease control. Second, the detection and characterization must be reliable and consistent. It must be feasible in the clinical setting, analysis should be performed on easily available tissues or body fluids, and the marker must be able to be modulated by clinical interventions. Finally, the intermediate endpoint must be validated via measurement of a relevant clinical outcome, which is cancer incidence or cancer-related mortality in the case of cancer prevention.

To date, no intermediate endpoint marker has passed the required rigorous validation measurements. However, it is becoming clear that the complex molecular mechanisms that regulate tumor development involve a number of molecules and regulatory pathways controlling various cellular processes, including proliferation, differentiation, apoptosis, invasion of the basement membrane, and neoangiogenesis. Classes of molecules found to be altered in lung cancer and precancerous lesions include oncogenes, tumor suppressor genes, growth factors or their receptors, and nuclear retinoid receptors, in addition to the molecules regulating cellular immortality, immune defense and tumor-associated angiogenesis (Carbone 1997). Improved understanding of aberrantly functioning molecules associated with lung cancer development provides the opportunity to develop biomarkers which can be used in risk assessment as well as in monitoring response to chemopreventive or therapeutic interventions. Biomarkers associated with early stages of carcinogenesis could be of great value for early detection of lung cancer and precancerous lesions. In addition, biomarkers that regulate molecular pathways critically important in lung carcinogenesis may also serve as targets for novel therapies.

New Directions

In addition to issues of drug development and intermediate endpoint identification, there are several emerging concepts that may have a major impact on how lung cancer chemoprevention trials are conducted. While identifying the appropriate and specific molecular targets for intervention is a high priority, maximizing the therapeutic effectiveness while minimizing toxicity remains a major hurdle. Regional drug delivery to the lung via inhalation offers a major opportunity to minimize systemic toxicity. For instance, systemic corticosteroids have potent lung cancer chemopreventive properties in carcinogen treated mice, but systemic side effects preclude such a strategy in human beings (Estensen and Wattengerg 1993). Wattenberg et al. showed that aerosolized steroids could reduce tumor burden in carcinogen treated mice by 60%, without systemic side effects (Wattenberg et al. 2000). This strategy is currently being employed in an ongoing chemoprevention trial using inhaled budesonide in the treatment of subjects with bronchial dysplasia.

Similarly, the use of combinations of agents offers another strategy to maximize the benefit to risk ratio. Agents that target the same or complementary pathways may increase the efficacy of interventions or allow for the use of lower doses that decrease the side effects. Examples of such strategies in preclinical models includes the concurrent treatment of carcinogen-exposed mice with COX and LOX inhibitors, decreasing the tumor burden in animals treated with the combination compared with animals treated with either agent alone (Rioux and Castonguay 1998b). Similarly, the addition of dietary myo-inositol to inhaled budesonide improved the inhibition of tumor burden from 60% to 79% in carcinogen-treated mice at higher doses of budesonide, giving greater efficacy (Wattenberg et al. 2000). In parallel experiments, the addition of myo-inositol to lower doses of budesonide improved the reduction in tumor formation from 34% to 60%, giving the same efficacy as the higher doses of budesonide alone. Thus, in animal models, combination treatment can increase the effectiveness of interventions. Translation of these concepts to human clinical studies will be an important future endeavor.

As noted previously, the large phase III lung chemoprevention trials using β-carotene and isotretinoin showed an adverse outcome in ongoing smokers. Currently, half of all lung cancers occur in former smokers (Tong et al. 1996), and a significant number of former smokers continue to have persistent genetic abnormalities in the bronchial epithelium (Mao et al. 1997). There are biologic differences between current and former smokers that have yet to be fully elucidated. By targeting a population that does not have ongoing DNA damage from persistent carcinogen exposure, chemoprevention trials in former smokers may uncover a benefit that is hidden in a mixed population. The National Cancer Institute is currently sponsoring several trials aimed specifically at former smoker cohorts.

Although chemoprevention of lung cancer remains a challenge, the dismal survival after the diagnosis of lung cancer requires efforts to prevent or detect the disease at early stages. A comprehensive research program focusing on smoking cessation, early detection, and chemoprevention offers hope that progress can be made in curtailing this disease.

References

Achiwa H, Yatabe Y, Hida T, et al (1999) Prognostic significance of elevated cyclooxygenase 2 expression in primary, resected lung adenocarcinomas. Clin Cancer Res 5:1001–1005

Alpha-Tocopherol, Beta Carotene Cancer Prevention Study Group. (1994) The effect of vitamin E and beta carotene on the incidence of lung cancer and other cancers in male smokers. N Eng J Med 330:1029–1035

Arnold AM, Browman GP, Levine MN, et al (1992) The effect of the synthetic retinoid etretinate on sputum cytology: results from a randomised trial. Br J Cancer 65:737–743

Avis IM, Jett M, Boyle T, et al (1996) Growth control of lung cancer by interruption of 5-lipoxygenase-mediated growth factor signaling. J Clin Invest 97:806–813

Carbone DP (1997) The biology of lung cancer. Semin Oncol 24:388–401

Castonguay A, Rioux N, Duperron C, et al (1998) Inhibition of lung tumorigenesis by NSAIDs: A working hypothesis. Exp Cell Res 24:605–615. 1998

Clark LC, Combs GF, Turnbull BW, et al (1996) Effects of selenium supplementation for cancer prevention in patients with carcinoma of the skin. JAMA 276:1957–1963

Druker BJ, Talpaz M, Resta D, et al (2001) Efficacy and safety of a specific inhibitor of the Bcr-Abl tyrosine kinase in chronic myeloid leukemia. N Eng J Med 344:1031–1037

Estensen RD and Wattenberg LW. (1993) Studies of chemopreventive effects of myo-inositol on benzo[a]-pyrene-induced neoplasia of the lung and forestomach of female A/J mice. Carcinogenesis (Lond) 14:1975–1977

Fisher B, Costantino JP, Wickerham DL, et al (1998) Tamoxifen for prevention of breast cancer: Report of the National Surgical Adjuvant Breast and Bowel Project P-1 Study. J Natl Cancer Inst 90:1371–1388

Greenlee RT, Hill-Harmon MB, Murray T, et al (2001) Cancer statistics 2001. CA Cancer J Clin 51:15–36

Hida T, Yatabe Y, Achiwa H, et al (1998) Increased expression of cyclooxygenase 2 occurs frequently in human lung cancers, specifically in adenocarcinomas. Cancer Res 58:3761–3764

Hong WK, Endicott J, Itri LM, et al (1986) 13-cis-retinoic acid in the treatment of oral leukoplakia. N Eng J Med 315:1501–1505

Hong WK, Lippman SM, Itri LM, et al (1990) Prevention of second primary tumors with isotretinoin in squamous-cell carcinoma of the head and neck. N Eng J Med 323:795–801

Khuri FR, Wu H, Lee JJ, et al (2001) Cyclooxygenase-2 overexpression is a marker of poor prognosis in stage I non-small cell lung cancer. Clin Cancer Res 7:861–867

Kurie JM, Lee JS, Khuri FR, et al (2000) N-(4-hydroxyphenyl)retinamide in the chemoprevention of squamous metaplasia and dysplasia of the bronchial epithelium. Clin Cancer Res 5:2973–2979

Kurie JM, Shin HJ, Lee JS, et al (1996) Increased epidermal growth factor receptor expression in metaplastic bronchial epithelium. Clin Cancer Res 2:1787–1793

Lee JS, Lippman SM, Benner SE, et al (1994) Randomized placebo-controlled trial of isotretinoin in chemoprevention of bronchial squamous metaplasia. J Clin Oncol 12:937–945

Lippman SM, Batsakis JG, Toth BB, et al (1993) Comparison of low-dose isotretinoin with beta carotene to prevent oral carcinogenesis. N Eng J Med 328:15–20

Lippman SM, Benner SE, Hong WK. (1994) Cancer chemoprevention. J Clin Oncol 12:851–873

Lippman SM, Lee JJ, Karp DD, et al (2001) Randomized phase III Intergroup trial of isotretinoin to prevent second primary tumors in stage I non-small-cell lung cancer. J Natl Cancer Inst 93:605–618

Lippman SM, Lee JS, Lotan R, et al (1990) Biomarkers as intermediate end points in chemoprevention trials. J Natl Cancer Inst 82:555–560

Lippman SM, Spitz MR (2001) Lung cancer chemoprevention: an integrated approach J Clin Oncol 19:74s–82s

Mao L, Lee JS, Kurie JM, et al (1997) Clonal genetic alterations in the lungs of current and former smokers. J Natl Cancer Inst 89:857–862

McLarty JW, Holiday DB, Girard, WM, et al (1995) β-carotene, vitamin A, and lung cancer chemoprevention: results of an intermediate endpoint study. Am J Clin Nutr 62:1431s–1438 s

Moody TR, Leyton J, Martinez A, et al (1998) Lipoxygenase inhibitors prevent lung carcinogenesis and inhibit non-small cell lung cancer growth. Exp Lung Res 24:617–628

Omenn GS (1998) Chemoprevention of lung cancer: The rise and demise of beta-carotene. Annu Rev Public Health 19:73–99

Omenn GS, Goodman GE, Thornquist MD, et al (1996) Effects of a combination of beta carotene and vitamin A on lung cancer and cardiovascular health. N Eng J Med 334:1150–1155

Parkin DM (2001) Global cancer statistics in the year 2000. Lancet Oncol 2:533–543

Pastorino U, Infante M, Maioli M, et al (1993) Adjuvant treatment of stage I lung cancer with high-dose vitamin A. J Clin Oncol 11:1216–1222

Raben D, Helfrich BA, Chan D, et al (2002) ZD1839, a selective epidermal growth factor receptor tyrosine kinase inhibitor, alone and in combination with radiation and chemotherapy as a new therapeutic strategy in non-small cell lung cancer. Sem Oncol 29:37–46

Rioux N and Castonguay A (1998a) Prevention of NNK-induced lung tumorigenesis in A/J mice by acetylsalicylic acid and NS-398. Cancer Res 58:5354–5360

Rioux N and Castonguay A (1998b) Inhibitors of lipoxygenase: A new class of cancer chemopreventive agents. Carcinogenesis 19:1393–1400

Saccomanno G, Archer VE, Auerbach O, et al (1974) Development of carcinoma of the lung as reflected in exfoliated cells. Cancer 33:256–270

Schreinemachers DM, Everson RB (1994) Aspirin use and lung, colon, and breast cancer incidence in a prospective study. Epidemiology 5:138–146

Shureiqi I, Lippman SM (2001) Lipoxygense modulation to reverse carcinogenesis. Cancer Res 61:6307–6312

Steele VE, Holmes CA, Hawk ET, et al (1999) Lipoxygenase inhibitors as potential cancer chemopreventives. Cancer Epidemiol Biomarkers Prev 8:467–483

Steinbach G, Lynch PM, Phillips RKS, et al (2000) The effect of celecoxib, a cyclooxygenase-2 inhibitor, in familial adenomatous polyposis. N Eng J Med 342:1946–1952

Szabo E, Shaw GL (1997) Intermediate markers and molecular genetics of lung carcinogenesis Cancer Control 4:109–117

Tong L, Spitz MR, Fueger JJ, et al (1996) Lung carcinoma in former smokers. Cancer 78:1004–1010

Van Zandwijk N, Dalesio O, Pastorino U, et al (2000) EUROSCAN, a randomized trial of vitamin A and N-acetylcysteine in patients with head and neck cancer or lung cancer. J Natl Cancer Inst 92:977–986

Watkins DN, Lenzo JC, Segal A, et al (1999) Expression and localization of cyclo-oxygenase isoforms in non-small cell lung cancer. Eur Respir J 14:412–418

Wattenberg LW, Wiedmann TS, Estensen RD, et al (2000) Chemoprevention of pulmonary carcinogenesis by brief exposures to aerosolized budesonide or beclomethasone dipropionate and by the combination of aerosolized budesonide and dietary myo-inositol. Carcinogenesis 21:179–182

Wolff H, Saukkonen K, Anttila S, et al (1998) Expression of cyclooxygenase-2 in human lung carcinoma. Cancer Res 58:4997–5001

Xu X-C (2002) COX-2 inhibitors in cancer treatment and prevention, a recent development. Anticancer Drugs 13:127–137

Key Issues in Lung Cancer Chemoprevention Trials of New Agents

Stephen Lam, Calum MacAulay, Jean C. LeRiche, Adi F. Gazdar

S. Lam (✉)
Lung Tumour Group, The British Columbia Cancer Agency and The University of British Columbia, West 10 Avenue, Vancouver, BC V5Z 4E6, Canada

Abstract

Lung cancer is a major health problem world-wide. Former heavy smokers retain a significant risk for lung cancer after smoking cessation. With a large population of current and former smokers at risk, an alternative cancer control strategy such as chemoprevention needs to be developed to reduce lung cancer mortality especially for smokers who have followed medical advice to give up smoking. Currently, there is no agent that has been shown to be effective in preventing lung cancer. Key issues that need to be addressed in phase II trials of promising chemopreventive agents include selection of high-risk subjects, potential variation in response due to differences in gender and smoking history as well as the choice of surrogate endpoint biomarkers. Sputum biomarkers such as image analysis of sputum cells and detection of aberrant methylation hold promise in identifying those at highest risk for chemopreventive intervention. Autofluorescence bronchoscopy is an effective method to localize dysplastic lesions to evaluate the efficacy of new chemopreventive agents. Novel imaging methods such as confocal micro-endoscopy and spiral CT-directed endoscopic biopsies are under development to evaluate the response of chemopreventive agents on peripheral pre-neoplastic lesions in small airways.

Abbreviations SEB, surrogate endpoint biomarkers; HFCWO, high-frequency chest wall oscillation; ROC, receiver operating characteristic; CR, complete response; PD, progressive disease

Introduction

In the United States and Canada, lung cancer accounts for 28% of all cancer deaths. There are more patients who die from lung cancer than from breast,

Recent Results in Cancer Research, Vol. 163
© Springer-Verlag Berlin Heidelberg 2003

Table 1. Prevalence of premalignant lesions and cancer in heavy smokers ≥30 pack-years

Histopathology	Current smokers	Former smokers
–	n=640	n=279
Mild dysplasia	49%	32%
Moderate dysplasia	11%	11%
Severe dysplasia	3%	3%
Carcinoma in situ	0.5%	1.8%
Cancer	1%	1%

colon, and prostate cancers combined (Greenlee et al. 2001). The overall 5-year survival rate of lung cancer is 14% (Greenlee et al. 2001). Advances in the detection and treatment of this disease have not resulted in significant improvement in mortality rates. In the last 50 years, lung cancer incidence increased by 249% and the mortality by 259% (Welch et al. 2000).

Approximately 85% of all lung cancers are related to tobacco smoking. The risk of lung cancer varies with the number of cigarettes smoked per day, the duration of smoking and the age at which the individual began smoking. Individuals who stop smoking after the age of 50 retain a substantial risk for lung cancer life-long (Peto et al. 2001; Halpern et al. 1993). Our studies showed that although the prevalence of mild dysplasia may decline on smoking cessation, the prevalence of high-grade dysplasia, carcinoma in situ or invasive cancer is similar in current and former smokers 45 years of age or older (Lam et al. 1999; Table 1).

In addition, no differences were noted between the patterns of molecular changes in current and former smokers (Wistuba et al. 1997). Approximately half of all the newly diagnosed lung cancer cases are former smokers (Tong et al. 1996). Currently, in the United States and Canada alone, there are approximately 50 million former smokers and 50 million current smokers. With this large population of people at risk, an alternative cancer control strategy such as chemoprevention needs to be developed to reduce lung cancer mortality especially for smokers who have followed medical advice to give up smoking.

Proof-of-principle studies by Ki Hong and co-workers (Hong et al. 1986, 1990) showed that chemoprevention could prevent cancer in the upper aerodigestive tract. However, chemoprevention of lung cancer is proving difficult and frustrating (Omenn 1999). The results of lung cancer chemoprevention trials have been disappointing (van Zandwijk et al. 2000; Hennekens et al. 1996; The Alpha-Tocopherol, Beta Carotene Cancer Prevention Study Group 1994; Omenn et al. 1996; Xu et al. 1999; Lee et al. 1994; Lippman et al. 2001; Arnold et al. 1992; Kurie et al. 2000; Mclarty et al. 1995; Pastorino et al. 1993). Several large-scale chemoprevention trials have been performed, including the EUROSCAN Trial (van Zandwijk et al. 2000), the Physicians Health Study (Hennekens et al. 1996), the Alpha-Tocopherol and Beta-Carotene (ATBC) trial (The Alpha-Tocopherol, Beta Carotene Cancer Prevention Study Group 1994), and the Beta-Carotene and Retinol Efficacy Trial (CARET) (Omenn et al. 1996), which involved thousands of active smokers followed up for over

10 years. These studies demonstrated no protective effect of treatment on lung cancer incidence. In fact, beta-carotene treatment appeared to act as a cocarcinogen, enhancing lung cancer incidence in active smokers (The Alpha-Tocopherol, Beta Carotene Cancer Prevention Study Group 1994; Omenn et al. 1996). A recently completed Intergroup Lung Second Primary Tumor Prevention Trial of isotretinoin also demonstrated no overall treatment effect and may be harmful in active smokers (Lippman et al. 2001). Phase III chemoprevention trials typically involve over 20,000 people and take 7–10 years to complete (van Zandwijk et al. 2000; Hennekens et al. 1996; The Alpha-Tocopherol, Beta Carotene Cancer Prevention Study Group 1994; Omenn et al. 1996; Lippman et al. 2001). Even phase II trials require considerable resources and take more than 2 years to complete. Thus, we need to examine the methods used in phase II evaluation of promising agents before proceeding to phase III clinical trials.

Key issues that need to be addressed in phase II trials of new chemopreventive agents include selection of high-risk subjects, potential variation in response due to differences in gender and smoking history as well as the choice of surrogate endpoint biomarkers (SEB).

Identification of Individuals with Premalignant Bronchial Lesions

The life-time risk for lung cancer in smokers is approximately 16% (Peto et al. 2001). In the ATBC study of 29,133 smokers age 50–69, who smoked an average of 36 pack-years, 3% developed lung cancer over 6 years (The Alpha-Tocopherol, Beta Carotene Cancer Prevention Study Group 1994). In the CARET study of 18,314 smokers age 45–69 who smoked an average of 45 pack-years, 2.1% developed lung cancer over 4 years (Omenn et al. 1996). Early detection studies involving self-selected, older smokers with a heavier smoking history, some of which had asbestos exposure, showed a prevalence of 2.7% (Henchke et al. 1999). Thus, at a given point in time, the proportion of smokers harboring cancer or premalignant lesions that will progress to cancer is small. The challenge, therefore, is to have the means to identify the minority of smokers who would benefit from chemoprevention.

Currently, the only noninvasive method for detecting premalignant lesions in the lower respiratory tract is by examination of sputum cells. Although conventional sputum cytology is quite specific, it is not sensitive for the detection of early lung cancer or high-grade premalignant lesions. Using nongenomic nuclear changes measurable by quantitative microscopy in morphologically normal cells with a normal DNA index (Macaulay et al. 1995; Payne 1997; Wilton 1997), we were able to show that a sensitivity of 70%–80% at a specificity of 90% to detect early stage (stage 0/I) lung cancer including peripheral adenocarcinoma (Payne et al. 1997; Lam et al. 2000). The image analysis algorithm was developed to distinguish malignant versus nonmalignant sputum samples. However, in chemoprevention trials where premalignant lesion is the endpoint, we need to have a means not only to exclude individuals who already have lung cancer from entering the trial, but also a way to identify those harboring premalignant lesions who might benefit from the chemopreventive intervention.

Sputum Collection, Processing and Analysis Methods for SEB Studies

To perform sputum biomarker studies, it is important to be able to obtain adequate specimens. However, cough and sputum production decrease significantly or stop within several months of smoking cessation. Therefore, special methods are needed to collect, process and analyze sputum cells. We investigated several collection methods such as 3 day pooled, induction with ultrasonic nebulization of 3% saline, simultaneous hypertonic saline induction and high frequency chest wall oscillation (HFCWO) using the ThAIRapy Vest (Advanced Respiratory Inc., St. Paul, Minn., USA) in 312 heavy smokers 45 years of age or older. The proportion of unsatisfactory samples as assessed by standard cytology criteria (presence of dust cells/alveolar macrophages) are shown in Table 2.

As expected, and in keeping with published data, the unsatisfactory sample rates were much higher in former smokers than current smokers with all methods. HFCWO improved the adequacy rate in former smokers. By coupling hypertonic saline induction with HFCWO, followed by half day pooled sputum collection, the unsatisfactory rate could be reduced to only 3% or less and hence is the optimal method for collection of sputum cells.

To detect the presence of atypical or malignant cells, the sputum cells were stained with a quantitative DNA stain (thionine) after ethanol fixation. Quantitative nuclear morphometry was performed using an automated image cytometer (Garner et al. 1994; Doudkine et al. 1995).

ROC analysis showed that using a single feature (the frequency of cells with a DNA index greater than 1.25), over 75% of those harboring one or more sites of bronchial dysplasia could be detected (Fig. 1). If bronchial dysplasia is used as the surrogate endpoint biomarker for the chemoprevention trial, the number of subjects that need to be bronchoscoped for confirmation of the

Table 2. Collection method and percent unsatisfactory sputum specimens in current versus former smokers

Collection method	No. of subjects	Current smokers	Former smokers
3-Day pooled	817	19%	34%
Hypertonic saline	440	12%	30%
Hypertonic saline+HFCWO	1,559	14%	24%
Hypertonic saline+HFCWO+1/2 D pooled	306	3%	1%

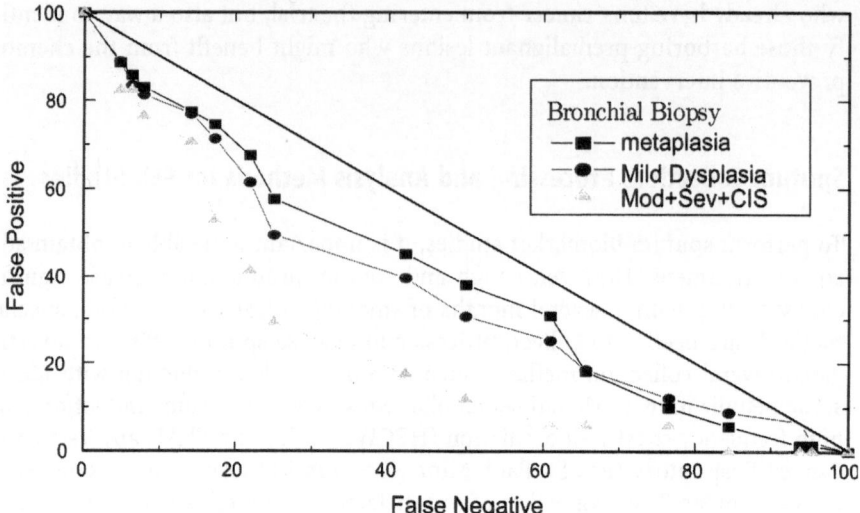

Fig. 1. ROC curve of image analysis of sputum cells for detection of bronchial dysplasia and cancer

presence of bronchial dysplasia could be reduced by more than 50% by using image analysis of sputum cells as the first-step screening method.

Choice of Surrogate Endpoint Biomarker

To evaluate new chemopreventive agents in phase II studies, it is important to have SEBs that will reflect the outcome of phase III studies. The criteria for an ideal, validated SEB for phase II clinical trials set forth by the NCI include: statistical association with cancer or pre-cancer in prospective studies, differential expression in normal and high-risk tissue, presence in a reasonable proportion of at-risk population to be studied, ease of sampling, ability to quantitate the biomarker, and alteration of cancer risk with modulation of the biomarker.

The cytologic and histopathologic alterations of premalignant lesions are associated with changes in cellular population dynamics (proliferation and apoptosis); cell–cell and cell–matrix communications (levels of growth factors and growth factor receptors), and changes in nuclear/nucleolar morphology. At earlier and subcellular levels of lung carcinogenesis, multiple abnormalities in structure and function have been described including activation of oncogenes (e.g., ras, myc, erb families), losses of tumor suppressor activity/physical loci (e.g., p53, Rb, 3p, 9p, 5q), suppression of genetic expression (e.g., through abnormalities of DNA methylation), cell cycle abnormalities (e.g., cyclins), multiple enzyme alterations (e.g., GSTs, telomerase activity) signal transduction abnormalities (e.g., RARs, RXRs), and additional alterations that may lie at the interface of dynamic structure/function changes, such as those involving the cellular/nuclear matrix (Wistuba and Gazdar 1999; Wistuba et al. 1999). Neoplastic progression from an "initiating" lesion to invasive bronchopulmonary malignancy appears to be a cumulative time- and lesion-dependent process. Despite extensive research, the key "gate-keeping" genes unique to the development of lung cancer have not been identified. Thus, although molecular biomarkers hold promise as surrogate endpoints (Xu et al. 1999; Thieberville et al. 1997; Mao et al. 1998), their use for evaluation of new agents requires further investigation. The risk of development of lung cancer for a single or a combination of molecular biomarkers has not been determined in animal or human studies. Widespread molecular damage in the bronchial epithelium has been shown even in histologically normal bronchial epithelium in both current and former smokers (Wistuba 1997; Mao et al. 1997). Many of the clonal patches are very small. They are difficult to localize with current imaging methods. Furthermore, the clonal patches may have different genetic alteration (Park et al. 1999). Disappearance or appearance of molecular markers after chemoprevention treatment could well be due to sampling and may have no bearing on regression or progression of the pre-treatment sites.

Since molecular damage is widespread, it may not be realistic to aim for complete reversal of molecular damage with chemopreventive intervention. Other commonly used biomarkers such as RARβ, Ki67 contribute to a better understanding of the mechanism of action of chemopreventive agents (Xu et al. 1999; Shin et al. 2000); however, there is currently no evidence to show that modulation of these biomarkers correlates with an altered risk for lung cancer.

Bronchial Dysplasia as SEB

At the present time, bronchial dysplasia is one of the best surrogate endpoint biomarker to assess the effect of new chemopreventive agents for the following reasons:

1. The carcinogenesis sequence has been defined for squamous cell carcinomas, although it is less understood for other cell types. The development of squamous cell carcinoma of the lung has been studied in animal models (Nasiell et al. 1987) and in humans (Nasiell et al. 1987; Saccomanno 1982; Saccomanno et al. 1974; Auerach et al. 1978; Risse et al. 1988; Frost et al. 1986; Band et al. 1986; Melamed and Zaman 1982). Serial sputum cytology examinations in uranium miners and in smokers showed that invasive lung cancer develops through a series of stages from mild, moderate, and severe atypia, carcinoma in situ and then invasive cancer (Saccomanno 1982; Frost et al. 1986).

2. The morphological criteria for preinvasive lesions have been defined in the recent WHO classification (Travis et al. 1999). Grading of squamous preinvasive lesions was found to be very reproducible for high-grade lesions in an internet study conducted by one of us (Gazdar) in collaboration with a

Table 3. Smoking history and prevalence of dysplasia and cancer

–	Smoking history (pack-years)		
Pathology	20–29	30–39	≥40
–	n=30	n=206	n=403
Mild dysplasia	27%	44%	53%
Moderate dysplasia	27%	15%	8%
Severe dysplasia	0%	2%	4%
Carcinoma in situ	0%	0%	0.7%
Invasive cancer	0%	0.5%	1.2%

panel of experienced pulmonary pathologists (A.F. Gazdar, unpublished data) for high-grade lesions in keeping with other studies (Venmans et al. 2000; Nicholson et al. 2001). The correlation is not as good for metaplasia and mild dysplasia (Lam and Macaulay 1998; Venmans et al. 2000), but the accuracy can be improved with quantitative microscopy (Lam and Macaulay 1998).

3. The prevalence of bronchial dysplasia and carcinoma in situ correlates with the smoking history (Auerbach et al. 1961; Table 3). In very heavy smokers (≥40 pack-years) with chronic obstructive pulmonary disease, the prevalence of mild, moderate, or severe atypia and carcinoma in situ on sputum cytology examination was found to be 48%, 25%, 0.8%, and 0.9%, respectively (Kennedy et al. 1996). A similar high prevalence of premalignant and malignant lesions was found by us using autofluorescence bronchoscopy-directed bronchial biopsies in 919 current and former smokers 45–79 years of age with ≥30 pack-years smoking history (Table 1). In addition, the prevalence of high-grade dysplasia, carcinoma in situ or cancer are similar between current and former smokers (Lam et al. 1999; Table 1), explaining the persistent risk of lung cancer in long-term heavy smokers despite smoking cessation (Peto et al. 2001; Halpern et al. 1993).

4. In humans, the presence of dysplastic cells in sputum cytology or dysplastic lesions in bronchial biopsy and the severity of abnormality correlate with the risk of development of invasive lung cancer in prospective studies similar to what is known from cancer progression models in animals. The proportion of individuals with mild, moderate, or severe sputum cell atypia who will develop invasive lung cancer within 10 years was found to be 4%, 10%, and 40% respectively (Risse et al. 1988; Frost et al. 1986). Serial bronchoscopy and biopsy in patients with bronchial dysplasia showed that approximately 25% of the dysplastic lesions progress to invasive cancer over a mean period of 36 months. The dysplastic lesions were found to persist in another 42% (Sato et al. 1999; Shibuya et al. 2001). Over 50% of patients with carcinoma in situ were found to progress to invasive cancer within 30 months (Thiberville et al. 1997; Venmans et al. 2000). These numbers are probably low, since small lesions might have been removed by the biopsy procedure.

5. The morphological changes of bronchial dysplasia can be quantitated using nuclear morphometry to minimize interobserver variation (Lam and Macaulay 1998; Boone et al. 1992, 1997). We observed that the "spontaneous" regression rate of dysplastic lesions was significantly lower for lesions that were classified as dysplastic on conventional histopathology criteria and nuclear morphometry compared to histopathology alone. The regression rate was 19.5% versus 33.2% respectively.
6. Reversal of dysplasia with successful modulation is associated with reduced cancer risk (Boone et al. 1992, 1997).

Quantitative Autofluorescence Bronchoscopy

Bronchial dysplasia is usually invisible by white-light bronchoscopy. The usefulness of autofluorescence bronchoscopy to localize small, premalignant bronchial lesions has been confirmed in multiple studies. Worldwide experience in over 1,700 reported cases showed that autofluorescence bronchoscopy using the LIFE-Lung device is a very sensitive method to localize areas of dysplasia and carcinoma in situ (Lam et al. 2000).

In collaboration with Xillix Technologies (Richmond, BC, Canada), we have developed special software for the LIFE-Lung device that can quantitate the degree of abnormal fluorescence as well as to measure the size of abnormal fluorescence patches. Quantitation removes subjective assessment of color changes and improves the sensitivity and specificity of detection of premalignant lesions.

The anatomy of the tracheobronchial tree provides a unique opportunity to evaluate the effect of chemopreventive agents by sequential biopsy of the same sites before and after chemopreventive intervention. Each of the segmental and submental bronchi accessible by fiberoptic bronchoscopy are named and thus provide a landmark for longitudinal observation. A biopsied site also has a different fluorescence than previously unbiopsied areas, thus allowing precise rebiopsy of the same lesions before and after treatment. The ability to localize the site and count the number of dysplastic lesions before and after chemopreventive intervention allows measurement of the effect of chemoprevention.

Evaluation of Response to Treatment

To evaluate the efficacy of new chemopreventive agents in phase II studies, it is important to have SEBs that will correlate with the outcome of phase III studies.

A previous NCI-sponsored phase II chemoprevention trial (NCI grant U01-CA68381 – A randomized, double-blind placebo trial of retinol versus placebo), provided us with the opportunity to establish response criteria since we now know from phase III clinical trials that retinol is not an effective chemopreventive agent for lung cancer (van Zandwijk et al. 2000; Omenn et al. 1996).

On a participant level, if we define complete response (CR) as regression of all dysplastic lesions found at baseline to no higher than hyperplasia at 6 months and no appearance of new dysplastic lesions that are mild dysplasia or worse, and progressive disease (PD) as progression of one or more sites by two or more grades or appearance of new dysplastic lesions that are mild dysplasia or worse, retinol is not an effective chemopreventive agent (Fig. 2). However, in the lesion-specific analysis, retinol was found to have a borderline effect in regression of dysplastic lesions versus placebo (43.6% versus 29.9% respectively, P=0.051) as well as reducing the progression rate (11.3% retinol

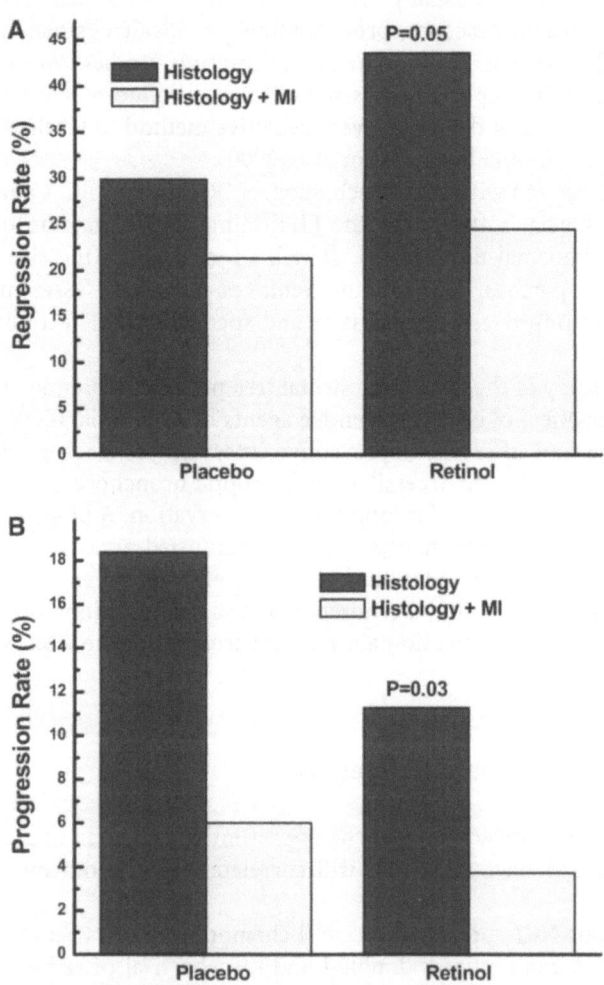

Fig. 2A,B. Effect of retinol on bronchial dysplasia compared to placebo. **A** Lesion-specific analysis. **B** Person-specific analysis

versus 18.4% placebo, $P=0.03$). By combining histopathology and nuclear morphometry, no significant effect was observed with retinol compared to placebo (Fig. 2). Thus, nuclear morphometry alone or in combination with histopathology may be a more precise SEB to assess the efficacy of new chemopreventive agents. The usefulness of quantitative microscopy to evaluate the effect of chemopreventive agents has also been reported by Boone and co-workers (Boone et al. 1992, 1997). Using this approach, we have identified two potentially useful chemopreventive agents in phase IIa trials. One of these is anethole dithioethione (Lam et al. 2001). Another inhaled budesonide (Lam et al. 2000; Wattenberg et al. 1997; Wattenberg and Estensen 1997), is being further investigated in a double-blind, randomized, placebo controlled trial (NCI contract N01-CN-85188). The result of this trial is expected at the end of 2002.

Future Directions

The small size of the histopathological lesions and clonal patches of molecular changes (usually smaller than a bronchial biopsy) presents problems for monitoring of the effect of the chemopreventive intervention by sequential biopsies. Development of in vivo optical imaging methods such as confocal microscopy or optical coherence tomography may allow more accurate outcome assessment without removal of the premalignant lesions by the biopsy procedure. Currently, we do not have the means to study the effect of chemoprevention of peripheral adenocarcinoma. Coupling low-dose spiral CT with optical imaging methods via fiberoptics to detect and to characterize small lung nodules may allow the use of atypical adenomatous hyperplasia as the SEB. Other promising biomarkers such as methylation markers in sputum cells or bronchoalveolar lavage fluid (Palmisano et al. 2000; Belinsky et al. 1998; Gazdara et al. 2001) need to be studied further to validate their usefulness as SEB. Successful chemoprevention may be more difficult to achieve in current smokers who remain at continuous exposure to tobacco carcinogens. Different agents may be required for current smokers versus former smokers. Potential differences in the response of women versus men are poorly understood and need to be investigated further as well.

References

Arnold AM, Brownmann GP, Levine MN, et al (1992) The effect of the synthetic retinoid etretinate on sputum cytology: results from a randomized trial. Br J Cancer 65:737–743

Auerbach O, Stout AP, Hammond EC, Garfinkel L (1961) Changes in bronchial epithelium in relation to cigarette smoking and in relation to lung cancer. New Engl J Med 265:253–267

Auerbach O, Saccomanno G, Kuschner M, Brown RD, Garfinkel L (1978) Histologic findings in the tracheobronchial tree of uranium miners and nonminers with lung cancer. Cancer 42:483–489

Band PR, Feldstein M, Saccomanno G (1986) Reversibility of bronchial marked atypia. Implication for chemoprevention. Cancer Detect Prev 9:157–160

Belinsky SA, Nikula KJ, Palmisano WA, Michels R, Saccomanno G, Gabrielson E, et al (1998) Aberrant methylation of p16(INK4a) is an early event in lung cancer and a potential biomarker for early diagnosis. Proc Natl Acad Sci USA 95:11891–11896

Boone CW, Kelloff GJ, Steele VE (1992) Natural history of intraepithelial neoplasia in humans with implications for cancer chemoprevention strategy. Cancer Res 52:1651–1659

Boone CW, Bacus JW, Bacus JV, Steele VE, Kelloff GJ (1997) Properties of intraepithelial neoplasia relevant to the development of cancer chemopreventive agents. J Cell Biochem Suppl 28/29:1–20

Doudkine A, MacAulay C, Poulin N, Palcic B (1995) Nuclear texture measurements in image cytometry. Pathologica 87:286–289

Frost JK, Ball WC Jr, Levin ML, Tockman MS, Erozan YS, Gupta PK, Eggleston JC, Pressman NJ, Donithan MP, Kimball AW (1986) Sputum cytopathology: use and potential in monitoring the workplace environment by screening for biological effects of exposure. J Occup Med 28:692–703

Garner DM, Harrison A, MacAulay C, Palcic B (1994) Cyto-savant and its use in automated screening of cervical smears. In: Wied GL, Bartels PH, Rosenthal DL, Schenck U (eds) Compendium on the computerized cytology and histology laboratory. Tutorials of cytology, Chicago, pp 346–352

Gazdar AF, Zöchbauer-Müller S, Virmani A, Kurie J, Minna JD, Lam S (2001) Promoter methylation and silencing of the retinoic acid receptor-beta gene in lung carcinomas. J Natl Cancer Inst 93:67–68

Greenlee RT, Hill-Harmon MB, Murray T, Thun M (2001). Cancer statistics, 2001. CA Cancer J Clin 51:15–36

Halpern MT, Gillespie BW, Warner KE (1993) Patterns of absolute risk of lung cancer mortality in former smokers (see comments). J Natl Cancer Inst 85:457–64

Hennekens CH, Buring JE, Manson JE, Stampfer M, Rosner B, Cook NR, Belanger C, LaMotte F, Gaziano JM, Ridker PM, Willett W, Peto R (1996) Lack of effect of long-term supplementation with beta carotene on the incidence of malignant neoplasms and cardiovascular disease. N Engl J Med 334:1145–1149

Henschke CI, McCauley DI, Yankelevitz DF, Naidich DP, et al (1999) Early Lung Cancer Action Project: overall design and findings from baseline screening. Lancet 354:99–105

Hong W, Endicott J, Itri LM, Doos W, Batsakis JG, Bell R, et al (1986) 13-cis retinoic acid in the treatment of oral leukoplakia. N Engl J Med 315:1501–1505

Hong WK, Lippman SM, Itri LM, Karp DD, Lee JS, Byers RM, Schantz SP, Kramer AM, Lotan R, Peters LJ, Dimery IW, Brown BW, Goepfert H (1990) Prevention of second primary tumors with isotretinoin in squamous-cell carcinoma of the head and neck. N Engl J Med 323:795–801

Kennedy TC, Proudfoot SP, Franklin WA, Merrick TA, Saccomanno G, Corkill ME, Mumma DL, Sirgi KE, Miller YE, Archer PG, Prochazka A (1996) Cytopathological analysis of sputum in patients with airflow obstruction and significant smoking histories. Cancer Res 56:4673–4678

Kurie JM, Lee JS, Khuri FR, et al (2000) N-(4-Hydroxyphenyl)retinamide in the chemoprevention of squamous metaplasia and dysplasia of the bronchial epithelium. Clin Cancer Res 6:2973–2979

Lam S, MacAulay CE (1998) Endoscopic localization of preneoplastic lung lesions. In: Martinet Y, Hirsch FR, Martinet N, Vignaud J-M, Mulshine JL (eds) Clinical and biological basis of lung cancer prevention. Birkhauser Verlag, Basel, pp 231–237

Lam S, leRiche JC, Zheng Y, Coldman A, MacAulay CE, Hawk E, Kelloff G, Gazdar AF (1999) Sex-related differences in bronchial epithelial changes associated with tobacco smoking. J Natl Cancer Inst 91:691–696

Lam S, Palcic B, Garner D, Beveridge J, MacAulay C, leRiche JC, Coldman A (2000) Lung cancer control strategy in the new millennium. Lung Cancer 29(S2):145

Lam S, MacAulay CE, leRiche JC, Palcic B (2000) Detection and localization of early lung cancer by fluorescence bronchoscopy. Cancer 89:2468–2473

Lam S, MacAulay C, LeRiche JC, Dyachkova Y, Coldman A, Guillaud M, Hawk E, Christen MO, Gazdar AF (2002) A randomized phase IIb trial of anethole dithiolethione in smokers with bronchial dysplasia. J Natl Cancer Inst 94 (13):1001–1009

Lee JS, Lippman SM, Benner SE, Lee JJ, Ro JY, Lukeman JM, Morice RC, Peters EJ, Pang AC, Fritsche HA Jr, Hong WK (1994) Randomized placebo-controlled trial of isotretinoin in chemoprevention of bronchial squamous metaplasia. J Clin Oncol 12:937–945

Lippman SM, Lee JJ, Karp DD, Vokes EE, Benner SE, Goodman GE, Khuri FR, Marks R, Winn RJ, Fry W, Graziano SL, Gandara DR, Okawara G, Woodhouse CL, Williams B, Perez C, Kim HW, Lotan R, Roth JA, Hong WK (2001) Randomized phase III intergroup trial of isotretinon to prevent second primary tumors in stage I nonsmall cell lung cancer. J Natl Cancer Inst 93:605–618

MacAulay C, Lam S, Payne PW, leRiche JC, Palcic B (1995) Malignancy-associated changes in bronchial epithelial cells in biopsy specimens. Anal Quant Cytol Histol 17:55–61

Mao L, Lee JS, Kurie JM, Fan YH, Lippman SM, Lee JJ, Ro JY, Broxson A, Yu R, Morice RC, Kemp BL, Khuri FR, Walsh GL, Hittelman WN, Hong WK (1997) Clonal genetic alterations in the lungs of current and former smokers. J Natl Cancer Inst 89:857–862

Mao L, El-Naggar AK, Papadimitrakopoulou V, Shin DM, Shin HC, Fan Y, Zhou X, Clayman G, Lee JJ, Lee JS, Hittelman WN, Lippman SM, Hong WK (1998) Phenotype and genotype of advanced premalignant head and neck lesions after chemopreventive therapy. J Natl Cancer Inst 90:1545–1551

McLarty JW, Holiday DB, Girard WM, et al (1995) Beta-carotene, vitamin A and lung cancer chemoprevention: results of an intermediate endpoint study. Am J Clin Nutr 62:14315–14385

Melamed MR, Zaman MB (1982) Pathogenesis of epidermoid carcinoma of lung. In: Shimosato Y, Melamed MR, Nettesheim P (eds) Morphogenesis of lung cancer, vol I. CRC Press, Boca Raton, pp 37–64

Nasiell M, Auer G, Kato H (1987) Cytological studies in man and animals on the development of bronchogenic carcinoma. In: McDowell EM (ed) Lung carcinomas. Churchill Livingstone, Edinburgh, pp 207–242

Nicholson AG, Perry LJ, Cury PM, Jackson P, McCormick CM, Corrin B, Wells AU (2001) Reproducibility of the WHO/IASLC grading system for preinvasive squamous lesions of the bronchus: a study of the interobserver and intra-observer variation. Histopathology 38:202–208

Omenn GS (1999) Chemoprevention of lung cancer is proving difficult and frustrating, requiring new approaches. J Natl Cancer Inst 92:959–60

Omenn GS, Goodman G, Thornquist M, Barnhart S, Balmes J, Cherniack MG, Cullen M, Glass A, Keogh J, Liu D, Meyskens Jr F, Perloff M, Valanis B, Williams Jr J (1996) Chemoprevention of lung cancer: the β-Carotene and Retinol Efficacy Trial (CARET) in high-risk smokers and asbestos-exposed workers. IARC Sci Publ 136:67–85

Palmisano WA, Divine KK, Saccomanno G, Gilliland FD, Baylin SB, Herman JG, et al (2000) Predicting lung cancer by detecting aberrant promoter methylation in sputum. Cancer Res 60:5954–5958

Park IW, Wistuba II, Maitra A, Milchgrub S, Virmani AK, Minna JD, Gazdar AF (1999) Multiple clonal abnormalities in the bronchial epithelium of patients with lung cancer. J Natl Cancer Inst 91:1863–1868

Pastorino U, Infante M, Maioli M, et al (1993) Adjuvant treatment of stage I lung cancer with high dose vitamin A. J Clin Oncol 1:1216–1222

Payne PW (1997) Cytometric detection of nuclear features associated with pre-malignancy or malignancy in human bronchial specimens. Cytometric detection of nuclear features associated with pre-malignancy or malignancy in human bronchial specimens. PhD Thesis, University of British Columbia

Payne PW, Sebo TJ, Doudkine A, Garner D, MacAulay C, Lam S, leRiche JC, Palcic B (1997) Sputum screening by quantitative microscopy: a reexamination of a portion of the National Cancer Institute Cooperative Early Lung Cancer Study. Mayo Clin Proc 72:697–704

Peto R, Darby S, Deo H, Silcocko P, Whitley E, Doll R (2001) Smoking, smoking cessation, and lung cancer in the UK since 1950: combination of national statistics with two case-control studies. Lancet 321:323–329

Risse EKJ, Vooijs GP, van't Hof MA (1988) Diagnostic significance of "severe dysplasia" in sputum cytology. Acta Cytologica 32:629–634

Saccomanno G (1982) Carcinoma in situ of the lung: its development, detection, and treatment. Semin Resp Med 4:156–160

Saccomanno G, Archer VE, Auerbach O, Saunders RP, Brennan, LM (1974) Development of carcinoma of the lung as reflected in exfoliated cells. Cancer 33:256–270

Sato M, Minowa M, Sagawa M, Saito Y, Sakurada A, Okada Y, Takahashi H, Matsumura Y, Ono S, Tanita T, Kondo T, Fujimura S (1999) Diagnosis of roentgenographically occult lung cancer in patients with positive or suspected positive sputum cytology by the LIFE-lung system and follow-up study of dysplastic lesions of the bronchi. First Chiba International Workshop on Lung Cancer – Early Detection. Chiba, Japan, February 12–13, p 16

Shibuya K, Fujisawa T, Hoshino H (2001) A follow-up study of squamous dysplasia. J Clin Exp Med 199:593–596

Shin DM, Mao L, Papadimitrakopoulou VM, Clayman G, El-Naggar A, Shin HJC, Lee JJ, Lee JS, Gillenwater A, Myers J, Lippman SM, Hittelman WN, Hong, WK (2000) Biochemo-preventive therapy for patients with premalignant lesions of the head and neck and p53 gene expression. (Brief Communication) J Natl Cancer Inst 92:69–73

The Alpha-Tocopherol, Beta Carotene Cancer Prevention Study Group (1994) The effect of vitamin E and beta carotene on the incidence of lung cancer and other cancers in male smokers. N Engl J Med 330:1029–1035

Thieberville L, Payne P, Metayer J, Vielkinds J, LeRiche J, Palcic B, Lam S (1997) Molecular follow-up of a preinvasive bronchial lesion treated by 13-cis-retinoic acid. Hum Pathol 28:108–10

Thiberville L, Metayer J, Raspaud C, Nouvet G (1997) A prospective, short term follow-up study of 59 severe dysplasias and carcinoma in situ of the bronchus using autofluorescence endoscopy. Eur Respir J 10:425S

Tong L, Spitz MR, Fueger JJ, Amos CA (1996) Lung cancer in former smokers. Cancer 78:1004–1010

Travis WD, Colby TV, Corrin B, Shimosato Y, Brambilla E (1999) Histologic and graphical text slides for the histological typing of lung and pleural tumors. In: International histological classification of tumors, 3rd edn. World Health Organization Pathology Panel, Springer Verlag, Berlin, p 5

Venmans BJ, Linder van der HC, Elbers HR (2000) Observer variability in histopathologic reporting of bronchial biopsy specimens. Influence on the results of autofluorescence bronchoscopy in detection of preinvasive bronchial neoplasia. J Bronchology 7:210–214

Welch HG, Schwartz LM, Woloshin S (2000) Are increasing 5-year survival rates evidence of success against cancer? JAMA 283:2975–78

van Zandwijk N, Pastorino U, de Vries N, et al (2000) EUROSCAN: a randomized trial of vitamin A and N-Acetylcysteine in patients with head and neck cancer or lung cancer. J Natl Cancer Inst 92:977–986

Venmans BJ, van der Linden HC, Elbers HR, Boxem TJ, Smit EF, Postmus PE, Sutedka TG (2000) Observer variability in histopathologic reporting of bronchial biopsy specimens. J Bronchol 7:210–214

Venmans BJW, van Boxem AJM, Smit EF, Postmus PE, Sutedja TG (2000) Outcome of bronchial carcinoma in situ. Chest 117:1572–1576

Wattenberg LW, Estensen RD (1997) Studies of chemopreventive effects of budenoside on benzo[a]pyrene- induced neoplasia of the lung of female A/J mice. Carcinogenesis 18:2015–7

Wattenberg LW, Wiedmann TS, Estensen RD, Zimmerman CL, Steele VE, Kelloff GJ (1997) Chemoprevention of pulmonary carcinogenesis by aerosolized budesonide in female A/J mice. Cancer Res 57:5489–92

Wilton DW (1997) The mechanism of malignancy associated changes. MSc Thesis, University of British Columbia

Wistuba II, Gazdar AF (1999) Molecular abnormalities in the sequential development of lung carcinoma. In: Srivastava S, Henson DE, Gazdar AF (eds) Molecular pathology of early cancer. IOS Press, Amsterdam, pp 265–276

Wistuba II, Lam S, Behrens C, Virmani AK, Fong KM, LeRiche JC, Samet J, Srivastava S, Minna JD, Gazdar AF (1997) Molecular damage in the bronchial epithelium of current and former smokers. J Natl Cancer Inst 89:1366–1373

Wistuba II, Behrens C, Milchgrub S, Bryant D, Hung J, Minna JD, Gazdar AF (1999) Sequential molecular abnormalities are involved in the multistage development of squamous cell lung carcinoma. Oncogene 18: 643–650

Xu XC, Lee JS, Lee J, Morice RC, Liu X, Lippman SM, Hong WK, Lotan R (1999) Nuclear retinoid receptor beta in bronchial epithelium of smokers before and during chemoprevention. J Natl Cancer Inst 91:1317–1721

Prevention and Screening **6**
of Prostate Cancer

Prevention of Prostate Cancer

Claude C. Schulman, Alexandre R. Zlotta

C.C. Schulman (✉)
Department of Urology, Erasme Hospital, University Clinics of Brussels,
808 route de Lennik, 1070 Brussels, Belgium

Abstract

Prostate cancer is an ideal candidate for chemoprevention because of its high prevalence, long latency time, hormone dependency, precursor lesions, and its unique serum marker, PSA. Chemoprevention is the administration of drugs or other agents which aim to prevent the induction or inhibit/delay cancer progression. Large-scale studies favor environmental rather than genetic factors as key determinants of prostate cancer development. Among these environmental factors, nutrition certainly has a leading role. Numerous basic science studies but also clinical studies indicate that dietary compounds or diet modifications may ultimately play a major role in prostate cancer promotion and inhibition. Definitive proofs are often difficult because of methodological problems and complex triggering cascades. New pharmaceutical drugs with minimal toxicity are also currently evaluated.

Introduction

Prostate cancer lends itself ideally to chemoprevention due to a number of particularities specific to this disease. These include a high prevalence, long latency time, hormone dependency, the availability of an ideal marker [prostate-specific antigen (PSA)], and last, but not least, the availability of a defined precursor lesion [prostatic intraepithelial neoplasm (PIN)] among the pathways leading to clinical disease (Schulman et al. 2001).

The large variability of the tumor in different geographical regions suggests the possibility of nutritional influences regarding the stimulation and/or inhibition of clinical cancer, since there is a similar prevalence worldwide of the precursor lesion.

A significant number of publications have dealt with a number of nutritional concepts including fat, phyto-estrogens, vitamins (especially vitamin E), and minerals like selenium and calcium. Although there is a growing body of evidence underlying a link between diet, lifestyle, several compounds, and prostate cancer, so far there are no conclusive results or study outcomes to achieve the scientific bases of our accepted standards of evidence.

Ongoing studies on nutrition and prostate cancer might bring the needed evidence to what is still often a hypothesis only.

The epidemiology of prostate cancer gives some indications that its etiology is likely both environmental and genetic. Indeed, large international variations in not only rates of prostate cancer incidence but also mortality suggest that environmental factors have an influence on the development of the first neoplasm in man (Parkin and Muir 1992; Brawley 1994).

Variations in international rates of prostate cancer are considerable. These variations in incidence of prostate cancer range from 0.5 per 100,000 in Qidong (China) to 102.1 per 100,000 in the United States, to 135.5 per 100,000 in Sweden (Heber et al. 1998).

Pathological studies on prostatic tissue from various populations support the fact that noninfiltrating lesions have similar distributions, whereas small infiltrating lesions discovered incidentally at autopsy follow global distributions of invasive disease. The implication of this observation is that invasive cancer has a distinct etiologic basis and it is believed diet plays a key role in its development.

Strong support of the relationship between diet and cancer is, however, found in studies of migrants moving from countries of birth like China and Japan through Hawaii to North America, where the incidence of prostate cancer increases from an initial low rate to one almost equal that of the indigenous population within a few generations (Muir et al. 1991; Denis et al. 1999). There is growing scientific evidence that several of these dietary compounds demonstrate antineoplastic activities.

In order to establish the role of a dietary compound on prostate cancer genesis or promotion, clinical, epidemiological data, and finally large-scale prospective trials should further support experimental data.

Diet

Energy Intake and Fat

The risk of prostate cancer was found to be about 70% greater in men in the upper quartile of energy intake than those in the lower quartile (Rohan et al. 1995). The results of a number of dietary intake surveys support the concept that high-fat diet and especially animal fat may increase the risk of clinically significant prostate cancer. Animal dietary fat presumably is converted to androgens with resultant increased androgenic stimulation of the prostate.

Sources of *polyunsaturated* fats (e.g., *linolenic acid*) include corn oil and sunflower oil. These fats are thought to have a damaging effect on DNA and other cell components, affect cell proliferation, immune defenses, tissue invasiveness, and tumor metastatic spread. They have equally been shown to alter 5-α reductase activity (Montironi et al. 1999).

Polyunsaturated and vegetable fats have been investigated equally in cohort studies. These authors observed an increased risk of prostate cancer in men with higher intakes of α-linolenic acid, with adjusted relative risk of 3.4 ($p=0.002$ for trend). α-Linolenic acid is present primarily in red meat, butter, and vegetable oils (soya bean oil, rapeseed oil).

Consistent evidence on the possible association of high monounsaturated and polyunsaturated fat intakes with prostate cancer is yet to be reported (Bairati et al. 1998).

Omega-3 fatty acids have been shown to inhibit prostate cancer cell lines. Omega-3 fatty acids obtained primarily from fatty fish and eicosanoid synthesis inhibitors are found to block cancer cell invasion by regulating tumor cell proteolytic enzyme activity in vitro (Pandali et al. 1996).

Acids measured before diagnosis in the donors' serum were examined. Data showed no definitive conclusion can be drawn at this point.

Vitamins and Micronutrients

Carotenoids

This is a group of complex unsaturated hydrocarbons occurring as pigments in plants, e.g., carrot. (Tables 1 1, 2). Some carotenoids are precursors of vitamin A, whereas others, for instance lycopene, have a different structure not convertible into vitamin A. These compounds have been shown to have anti-

Table 1. Vitamins and prostate cancer (adapted from Kelloff et al. 1999)

Dietary constituent	Source	Evidence	Mechanism
Caroteroids			
β-carotene	Carrots	Insufficient	Unclear
α-carotene	Carrots	No association	
Lycopene	Tomatoes	Inhibition	Unclear
Vitamin C	Fruits Vegetables	Insufficient	Antioxidant
Retinoids (retinol, retinoin, isotretinoin, fenretinide)	Vegetables Synthetic		Inhibit cell proliferation
Vitamin E (α-tocopherol)	Lettuce, water cress	Inhibition	Inhibition of tumor progression (prolong latent phase)
	Cotton seed oil, hemp seed oil		
Vitamin D (1,25(OH_2 D_3))	Vegetables Milk UV radiation	Inhibition	$\downarrow$ Cell proliferation $\uparrow$ Cell differentiation

Table 2. Minerals/trace elements and prostate cancer (adapted from Kelloff et al. 1999)

Element	Source	Evidence	Molecular target effect
Calcium	Milk Cheese	Promotion	Vitamin D synthesis inhibition
Zinc	Meat	Insufficient	
Selenium	Bread Cereals Fish Meat	Inhibition	Antioxidant Apoptosis inducer Catalase enhancer Cytochrome P450 modifier Immunostimulant
Isoflavonoids	Peas Beans Soy beans	Inhibition	Angiogenesis inhibition Antioxidant Apoptosis induction Oncogene expression inhibition EGFR inhibition Antioestrogens ODC synthesis inhibition ↓ Cholesterol and LDH
Fenretinide (4HPR)	Carrots	Inhibition	Antiproliferative Apoptosis induction Angiogenesis inhibition Cellular differentiation IGF-1 inhibition Immunostimulation ODC synthesis inhibition Protein kinase C inhibition

oxidant potential, particularly marked with lycopene (Giovannucci et al. 1995; Krisnsky 1998).

A population-based case-control study carried out in Auckland, New Zealand, in 1996–1997 and recruiting 317 prostate cancer cases and 480 controls investigated associations between prostate cancer risk and dietary intake of the carotenoids β-carotene and lycopene and their major plant food sources, including carrots, green leafy vegetables, and tomato-based foods. Dietary intake of β-carotene and its main vegetable sources was largely unassociated with prostate cancer risk, whereas intake of lycopene and tomato-based foods was weakly associated with a reduced risk (Norris et al. 2000).

A prospective study was designed to examine the relationship between plasma concentrations of several major antioxidants and risk of prostate cancer, using plasma samples obtained in 1982 from healthy men enrolled in the Physicians' Health Study, a randomized, placebo-controlled trial of aspirin and β-carotene. Subjects included 578 men who developed prostate cancer within 13 years of follow-up and 1,294 age- and smoking status-matched controls.

Lycopene was the only antioxidant found at significantly lower mean levels in cases than in matched controls ($p=0.04$ for all cases). There was no evidence for a trend among those assigned to β-carotene supplements. None of the associations for lycopene were confounded by age, smoking, body mass index, exercise, alcohol, multivitamin use, or plasma total cholesterol level (Gann et al. 1999).

The current literature regarding intake of tomatoes and tomato-based products and blood lycopene (a compound derived predominantly from tomatoes) level in relation to the risk of various cancers was recently reviewed (Giovannucci 1999). Among 72 studies identified, 57 reported inverse associations between tomato intake or blood lycopene level and the risk of cancer at a defined anatomic site; 35 of these inverse associations were statistically significant.

Lycopene may account for or contribute to these benefits, but this possibility is not yet proven and requires further study. Numerous other potentially beneficial compounds are present in tomatoes, and, conceivably, complex interactions among multiple components may contribute to the anticancer properties of tomatoes.

Vitamin C

Vitamin C is a water-soluble antioxidant obtained from fruits and vegetables in food. Most recent cohort and case-control studies showed no significant association between vitamin C intake and risk of prostate cancer (Eichholzer 1996; Fair et al. 1997).

The lack of activity of vitamin C, which is known as a powerful antioxidant, underlines the complexity of prostate cancer biology and prevention.

Retinoids (Retinol or Vitamin A)

Vitamin A (retinol) is found in foods of animal origin such as animal liver and fish oil, with eggs and milk being low concentration sources. The precursor β-carotene is found in carrots and green vegetables (spinach, broccoli) and transformed into vitamin A in the gut (Peto et al. 1981; Machlin and Bendich 1987).

Cohort and case-control studies have shown differences in risk estimates between younger and older men based on dietary retinoid levels with an association in some reports and a protective role in others. The major setbacks to the use of these agents in clinical trials reside in their dose-related side effects, including hepatotoxicity, central nervous system changes, and mucocutaneous dryness (Heinonen et al. 1998).

Vitamin E (α-Tocopherol)

Vitamin E is one of the most researched compounds in medicine. Vitamin E is actually a general name for different compounds, so supplements can contain several forms (Moyad 1999). Vitamin E in the diet also differs from the form found over the counter. There has been a strong interest in this supplement in the prostate cancer arena primarily because of a Finnish study that demonstrated a lower morbidity and mortality from this disease in men taking 50 mg of synthetic (α-tocopherol) vitamin E daily (Heinonen et al. 1998; Bonn 1998). A trial of 29,133 lung cancer subjects aged 58–69 years in Finland, with α-tocopherol 50 mg and/or β-carotene 20 mg daily for 5–8 years, unexpectedly showed a 32% decrease in incidence of prostate cancer among men receiving α-tocopherol (Heinonen et al. 1998). It is noteworthy that β-carotene when given alone was shown to be associated with 23% and 15% higher incidence and mortality, respectively.

In 1986, 47,780 United States male health professionals free from diagnosed cancer completed a dietary and lifestyle questionnaire; supplemental vitamin E and prostate cancer incidence were updated through 1996 (Chan et al. 1999).

Supplemental vitamin E was not associated with prostate cancer risk generally, but a suggestive inverse association between supplemental vitamin E and risk of metastatic or fatal prostate cancer among current smokers and recent quitters was consistent with the Finnish trial among smokers.

Caution should be exercised in interpreting data on the role of vitamin E because of a possible bias in the endpoint assessment with respect to the effect of α-tocopherol on prostate cancer, and differences in both diagnostic procedures and on the types of vitamin E analyzed.

Vitamin D

Studies have demonstrated an inverse correlation between ultraviolet radiation, the main source of vitamin D, and prostate cancer mortality (Hanchette and Schwarz 1992). Recent studies have suggested that vitamin D is an important determinant of prostate cancer risk, and inherited polymorphisms in the 3'-untranslated region (3'UTR) of the vitamin D receptor (VDR) gene are associated with the risk and progression of prostate cancer (Habuchi et al. 2000).

Clinical trials in patients with advanced hormone refractory prostate cancer showed a rapid drop in levels of PSA. In patients with minimal recurrence, tumor doubling time was increased by a mean of 45% during treatment with $1,25(OH_2)D_3$ assessed by PSA values (Peehl 1999; Konety et al. 1993).

Solid clinical and epidemiological data about the place of vitamin D in prostate cancer promotion and prevention are, however, lacking.

Fruit and Vegetable Intakes

Fruit and vegetable intake have been hypothesized to be associated with decreased risk of many cancers, but results for prostate cancer are sparse. A case-control study including over 1,200 patients has investigated the association between fruit and vegetables intake and prostate cancer risk. If no association was found between fruit intake and prostate cancer risk, high consumption of vegetables, particularly cruciferous vegetables (with four leaves) was associated with a reduced risk of prostate cancer (Cohen et al. 2000).

Calcium

It is hypothesized that dietary and supplemental calcium intakes or diets high in milk, the main source of calcium, are consistently associated with prostate cancer risk by lowering the serum levels of bioactive metabolites of vitamin D $(1,25 (OH)_2 D)$, which plays a role in reducing the development and/or progression of prostate cancer. Low serum calcium levels stimulate the secretion parathyroid hormone, which promotes the conversion of vitamin D into $1,25 (OH)_2 D$. A clinical study on 47,781 men found higher consumption of calcium to be related to risk of advanced prostate cancer (RR: 2.97) and metastatic cancer (RR: 4.57) (Giovannucci et al. 1998).

Selenium

Selenium is a trace element found in the soil as selenide, and is widely obtained from bread, cereals, fish, chicken, and meat. Differences in bioavailability of selenium reflect large geographical dietary intake variations. Selenium enters the food chain through plants (Nelson et al. 1999; Yip et al. 1999). Commercial sources of selenium come from copper ore refinement.

Selenium is a key component of a number of functional selenoproteins required for normal health, like glutathione peroxidase enzymes antioxidants that remove hydrogen peroxide, and damaging lipid and phospholipid hydroperoxides generated in vivo by free radicals.

A clinical double-blind study on 974 men in the United States showed that selenium reduced overall cancer incidence by 37% and that of prostate cancer by 50% (Clark et al. 1998).

The association between risk of prostate cancer and prediagnostic levels of selenium in toenails, a measure of long-term selenium intake, was investigated in 51,529 male health professionals aged 40–75 years. The selenium level in toenails varied substantially among men. When matched case-control data were analyzed, higher selenium levels were associated with a reduced risk of advanced prostate cancer. After additionally controlling for family history of prostate cancer, body mass index, calcium intake, lycopene intake, saturated fat intake, vasectomy, and geographical region, the OR was 0.35 ($p=0.03$) (Yoshizawa et al. 1998).

Given this significant reduction in prostate cancer incidence and mortality associated with selenium supplementation at initial daily dose of 250 µg reduced to 80–90 µg/daily as recommended doses, larger trials are on the way. High doses of selenium have been shown to be hepatotoxic and toxic to the nervous system in animals (Nelson et al. 1999).

Isoflavonoids, Flavonoids and Soy Proteins

One of the major difference in diet between Asian and Western countries is the consumption of soy-derived products. Soy bean plant has been cultivated by the Chinese for at least 4,500 years and there are more than 2,500 known varieties (Miller 2000). Soy is a well-recognized source of phyto-estrogens, also known as isoflavones. A limited amount of clinical evidence points to a beneficial role of soy in reducing hormonal levels and exhibiting weak estrogen and antiestrogen-like qualities.

The beneficial effects of soy diet have been attributed to isoflavonoids. Isoflavonoids are compounds or plant pigments found in legumes (peas, beans) with soya bean as a major source. *Genistein* and *daidzein* are the major isoflavones shown to inhibit the growth of prostate cancer cell lines. The lignan enterolactone and the soya-derived isoflavone genistein are inhibitors of several steroid metabolizing enzymes such as aromatase or 5 α-reductase.

Although there are many experimental data regarding the antitumoral effects of several soy-derived products, large-scale epidemiological studies are sparse. A recently published work aimed at identifying variables for prostate cancer mortality from data collected in 59 countries. Prostate cancer was inversely associated with estimated consumption of cereals, nuts and oil-seeds, fish, and above all soy products. The effect size per calories for soy products was at least four times as large as for any other dietary factor (Hebert et al. 1998).

Common Concepts of Cancer Chemoprevention

Chemoprevention consists of the administration of drugs or other agents aimed at preventing induction or inhibiting or delaying progression of cancer. Development of chemopreventive strategies requires proper knowledge of the mechanisms of carcinogenesis in prostate disease and identification of agents that can interfere with these mechanisms.

Prostate cancer represents a prime target for chemoprevention studies because known risk factors, hormonal dependency, and precursor lesions such as PIN are well documented (Kelloff et al. 1999; Montironi and Schulman 1996).

Table 3. Prostate cancer chemoprevention and chemoactive target population (adapted from Montironi et al. 1999)

Target population	Major advantage	Major disadvantage
Chemoprevention		
1. Healthy men	Applicable to general population	Requires large number of subjects Requires long study period Expensive May require biopsy at end of study to establish status
2. High-risk groups (e.g., strong family history)	Findings directly applicable to the high-risk group studied	Findings may not be applicable to general population
3. High-grade PIN	Greatly decreases required sample size, study time, and expense Easily identified on subsequent biopsies	Possibility of coexisting malignancy may be decreased by requiring second biopsy before randomization Findings may not be applicable to general population
Chemoactive		
1. Cancer on biopsy (treated during 3–12-week period before radical prostatectomy)	Ability to evaluate whole mounted pathology specimen	Only stable to evaluate short term effects of the chemopreventive agent
2. Cancer on biopsy treated by watchful waiting	Results would evaluate long-term effects of the chemopreventive agent on malignancy	Would require subsequent biopsies Findings may not be applicable to general population Findings may confound the heterogeneity of prostate cancer

Table 4. Differences between trials for chemoprevention and therapy of cancer (adapted from Thompson and Coltman 2000)

Characteristic	Chemoprevention	Therapy
Population	Healthy men	Men with disease
Study sample size	Very large (often tens of thousands)	Large (perhaps 500 to 2,000)
Acceptable toxicity of intervention	None to minimal	Moderate to large
Cost of trial	Very expensive	Expensive
Duration of accrual and follow-up	Very long (often 10–20 years)	Intermediate length

Chemotherapeutic agents need to be given basically for short periods of time or in precise cycles to patients under physician care to allow early evaluation and management of their side effects (Kelloff et al. 1999; Tables 3, 4).

Chemopreventive agents are usually intended for relatively healthy subjects, many without detectable histological lesions, thus without evident clinical benefits at evaluation of intervention. Cancer incidence is not usually a feasible endpoint for chemoprevention trials because long time periods for carcinogenesis and large cohorts are needed for assessable studies. The identification and characterization of intermediate biomarkers and their validation as surrogate endpoints for cancer incidence in clinical chemoprevention trials are significant components in the development of chemoprevention agents and strategies.

Several biomarkers can be used to monitor carcinogenesis in the prostate such as PSA, PIN, nuclear and nucleolar morphometry, DNA ploidy, etc.

Other potentially useful biomarkers associated with cellular proliferation kinetics (proliferating cell nuclear antigen and apoptosis) include: differentiation (blood group antigens, vinentins); genetic damage (loss of heterozygosity on chromosome 8); signal transduction [tumor growth factor (TGF-α, TGF-β), insulin-like growth factor-I, c-erb B-2 expression]; angiogenesis and biochemical changes (PSA changes) (Kelloff et al. 1999).

A significant proportion of the promising chemopreventive agents for the prostate used in chemoprevention trials are phytonutrients in food, anticancer effects of which have been demonstrated in a variety of tumor types.

Cohorts in clinical trials should be suitable for measuring chemopreventive activity and efficacy of the agents as well as assessment of the intermediate biomarker.

Chemoprevention might also be considered in patients with rising PSA levels after radical surgery. Results from the first ever randomized double-blind placebo-controlled study of dietary supplements in tertiary prevention of prostate using a soy extract, tea extract, carotenoids, phytosterols, selenium, and vitamin E were recently revealed. The slope of the normal PSA significantly improved in the nutritional supplement group with a delay in PSA rise of 8 weeks with a 6 week course of supplements (Schröder et al. 2000).

Conclusion

Preventing rather than treating already established neoplasms is an attractive concept in oncology. Primary chemoprevention of prostate cancer is a relatively new concept and could be a promising strategy for preventing and arresting the development of the first neoplasm in men.

Chemoprevention could be performed using new pharmaceutical drugs with minimal long-term toxicity; however, each year it becomes more evident that diet plays a major role in prostate cancer promotion or inhibition.

Indeed, large-scale studies tend to favor environmental rather than genetic factors as key determinants of the development of prostate cancer (Lichtenstein et al. 2000) and among these environmental factors nutrition has a leading role.

Definitive proofs of the direct link between nutrition and prostate cancer are sometimes difficult to firmly establish because of methodological problems and because etiologies are obviously complex and multifactorial.

Retrospective studies are much more numerous than prospective trials and of course can be fraught with unsuspected confounding factors.

To firmly establish the influence of dietary compounds on prostate cancer biology and behavior, we urgently need well-performed, adequately large-scale prospective trials. We also need experimental research laboratory work which support unequivocally the influence of a dietary product on prostate cancer biology.

We also have to address the patient population itself, since mentalities have to be changed. A growing subset of the population is aware of the potential link between dietary habits and prostate cancer, but it is not obvious that they are necessarily ready to change their lifestyle (Demark-Wahnefried et al. 2000).

When all these issues are addressed, ultimately the fate of millions of individuals may be changed in the future.

References

Bairati I, Meyer F, Fradet Y, Moore L (1998) Dietary fat and advanced prostate cancer. J Urol 159:1271–1275

Bonn D (1998) Vitamin E may reduce prostate cancer incidence. Lancet 351:961

Brawley OW, Thompson IM (1994) Chemoprevention of prostate cancer. Urology 43:594–599

Chan JM, Stampfer MJ, Ma J, Rimm EB, Willett WC, Giovannucci EL (1999) Supplemental vitamin E intake and prostate cancer risk in a large cohort of men in the United States. Cancer Epidemiol Biomarkers Prev 8:893–899

Clark LC, Dalkin B, Krongrad A, Combs GF Jr, Turnbull EW, Slate EH, Witherington R, Herlong JH, Janosko E, Carpenter D, Borosso C, Falk S, Rounder J (1998) Decreased incidence of prostate cancer with selenium supplementation: results of a double-blind cancer prevention trial. Br J Urol 81:730–734

Cohen JH, Kristal AR, Stanford JL (2000) Fruit and vegetable intakes and prostate cancer risk. J Natl Cancer Inst 92:61–68

Demark-Wahnefried W, Peterson B, McBride C, Lipkus I, Clipp E (2000) Current health behaviors and readiness to pursue life-style changes among men and women diagnosed with early prostate and breast carcinomas. Cancer 88:674–684

Denis L, Morton MS, Griffiths K (1999) Diet and its preventive role in prostatic disease. Eur Urol 35:377–387

Eichholzer (1996) Prediction of male cancer mortality by plasma levels of interacting vitamins: 17 years of follow-up of the prospective based study. Int J Cancer 66:145–150

Fair WR, Fleshner NE, Heston W (1997) Cancer of the prostate: a nutritional disease? Urology 50:840–848

Food, nutrition and prevention of cancer: a global perspective (1997) American Institute for Cancer Research pp 310–323

Gann PH, Ma J, Giovannucci E, Willett W, Sacks FM, Hennekens CH, et al (1999) Lower prostate cancer risk in men within elevated plasma lycopene levels: results of a prospective analysis. Cancer Res 59: 1225–1230

Giovannucci E (1999) Tomatoes, tomato-based products, lycopene, and cancer: review of the epidemiologic literature. J Natl Cancer Inst 91:317–331

Giovannucci E, Ascherio A, Rimm EB, Stampfer NJ, Colditz GA, Willett WC (1995) Intake of carotenoids and retinols in relation to risk of prostate cancer. J Natl Cancer Inst 87:1767–1776

Giovannucci E, Rimm EB, Wolk A, Ascherio A, Stampfer MJ, Colditz GA, Willett NC (1998) Calcium and fructose intake in relation to risk of prostate cancer. Cancer Res 58:442–447

Habuchi T, Suzuki T, Sasaki R, Wang L, Sato K, Satoh S, et al (2000) Association of vitamin D gene polymorphism with prostate cancer and benign prostatic hyperplasia in Japanese population. Cancer Res 60:305–308

Hanchette CL, Schwarz GG (1992) Geographic patterns of prostate cancer mortality: evidence for a preventive effect of ultraviolet radiation. Cancer 70:2861–2869

Heber D, Fair WR, Ornish D (1998) Nutrition and prostate cancer: A monograph from the CAPSURE nutrition project. 2nd edn. Cap Cure, Santa Monica, California

Hebert JR, Hurley TG, Olendzki BC, Teas J, Ma Y, Hampl JS (1998) Nutrition and socioeconomic factors in relation to prostate cancer mortality: a cross-national study. J Natl Cancer Inst 90:1637–1647

Heinonen OP, Albanes D, Virtano J, Huttunen JK, Taylor PR, Hartman AM (1998) Prostate cancer and supplementation with α-tocopherol and β-carotene: incidence and mortality in a controlled trial. J Nat Cancer Inst 90:440–446

Kelloff GJ, Lieberman R, Steele VE, Boone CN, Kopelovitch L, Malone WA, et al (1999) Chemoprevention of prostate cancer: concepts and strategies. Eur Urol 35:342–350

Konety BR, Johnson CS, Trump DL, Getzenberg RH (1993) Vitamin D in the prevention and treatment of prostate cancer. Sem Urol Oncol 17:77–84

Krisnsky NI (1998) Overview of lycopene, carotenoids and disease prevention. Proc Soc Exp Biol Med 218:95–97

Lichtenstein P, Holm NV, Verkasalo PK, Iliadou A, Kaprio J, Koskenvuo M, Pukkala E, Skytthe A, Hemminki K (2000) Environmental and heritable factors in the causation of cancer – analyses of cohorts of twins from Sweden, Denmark, and Finland. N Engl Med 343:135–136

Machlin LJ, Bendich A (1987) Free radical tissue damage: protective role of antioxidant nutrients. FASEB J 1:441–445

Miller GJ (2000) Prostate cancer among the Chinese: pathologic, epidemiologic and nutritional considerations. In: Resnick MI, Thompson IM (eds) Advanced therapy of prostate disease. BC Decker Inc. Hamilton, London, pp 18–27

Montironi R, Mazzucchelli R, Marshall JR, Bartels PH (1999) Prostate cancer prevention: review of target populations, pathological biomarkers, and chemopreventive agents. J Clin Pathol 52:793–803

Montironi R, Schulman CC (1996) Precursors of prostatic cancer: progression, regression and chemoprevention. Eur Urol 30:133–137

Moyad MA (1999) Soy, disease, prevention and prostate cancer. Sem Urol Oncol 17:97–102

Muir CS, Nectoux J, Staszewski J (1991) The epidemiology of prostatic cancer: geographical distribution and time trends. Acta Oncol 30:133–140

Nelson MA, Porterfield BW, Jacobs ET, Clark LC (1999) Selenium and prostate cancer prevention. Sem Urol Oncol.7:91–96

Norris AE, Jackson RT, Sharpe SJ, Skeaff CM (2000) Prostate cancer and dietary carotenoids. Am J Epidemiol 151:119–123

Pandali PK, Pilat MJ, Yamazaki K, Naik H, Pienta KJ (1996) The effects of Omega-3 and Omega-6 fatty acids on in vitro prostate cancer growth. Anticancer Res 16:815–820

Parkin DM, Muir CS (1992) Cancer incidence in five continents: comparability and quality of data. IARC Sci Publ 120:45–173

Peehl DM (1999) Vitamin D and prostate cancer risk. Eur Urol 35:392–394

Peto R, Doll R, Buckley JB, Sporn MB (1981) Can dietary beta-carotene materially reduce human cancer rates? Nature 290:201–208

Rohan TE, Howe GR, Burch JD, Jain M (1995) Dietary factors and risk of prostate cancer: a case-control study in Ontario, Canada. Cancer Causes Control 6:145–154

Schulman CC, Ekane S, Zlotta AR (2001) Nutrition and Prostate Cancer: Evidence or Suspicion? Urol 58:318–334

Schröder FH, Kranse R, Dijk MA, Blom MJ, Tijburg LM, Westrate JA, et al (2000) Tertiary prevention of prostate cancer by dietary intervention: results of a randomized double blind, placebo controlled, cross-over study. Eur Urol 37:A96

Thompson IA, Coltman CA (2000) Chemoprevention of prostate cancer. In: Resnick MI, Thompson IM (eds) Advanced therapy of prostate disease. BC Decker Inc. Hamilton, London, pp 428–445

Yip I, Heber D, Aronson W (1999) Nutrition and prostate cancer. Urol Clin North Am 26:403–411

Yoshizawa K, Willett WC, Morris SJ, Stampfer MJ, Spiegelman D, Rimm EB, et al (1998) Study of prediagnostic selenium level in toenails and the risk of advanced prostate cancer. J Natl Cancer Inst 90:1219–1224

Clinical Models for Testing Chemopreventative Agents in Prostate Cancer and Overview of SELECT: The Selenium and Vitamin E Cancer Prevention Trial

Eric A. Klein

E.A. Klein (✉)
Section of Urologic Oncology, Urologic Institute,
Cleveland Clinic Foundation, Desk A100, 9500 Euclid Avenue, Cleveland,
OH 44195, USA

Abstract

Target populations for chemoprevention trials should include those at higher than average risk for the development of prostate cancer as defined by explicit epidemiologic and genetic criteria. Such populations include a "primary prevention" group without histologic or clinical evidence of cancer, and several clinical models of "secondary prevention," including those with clinically evident disease prior to definitive therapy and those at high risk of recurrence after therapy based on histology and/or biochemical status. Each risk group and clinical model has potential advantages and disadvantages, and the mechanisms which underlie disease development and progression in each group may be unique. These observations give rise to many potential clinical trials of specific agents. These trials should also include collection of data on potentially confounding influences on disease development and progression. Preclinical, epidemiologic, and Phase II data suggest that both selenium and vitamin E have potential efficacy in prostate cancer prevention. The experience of the Prostate Cancer Prevention Trial (PCPT) demonstrates the interest and dedication of healthy men to long-term studies of cancer prevention. SELECT, the Selenium and Vitamin E Cancer Prevention Trial, is an intergroup phase III, randomized, double-blind, placebo-controlled, population-based clinical trial designed to test the efficacy of selenium and vitamin E alone and in combination in the prevention of prostate cancer which builds on secondary analyses of large-scale chemoprevention trials for other cancers and the lessons of PCPT.

Introduction

The identification and recruitment of high-risk study populations is necessary for the formulation and conduct of prostate cancer prevention trials. Specific clinical situations or models also need to be identified to allow for explicit selection criteria and to identify appropriate clinical and surrogate endpoints [1]. Based on the hypothesis that the specific molecular mechanisms which underlie the development and/or progression of disease in each risk group and model may be unique and that different agents may be useful for each situation, it seems apparent that multiple potential chemopreventative agents should be tried in all risk groups and clinical models to best define which agents appear promising for large-scale studies.

Potential Target Populations for Chemoprevention

Target populations appropriate for study can be subdivided into those with low- intermediate- and high-risk of developing prostate cancer based on current epidemiologic evidence [2–5]. Subgroup stratification, advantages, and disadvantages of each target group are compiled in Table 1. Several potential confounds in subgroup definitions are evident. For example, other than self-description, there is no clear agreement on what constitutes a specific racial group and use of this definition could be confounded by lack of clear criteria for inclusion. Furthermore, emerging evidence suggests that specific genetic profiles which predispose to prostate cancer may be more prevalent within specific groups, further blurring the categorical distinctions [6]. Finally, histologic criteria for the definition of risk are prone to vagaries associated with subjective interpretation of biopsy specimens and to sampling error.

Clinical Models

Testing of potentially active agents for prevention of prostate cancer in clinical models of patients with active disease is also appropriate. Collectively these models of "secondary prevention" should be considered fertile ground for identifying promising agents which may have activity in true chemoprevention trials, although they may also yield useful information on the management of patients with disease in specific clinical situations. The molecular mechanisms which underlie disease progression is likely to be different for each model, and the results for a particular model may not be generalizable. The presurgical model allows for pre-and posttreatment tissue biopsies for molecular assessment of the tumor microenvironment as modulated by an agent, making it an attractive and potentially very powerful model system both for identifying a clinical effect and for generation of new biological hypotheses. The other models rely only on clinical outcomes such as PSA progression rates, about which there is more uncertainty and less agreement as a potentially useful endpoint [7]. The advantages and disadvantages of these models are listed in Table 2.

Table 1. Target populations

Risk group	Specific population	Advantages	Disadvantages
Low	General population	Easily definable Readily available Results widely applicable	Rate of progression slow Requires large study population and long follow-up interval Studies costly
Intermediate	African Americans	Higher risk than general population	Difficult to define Difficult to recruit because of perceived bias
	Genetic Family History	Double or greater the risk of prostate cancer	Ascertainment bias Risk varies with number of affected family members, age of onset, and degree of relatedness Likely to be genetically heterogeneous
	HPC-1 linked	Genetically homogeneous	Identification invasive and costly Affected subjects rare
	Other genes	Genetically homogeneous	Identification invasive and costly Affected subjects rare Risk of progression undefined
High	High-grade PIN	Highest known risk	Sampling error Diagnosis subjective Uncommon

Table 2. Models of secondary prevention

Model	Advantages	Disadvantages
Presurgical	Early stage disease Readily available study population Pre- and posttreatment tissue available for biologic study	Treatment period short
Elevated PSA/negative biopsy	Well-defined histologic endpoint	Risk of progression undefined Sampling error
Adverse pathology after RP	High risk of progression	More advanced disease Clinical endpoint
Rising PSA after RP or RT	High risk of progression	Most advanced disease Clinical endpoint

RP, radical prostatectomy; RT, radiation therapy.

Identification of Other Risk Groups

Recognizing the limitations of current risk stratification, other additional risk groups can be defined. A useful adjunct would be the construction of a prostate-cancer specific multifactorial Gail-like model as used in chemoprevention trials of breast cancer for prediction of individual risk [8]. If validated, such a model could reduce the number of subjects needed for a large-scale prevention trial while still generating results which are widely applicable to the general population. Accumulating evidence suggests both individual and population-based variations in the metabolism of testosterone and other androgens necessary for the development of prostate cancer [9, 10], and it appears that simple biochemical tests could also be applied to individual subjects to define new risk groups. Other potential risk groups include the identification of genetically isolated populations with unique clinical characteristics, and definition of risk based on dietary and other personal habits, recognizing that no or limited data currently exists to support the existence of these groups.

Potential Confounds Bearing on the Risk of Developing Prostate Cancer

There are numerous observations in the epidemiologic literature suggesting associations between various dietary, lifestyle, genetic, and nontraditional factors and the risk of developing prostate cancer [11]. It is recognized that it will not be practicable to quantitate most of these factors in the conduct of a large-scale prevention trial, but it is recommended that data relevant to these factors be collected for secondary analysis and analysis of potential confounds for unexpected results.

SELECT: The Selenium and Vitamin E Cancer Prevention Trial

Recent research suggests that selenium and vitamin E are promising candidates for prostate cancer prevention, based primarily on secondary analyses of large-scale chemoprevention trials for other cancers. [12, 13] SELECT, the Selenium and Vitamin E Cancer Prevention Trial, is an intergroup phase III, randomized, double-blind, placebo-controlled, population-based clinical trial designed to test the efficacy of selenium and vitamin E alone and in combination in the prevention of prostate cancer.

Rationale for Study Agents

Selenium

Selenium is a nonmetallic trace element recognized as a nutrient essential to human health. Selenium is an essential constituent of at least four extracellular and cellular glutathione peroxidases, three thyroidal and extra-thyroidal iodo-thyronine 5'deiodinases, thioredoxin reductase, and other selenoproteins. Typical dietary intake of selenium in the United States is 80–120 µg/day, and the recommended dietary allowance is 0.87 µg/kg [14].

Selenium inhibits tumorigenesis in a variety of experimental models [15]. Of the more than 100 reported studies in more than two dozen animal models, two-thirds have shown reductions in tumor incidence in response to selenium supplementation. There are a number of potential mechanisms proposed for the antitumorigenic effects of selenium, including antioxidant effects, enhancement of immune function, induction of apoptosis, inhibition of cell proliferation, alteration of carcinogen metabolism, cytotoxicity of metabolites formed under high-selenium conditions, and an influence on testosterone production.

Human Observational Studies

Epidemiologic evidence suggests that selenium status may be inversely related to the risk of at least some cancers, including GI malignancies and prostate cancer [15]. A recent nested case-control study found that the risk of advanced prostate cancer was reduced by one-half to two-thirds for men with the highest selenium status [16].

Controlled Intervention Trials

Two large, randomized trials have reported findings relevant to selenium supplementation and cancer [17, 18]. In the Nutrition Intervention Trial conducted among more than 29,000 individuals aged 40–69 from the general population in Linxian, China, selenium (50 µg/day) in combination with vitamin E (30 mg/day) and β-carotene (15 mg/day) led to a 13% reduction in mortality from cancers at all sites and a 21% reduction in mortality from stomach cancer. In the second trial, also conducted in Linxian, investigators tested the hypothesis that a multivitamin/mineral (including selenium, 50 µg/day) plus β-carotene (15 mg/day) would reduce the risk of esophageal/gastric cardia cancer in a population of more than 3,000 individuals with esophageal dysplasia [18]. In this population, total cancer mortality was 7% lower and esophageal cancer was 14% lower in the supplemented group. The independent effect of selenium and the impact of supplementation on prostate cancers could not be evaluated in these trials because of the trial design and the small numbers of cases in the study population.

Recent enthusiasm for selenium in the prevention of prostate cancer arose after publication of results of the clinical trial conducted by Clark et al. [13]. In this study, 1,312 subjects with a prior history of skin cancer were randomized to receive 200 µg/day of elemental selenium in the form of selenized yeast or placebo and followed for an average of 4.5 years for the development of basal or squamous cell carcinoma of the skin and other cancers. While no difference was noted in rates of skin cancer, further analysis found that prostate cancer incidence was reduced by two-thirds among those in the selenium supplemented group. Based on a small number of cases, additional stratified analyses suggested a greater reduction in prostate cancer in those having low baseline selenium blood levels, those less than 65 years old, and those with low serum PSA values [19]. There also were significant reductions in lung and colon cancer incidences in this trial [16].

Vitamin E (α-Tocopherol)

Vitamin E is a family of naturally occurring, essential, fat-soluble vitamin compounds. Vitamin E functions as the major lipid-soluble antioxidant in cell membranes; it is a chain-breaking, free-radical scavenger and inhibits lipid peroxidation, specifically, biologic activity relevant to carcinogen-induced DNA damage [20]. The most active form of vitamin E is α-tocopherol; it is also among the most abundant and is widely distributed in nature and the predominant form in human tissues [21, 22].

Alpha-tocopherol may influence the development of cancer through several mechanisms. It has a strong inherent potential for antioxidation of highly reactive and genotoxic electrophyles, such as hydroxyl, superoxide, lipid peroxyl and hydroperoxyl, and nitrogen radicals, thereby preventing propagation of free radical damage in biological membranes, and decreasing mutagenesis and carcinogenesis [20]. Vitamin E also blocks nitrosamine formation. Alpha-tocopherol inhibits protein kinase-C activity and the proliferation of smooth muscle cells and melanoma cells [23–26]. Vitamin E also induces the detoxification enzyme NADPH:quinone reductase in cancer cell lines, and inhibits arachidonic acid and prostaglandin metabolism [27, 28]. Effects on hormones which can increase cellular oxidative stress and proliferative activity and on cell-mediated immunity have also been reported [28].

Studies suggest that vitamin E can inhibit the growth of certain human cancer cell lines, including prostate, lung, melanoma, oral carcinoma, and breast, while animal experiments show prevention of various chemically-induced tumors, including hormonally mediated tumors [29–32]. In the same studies, vitamin E has been shown to slow the growth of prostate tumors in vitro and in vivo in rats receiving various doses of chemotherapeutic agents.

The average dietary vitamin E intake among men and women in the United States is estimated to be 10 mg/day and 7 mg/day, respectively [33]. The recommended dietary allowance from the National Research Council are set at 10 mg for men and 8 mg for women daily [34].

Human Observational Studies

Evidence currently suggests that vitamin E status or intake is inversely related to risk of lung and colorectal cancers. Observational studies are inconsistent with regard to a beneficial association between serum vitamin E and prostate cancer. These studies have assessed cancer risk through estimated dietary intake or through determination of plasma or serum α-tocopherol concentrations. Of the few prospective studies having a sufficient number of prostate cancers for analysis; two reported no dose-response association, and one reported a statistically significant protective association [35–37]. A study of 2,974 subjects over a 17-year follow-up period found low α-tocopherol to be associated with higher prostate cancer risk [38]. These studies all noted lower serum or plasma vitamin E concentrations among prostate cancer cases years before diagnosis [36, 37, 38]. In a cohort analysis, the associations between prostate cancer and baseline serum and dietary α-tocopherol differed significantly according to the α-tocopherol intervention status, with the suggestion of a protective effect for total vitamin E intake among those men who also received α-tocopherol supplementation [39]. One case-control study reported no association between vitamin E intake and risk of prostate cancer [40].

Controlled Intervention Trials

One large-scale randomized, placebo-controlled trial supports the role for vitamin E in the prevention of prostate cancer: the Alpha-Tocopherol, Beta-Carotene Cancer Prevention Trial (ATBC) Study conducted in Finland, and the Nutrition Intervention Trials I and II conducted in China. The ATBC Study was a randomized, double-blind, placebo-controlled trial of α-tocopherol (50 mg synthetic dl-α-tocopheryl acetate daily) and β-carotene (20 mg daily, alone or in combination) among 29,133 male smokers 50–69 years old at entry [12, 41]. During the median follow-up period of 6.1 years, there were 246 new cases of prostate cancer and 64 deaths from prostate cancer. Among those assigned to the α-tocopherol supplementation arm of the trial (n=14,564), there were 99 incident prostate cancers compared with 147 cases among those assigned to the non-α-tocopherol arm (n=14,569) [12]. This represented a statistically significant 32% reduction in prostate cancer incidence (95% confidence interval, 12%–47%; p=0.002). The observed preventive effect appeared stronger in clinically evident cases (i.e., stages B–D) where the incidence was decreased 40% in subjects receiving α-tocopherol (95% confidence interval, -20%–55%). Prostate cancer mortality data, though based on fewer events, suggested a similarly strong effect of 41% lower mortality (95% confidence interval, –1% to –64%). Although prostate cancer was prespecified as a *secondary* endpoint in this trial, these findings suggest a potentially substantial benefit of α-tocopherol in reducing the risk prostate cancer.

SELECT Study Design

SELECT is a double-blind, placebo-controlled, 2×2 factorial study (Fig. 1) of selenium and vitamin E alone and in combination in 32,400 healthy men with a digital rectal examination (DRE) not suspicious for cancer and a serum prostate specific antigen (PSA) $\leq$4 ng/ml (Table 3). Age eligibility is 55 years for Caucasians and 50 years for African-Americans, as African-Americans aged 50–55 have comparable prostate cancer incidence rates as Caucasians aged 55–60. Randomized men will be equally distributed among four study arms (Fig. 1). Intervention will consist of a daily oral dose of study supplement and/or matched placebo according to the randomization (Fig. 1). Study duration will be 12 years, with a 5-year uniform accrual period and a minimum of seven and maximum of 12 years of intervention depending on the time of randomization.

The study supplements include 200 µg of l-selenomethionine, 400 mg of racemic α-tocopherol, and an optional multivitamin containing no selenium or vitamin E. The racemic mix of α-tocopherol will include both the d and l-isomers.

Table 3. Eligibility criteria

Age
55 years for Caucasians
50 years for African-Americans
DRE not suspicious for prostate cancer
Total serum PSA <4.0 ng/ml
No prior history of prostate cancer or high-grade prostatic intraepithelial neoplasia (PIN)
No anticoagulation therapy, except low-dose aspirin
Normal blood pressure (systolic BP<150 mmHg and diastolic BP<90 mmHg)
Willing to restrict supplementation of selenium and vitamin E during participation

Table 4. Study endpoints

Primary	
	Incident prostate cancer as determined by routine clinical care
Secondary	Prostate cancer-free survival
	Overall survival
	Incidence and survival
	All cancers
	Lung cancer
	Colorectal cancer
	Serious cardiovascular events
Other	Quality of Life Measures
	Molecular epidemiology
	Dietary Nutrient Assessment
	Biomarker Studies

Study Endpoints

The primary endpoint for the trial is the clinical incidence of prostate cancer as determined by a recommended routine clinical diagnostic work-up, including yearly DRE and serum PSA level. A centrally reviewed histologic diagnosis of prostate cancer will be required in all cases, except for those based on a total PSA >50 ng/ml and a positive bone scan. Prostate biopsy will be performed at the discretion of study physicians according to local community standards. The study protocol recommends biopsy for study participants who have a DRE suspicious for cancer and/or for elevations in serum PSA. Unlike the PCPT, no biopsy will be required at the end of SELECT.

Secondary endpoints will include prostate cancer-free survival, all cause mortality, and the incidence and mortality of other cancers and diseases potentially impacted by the chronic use of selenium and vitamin E (Table 4). Other trial objectives will include periodic quality of life assessments, assessment of serum micronutrient levels and prostate cancer risk, and studies of the evaluation of biological and genetic markers with the risk of prostate cancer.

Statistical Considerations

Sample Size Calculation

The primary analysis of the study includes five prespecified comparisons:

- Vitamin E vs. placebo
- Selenium vs. placebo
- Combination (vitamin E + selenium) vs. placebo
- Combination vs. vitamin E
- Combination vs. selenium

Table 5. Differences between the PCPT and SELECT study designs

Variable	PCPT	SELECT
Agent	Finasteride	l-selenomethionine and α-tocopherol
Eligibility criteria		
Age	≥55 years	≥50 years for African Americans; ≥55 all others
DRE	Not suspicious	Not suspicious
Total PSA	≤3.0 ng/ml	≤4.0 ng/ml
Primary endpoint	7-year prevalence	Incidence
Placebo run-in	Yes	No
Follow-up intervals	Every 3 months	Every 3 months year 1, then every 6 months
Disease ascertainment	Biopsy required	Biopsy recommended per community standard
End-of-study biopsy	Yes	No
Central lab facility	All PSAs	None
Pathology review	All biopsies	Prostate cancers only
Quality of life studies	All participants	Subset only
Secondary endpoints	Prostate cancer and screening issues	All cancer issues
African American participation	4%	Projected 20%

The study design will permit detection of a 25% reduction in the incidence of prostate cancer for selenium or vitamin E alone, with an additional 25% reduction for the combination of selenium and vitamin E compared to either agent alone. The study allows for the potential interaction between vitamin E and selenium, and additional statistical analyses will include tests for vitamin E vs. no vitamin E, selenium vs. no selenium, and for interactions between the two agents.

The overall α level for the study is 5% (two-sided), with each of the five comparisons tested at the 1% level to maintain an overall 5% level for the study. With a sample size of 32,400, the estimated power for the comparison of a single agent vs. placebo is 96% and the power for the comparison of an effective single agent vs. the combination of selenium and vitamin E is 89%. The median time under observation is estimated to be 8.8 years.

Incidence Rate

Based on PCPT, expectations are that participants will have a mean age of 63 years at study entry. The yearly prostate cancer incidence figures used in the sample-size calculations are derived from observations of the PCPT and SEER databases. The estimated incidence of prostate cancer begins at 0% at randomization, reaches 0.14% at year 1, and rises steadily to 1.36% 12 years later. The number of prostate cancer cases expected is 533 in the placebo arm, 403 in the Selenium arm, 403 in the Vitamin E arm, and 304 in the Selenium + Vitamin E arm.

Medication Rate

Medication rate is an estimate of the percentage of participants who actually take the study supplements. It is quantified as the percent of full active drug dose taken by men in each arm. It is assumed that the medication rate will vary over time, with a decline from 100% after randomization to 51% at the end of 12 years of treatment. These estimates are based on observed rates in the PCPT. Compliance with daily medication use in SELECT may be higher than PCPT because finasteride has more side effects than is known for selenium or vitamin E.

Drop-in Rate

The drop-in rate, defined as the rate of those randomized to placebo who obtain and take selenium and/or vitamin E on their own is assumed to be constant at 10% for the 12 years of treatment. Recent Heart Outcomes Prevention Evaluation (HOPE) data support this estimate. A drop-in rate of 15% reduces the power to 92% for the comparison of placebo to either single agent and 82% for an effective single agent vs. the combination.

Competing Risks – Death and Loss

The cumulative competing risk is defined to be the estimated cumulative all-cause mortality rate plus the cumulative Lost-to-Follow-Up (LTFU) rate. The mortality rates used were taken from PCPT for the first 4 years of treatment and then adjusted upwards to the 1995 United States rates for all races. The LTFU rate was calculated to be 0.05% per year. The Cumulative loss (death + LTFU) is expected to be 0.8% at the end of the first year of the study and 33.2% by the end of year 12.

Other Factors

In contrast to finasteride, it is assumed that the drugs being tested in SELECT do not affect PSA or prostate size, either of which could bias the diagnosis of prostate cancer. PSA levels at baseline and after 2 years of vitamin E use were analyzed on a subsample of participants from the HOPE trial and after 3 years in the ATBC study. There was no evidence of an effect on the PSA concentrations in these studies.

Differences Between SELECT and PCPT

The experience with PCPT has influenced the design of SELECT. These differences include broader eligibility criteria, elimination of the placebo run-in period, less frequent follow-up contacts, and reliance on community standards for the diagnosis of prostate cancer (Table 5). These changes reflect the larger sample size for SELECT, the minimal side effects expected with the study agents, and an effort to simplify data management.

References

1. Zlotta AR, Schulman CC (1999) Chemoprevention of prostate cancer. Rev Urol 1:35–40
2. Landis SH, Murray T, Bolden S, Wingo PA (1999) Cancer statistics CA Cancer J Clin 49:8–31
3. Smith JR, Freije D, Carpten JD, Gronberg H, Xu J, Issacs S, Brownstein MJ, Bova GS, Guo H, Bujnovszky P, et al (1995) Major susceptibility locus for prostate cancer on chromosome 1 suggested by a genome-wide search. Science 274:1371–1374
4. Carter BS, Bova GS, Beaty T (1993) Hereditary prostate cancer: epidemiologic and clinical features. J Urol 150:797–802
5. Zlotta AR, Schulman CC (1999) Clinical evolution of prostatic intraepithelial neoplasia. Eur Urol 35:498–503
6. Eeles RA, Durocher F, Edwards S, Teare D (1998) Linkage analysis of chromosome 1q markers in 136 prostate cancer families. Am J Human Genet 62:653–658
7. Jhaveri FM, Zippe CD, Klein EA, Kupelian PA (1999)Biochemical failure does not predict overall survival after radical prostatectomy for localized prostate cancer: 10 year results. Urology 54:884–890
8. Costantino JP, Gail MH, Pee D, Anderson S, Redmond CK, Benichou J, Wieand HS (1999) Validation studies for models projecting the risk of invasive and total breast cancer incidence. J Natl Cancer Inst 91:1541–1548
9. Paris PL, Kupelian PA, Hall J, Levin HS, Klein EA, Casey G, Witte JS (1999) Association of a CYP3A4 genetic variant and clinical presentation in African-American prostate cancer patients. Cancer Epidemiol Biomarkers Prev 10:901–990
10. Makridakis NM, Ross RK, Pike MC, Crocitto LE, Kolonel LN, Pearce CL, Henderson BE, Reichardt JK (1999) Association of mis-sense substitution in SRD5A2 gene with prostate cancer in African-American and Hispanic men in Los Angeles, USA. Lancet 354:975–978
11. Platz EA, Kantoff PW, Giovannucci E (2000) Epidemiology and risk factors for prostate cancer. In: Klein EA (ed) Management of prostate cancer. Humana Press, Totowa, NJ, pp 19–46
12. Heinonen OP, Albanes D, Huttunen JK, et al (1998)Prostate cancer and supplementation with α-tocopherol and ß-carotene: incidence and mortality in a controlled trial. J Natl Cancer Inst 90:440–446
13. Clark LC, Combs GF Jr, Turnbull BW, et al (1996) Effects of selenium supplementation for cancer prevention in patients with carcinoma of the skin. A randomized controlled trial. Nutritional Prevention of Cancer Study Group. JAMA 276:1957–1963
14. National Academy of Sciences (1989) Recommended dietary allowances, 10th edn. National Academy Press, Washington, pp 217–24
15. Combs GF Jr. Clark LC (1997) Selenium and cancer. In: Garewal H (ed) Antioxidants and disease prevention. CRC Press, New York
16. Yoshizawa K, Willett WC, Morris SJ, et al (1998) Study of prediagnostic selenium level in toenails and the risk of advanced prostate cancer. J Natl Cancer Inst 90:1219–1224
17. Blot WJ, Li JY, Taylor PR, Guo W, Dawsey S, Wang GQ, Yang CS, Zheng SF, Gail M, Li GY, Yu Y, Liu BQ, Tangrea J, Sun YH, Liu F, Fraumeni JF Jr, Zhang YH, Li B (1993) Nutrition

intervention trials in Linxian, China: supplementation with specific vitamin/mineral combinations, cancer incidence, and disease-specific mortality in the general population. J Natl Cancer Inst 85:1483–1492

18. Li JY, Taylor PR, Li B, Dawsey S, Wang GQ, Ershow AG, Guo W, Liu SF, Yang CS, Shen Q, Wang W, Mark SD, Zou XN, Greenwald P, Wu YP, Blot WJ (1993) Nutrition intervention trials in Linxian, China: multiple vitamin/mineral supplementation, cancer incidence, and disease-specific mortality among adults with esophageal dysplasia. J Natl Cancer Inst 85:1492–1498

19. Clark LC, Dalkin B, Krongrad A, et al (1998) Decreased incidence of prostate cancer with selenium supplementation: results of a double-blind cancer prevention trial. Br J Urol 81:730–734

20. Burton GW, Ingold KU (1981) Autoxidation of biological molecules. 1. The antioxidant activity of vitamin E and related chain-breaking phenolic antioxidants in vitro. J Am Chem Soc 103:6472

21. Machlin LJ (1991) Vitamin E. In LJ Machlin (ed) Handbook of vitamins, 2nd edn. Marcel Dekker, New York

22. Pappas AM (1998) Vitamin E: tocopherols and tocotrienols. In: Pappas AM (ed) Antioxidant status, diet, nutrition, and health. CRC, Boca Raton, pp 150–155

23. Azzi A, Boscoboinik D, Marilley D, Ozer NK, Stauble B, Tasinato A (1995) Vitamin E: a sensor and an information transducer of the cell oxidation state. Am J Clin Nutr 62:1337s-1346s

24. Mahoney CW, Azzi A (1988) Vitamin E inhibits protein kinase C activity. Biochem Biophys Res Commun 154:694–697

25. Chatelain E, Boscoboinik DO, Bartoli GM, et al (1993) Inhibition of smooth muscle cell proliferation and protein kinase C activity by tocopherols and tocotrienols. Biochim Biophys Acta 1176:83–89

26. Ottino P, Duncan JR (1997) Effect of alpha-tocopherol succinate on free radical and lipid peroxidation levels in BL6 melanoma cells. Free Radic Biol Med 22:1145–1151

27. Mahoney CW, Azzi A (1988) Vitamin E inhibits protein kinase C activity. Biochem Biophys Res Commun 154:694–697

28. Wang W, Higuchi CM (1995) Induction of NAD(P)H:quinone reductase by vitamins A, E and C in Colo205 colon cancer cells. Cancer Lett 98:63–69

29. Traber MG, Packer L (1995) Vitamin E: beyond antioxidant function. Am J Clin Nutr 62:1501–1504

30. Israel K, Sanders BG, Kline K (1995) RRR-alpha-tocopheryl succinate inhibits the proliferation of human prostatic tumor cells with defective cell cycle/differentiation pathways. Nutr Cancer 24:161–169

31. Kishimoto M, Yano Y, Yajima S, Otani S, Ichikawa T, Yano T (1998) The inhibitory effect of vitamin E on 4-(methylnitrosamino)-1-(3-pyridyl)-1-butanone-induced lung tumorigenesis in mice based on the regulation of polyamine metabolism. Cancer Lett 24:173–178

32. Sigounas G, Anagnostou A, Steiner M (1997) dl-alpha-tocopherol induces apoptosis in erythroleukemia, prostate, and breast cancer cells. Nutr Cancer 28:30–35

33. Umeda F, Kato K-I, Muta K, Ibayashi H (1982) Effect of vitamin E on function of pituitary-gonadal axis in male rats and human studies. Endocrinol Jpn 29:287–292

34. USDA (U.S. Department of Agriculture) (1987) Nationwide food consumption survey continuing survey of food intake by individuals: men 19–50 years 1 day, 1985, Report No. 85-3, Nutrition and Monitoring Division, Human Nutrition Information Economic Research Service, U.S. Department of Agriculture, Hyattsville, MD

35. National Research Council (NRC) (1989) Recommended dietary allowances, 10th edn. National Academy Press, Washington

36. Doll R, Peto R (1981) The causes of cancer: quantitative estimates of avoidable risks of cancer in the United States. J Natl Cancer Inst 66:1192–1308

37. Comstock GW, Helzlsouer KJ, Bush TL (1991) Prediagnostic serum levels of carotenoids and vitamin E as related to subsequent cancer in Washington County, Maryland. Am J Clin Nutr 53:260S-264S

38. Knekt P, Aromaa A, Maatala J, et al (1988) Serum vitamin E and risk of cancer among Finnish men during a 10-year follow-up. Am J Epidemiol 127:28–41
39. Hsing AW, Comstock GW, Abbey H, Polk BF (1990) Serologic precursors of cancer; retinol, carotenoids, and tocopherol and risk of prostate cancer. J Natl Cancer Inst 82:941–946
40. Eichholzer M, Stahelin HB, Gey FK, et al (1996) Prediction of male cancer mortality by plasma levels of interacting vitamins: 17-year follow-up of the prospective Basel study. Int J Cancer 55:145–150
41. Hartman TJ, Albanes D, Pietinen P, et al (1998) The association between baseline vitamin E, selenium, and prostate cancer in the Alpha-Tocopherol, Beta-Carotene Cancer Prevention Study. Cancer Epidemiol Biomarkers Prev 7:335–340
42. Rohan TE, Howe GR, Burch ID, et al (1995) Dietary factors and risk of prostate cancer: a case-control study in Ontario, Canada. Cancer Causes Control 6:145–154

Problems with Prostate-Specific Antigen Screening: A Critical Review

Hans-Peter Schmid, Ladislav Prikler, Axel Semjonow

H.-P. Schmid (✉)
Department of Urology, Kantonsspital, 9007 St. Gallen, Switzerland

Abstract

The effect of population screening with regard to reduction of prostate cancer specific mortality and quality of life issues is not yet clear. Several national and international prospective studies are currently being conducted to answer these important questions. They include the trials in the Federal State of Tyrol, Austria and in the Quebec City area, Canada, as well as the Prostate, Lung, Colorectal and Ovarian (PLCO) trial in the United States and the European Randomized Study of Screening for Prostate Cancer (ERSPC). In the meantime, individual case finding (opportunistic screening) is recommended for men with a life-expectancy of at least 10 years.

Abbreviations PSA, prostate-specific antigen; EGTM, European Group on Tumor Markers; DRE, digital rectal examination; PLCO, Prostate, Lung, Colorectal and Ovarian Cancer Screening Project; ERSPC, European Randomized Study of Screening for Prostate Cancer.

Introduction

Prostate cancer is unique among malignant tumors due to its high prevalence and relatively slow natural history (Stamey et al. 1993). Prevention is not yet possible because none of the firmly established risk factors – advancing age, race, and familial aggregation – can be influenced. Thus, nowadays, early detection strategies are the focus of attention.

Population or mass screening is defined as examination of asymptomatic men (at risk). Usually, this procedure takes place within the framework of a trial or study and is initiated by a screener. Contrary to that, early detection or opportunistic screening represents individual case finding. It is initiated by the patient being screened.

Recent Results in Cancer Research, Vol. 163
© Springer-Verlag Berlin Heidelberg 2003

The main rationale for screening for prostate cancer is that early stage disease is asymptomatic and only organ confined cancer (T1–2 N0 M0) can be cured. The criteria of the World Health Organization for screening of disease are met to a great extent in case of prostatic carcinoma (Wilson and Jungner 1969).

It is argued that the effectiveness of treatment modalities (radical prostatectomy, external beam irradiation, brachytherapy) with regard to reduction of cancer specific mortality is not yet proven. The risk–benefit balance is unclear (side effects and costs of diagnostic and therapeutic procedures). There is a considerable risk for overdiagnosis of prostate cancer given the fact that the incidence-mortality ratio for the year 2000 in the United States was 6.3 (Greenlee et al. 2001).

The primary endpoint of screening is twofold: first, the reduction of prostate cancer specific *mortality*. The goal is not to detect more and more carcinomas, nor is survival the endpoint because survival is heavily influenced by lead-time. Secondly, *quality of life* is important as expressed by quality of life adjusted gain in life years (QUALYs). In a recent short-term evaluation of quality of life in radical prostatectomy and radiation treated patients, there were no relevant differences between screen-detected and clinically diagnosed cases (Madalinska et al. 2001).

The primary tool in screening for prostate cancer is prostate-specific antigen (PSA) and its derivatives (age-adjusted PSA levels, ratio of free to total PSA, complexed PSA). Guidelines on how to best use PSA have been established by the European Group on Tumor Markers (EGTM) (Semjonow et al. 1999). Serial PSA determinations (PSA velocity and PSA doubling time) will be important in the follow-up of screened and nonscreened populations (Semjonow and Schmid 2002).

Ongoing Screening Trials

Several national and international prospective studies are being conducted to address mass screening for prostate cancer (Table1).

Federal State of Tyrol, Austria

In 1993, a prospective "natural experiment" was initiated to compare prostate cancer mortality in Tyrol, where PSA testing was introduced at no charge, with the rest of Austria, where it was not introduced. In the first year, of 65,123 men aged 45–75 years, 32.3% underwent determination of PSA (Bartsch et al. 2001). At least two-thirds of all men in this age range have been tested at least once during the first 5 years of the trial. Digital rectal examination (DRE) was not part of the screening procedure. In the beginning, the indication for prostatic biopsy was based on age referenced PSA levels and a free/total PSA ratio of less than 22%. Later on, in order to increase the speci-

Table 1. Ongoing screening trials

Trial	Geographic area	Type of trial	Total number of partici- pants	Age group (years)
Tyrol	Federal State of Tyrol, Austria	Prospective, not randomized	65,123	45–75
Quebec	Quebec City area, Canada	Prospective, randomized	46,193	45–80
PLCO	United States	Prospective, randomized	74,000	60–74
ERSPC	Finland, Sweden, Netherlands, Belgium, Italy, Spain, Switzerland	Prospective, randomized	196,500	55–69[a]

PLCO, Prostate, Lung, Colorectal and Ovarian Cancer Screening Project; ERSPC, European Randomized Study of Screening for Prostate Cancer.

[a] Core age group

ficity of the test and to reduce the number of unnecessary biopsies, bisected PSA levels and a free/total PSA ratio of less than 18% were introduced. From 1993 to 1995, the standard sextant biopsy was performed, and from 1995 ten systematic biopsies were taken. Patients underwent treatment with curative intent and there was no policy of watchful waiting.

A significant stage migration toward lower stages has been observed since the introduction of the program in Tyrol. The trends in prostate cancer mortality rates since 1993 differ significantly between Tyrol and the rest of Austria (Vutuc et al. 2001). Based on age-specific death rates, the difference between the number of expected and observed deaths from prostate cancer in Tyrol was ten in 1996, 17 in 1997, 22 in 1998 and 18 the following year (Bartsch et al. 2001).

Trials that run over a longer period of time are susceptible to changes in the protocol. In the present series, indications for and techniques of biopsies are rather heterogenous, which will certainly influence the detection rate of cancer. Important issues like rate of unnecessary biopsies, costs, quality of life, and the potential hazard of overdiagnosis are not addressed. Most striking, however, is the fact that mortality rates decreased very shortly after widespread PSA testing became available. Considering a certain lead time, this phenomenon is more likely due to opportunistic screening (early detection with PSA and DRE) in the time period between 1988 and 1993.

Quebec City Area, Canada

A prospective randomized study from Quebec showed an improvement of 67% in the relative risk of dying from prostate cancer in a screened population (Labrie et al. 1999). However, this trial was methodologically flawed and, thus, heavily criticized. The compliance for screening was only 23% and the study did not fulfill all the criteria of a strictly randomized comparison.

Prostate, Lung, Colorectal and Ovarian, United States

The Prostate, Lung, Colorectal and Ovarian (PLCO) cancer screening project was initiated in the United States by the National Cancer Institute. 74,000 men aged 60–74 years were randomly assigned to either yearly prostate cancer screening for 3 years or to a control group (Gohagan et al. 1994). The trial is expected to be completed in 2009, at which time disease specific mortality and morbidity can be compared after 12 years of follow-up. It might well be that the age group is not appropriate and that follow-up is too short to detect differences in mortality. Furthermore, there is a considerable contamination of the control group by opportunistic screening; in 1988, contamination was only 0.9%, but in 1998 it was already 38% (Legler et al. 1998).

European Randomized Study, Europe

The European Randomized Study of Screening for Prostate Cancer (ERSPC) began in 1994 and plans to enroll a total of 196,500 men in seven countries (Finland, Sweden, Netherlands, Belgium, Italy, Spain, Switzerland). In the intervention group, prostatic biopsies were performed if the PSA was more than 4 ng/ml or DRE was positive. In 1997, DRE was abandoned and PSA was lowered to 3 ng/ml (Schröder et al. 2001). In the control group, men were managed according to current clinical practice. The study aims to detect a 20% difference in cancer specific mortality by the year 2008 with a statistical power of 90%.

Several problems may arise in such a large-scale, long-lasting trial. First, there is a considerable problem with *compliance* in the intervention group. Not every man who is randomized to screening will actually participate. Not every man with an elevated PSA will undergo biopsy and, finally, not every man with prostate cancer will be treated with curative intent. As a result, the statistical power of the test is diminished. Secondly, there is a considerable *contamination* rate in the control group. The original assumption in 1994 was 12%, but meanwhile it is up to 30% (see also the chapter by Paul D.P. Pharoah, this volume). This will further decrease the statistical power and it is questionable if the trial will detect a 20% difference in mortality if there was any at all.

Thirdly, the Norwegian Urological Cancer Group decided against participating in ERSPC for the above-mentioned reasons, but also because of *ethical concerns* (Fossa et al. 2001). Assuming a positive predictive value of an elevated PSA of only 6%, 16–17 healthy men require biopsies to detect one case of cancer.

Conclusions

The currently available data *suggest* a decrease in prostate cancer-specific mortality through the introduction of population screening. Scientific proof is pending and results from important prospective randomized trials are expected in only a few years. Data on quality of life and economic issues are lacking.

In the meantime, individual case finding (opportunistic screening) should be offered to men with a life-expectancy of at least 10 years according to the guidelines of the European Association of Urology (Aus et al. 2001). Patients should be well informed about the potential benefits and harms before PSA testing. In summary, the optimal strategy for early detection of prostate cancer with PSA still remains unknown and will be a matter of debate for many years.

References

Aus G, Abbou CC, Pacik D, Schmid H-P, van Poppel H, Wolff JM, Zattoni F (2001) EAU guidelines on prostate cancer. Eur Urol 40:97–101

Bartsch G, Horninger W, Klocker H, Reissigl A, Oberaiger W, Schönitzer D, Severi G, Robertson C, Boyle P (2001) Prostate cancer mortality after introduction of prostate-specific antigen mass screening in the federal state of Tyrol, Austria. Urology 58: 417–424

Fossa SD, Eri LM, Skovlund E, Tveter K, Vatten L, for the Norwegian Urological Cancer Group (2001) No randomised trial of prostate-cancer screening in Norway. Lancet Oncol 2:741–745

Gohagan JK, Prorok PC, Kramer BS, Cornett JE (1994) Prostate cancer screening in the prostate, lung, colorectal and ovarian cancer screening trial of the National Cancer Institute. J Urol 152:1905–1909

Greenlee RT, Hill-Harmon MB, Murray T, Thun M (2001) Cancer statistics, 2001. CA Cancer J Clin 51:15–36

Labrie F, Candas B, Dupont A, Cusan L, Gomez J-L, Suburu RE, Diamond P, Levesque J, Belanger A (1999) Screening decreases prostate cancer death: first analysis of the 1988 Quebec prospective randomized controlled trial. Prostate 38:83–91

Legler JM, Feuer EJ, Potosky AL, Merrill RM, Kramer BS (1998) The role of prostate-specific antigen (PSA) testing patterns in the recent prostate cancer incidence decline in the United States. Cancer Causes Control 9:519–527

Madalinska JB, Essink-Bot ML, de Koning HJ, Kirkels WJ, van der Maas PJ, Schröder FH (2001) Health-related quality-of-life effects of radical prostatectomy and primary radiotherapy for screen-detected or clinically diagnosed localized prostate cancer. J Clin Oncol 19:1619–1628

Schröder FH, Roobol-Bouts M, Vis AN, van der Kwast T, Kranse R (2001) Prostate-specific antigen-based early detection of prostate cancer validation of screening without rectal examination. Urology 57:83–90

Semjonow A, Schmid H-P (2002) The rise and fall of PSA: clinical implications of prostate specific antigen kinetics. Urol Res 30:85–88

Semjonow A, Albrecht W, Bialk P, Gerl A, Lamerz R, Schmid H-P, Van Poppel H (1999) Tumour markers in prostate cancer: EGTM recommendations. Anticancer Res 19:2799–2801

Stamey TA, Freiha FS, McNeal JE, Redwine EA, Whittemore AS, Schmid H-P (1993) Localized prostate cancer: relationship of tumor volume to clinical significance for treatment of prostate cancer. Cancer 71:933–938

Vutuc C, Waldhoer T, Madersbacher S, Micksche M, Haidinger G (2001) Prostate cancer in Austria: impact of prostate-specific antigen test on incidence and mortality. Eur J Cancer Prev 10:425–428

Wilson JMG, Jungner G (1969) Principles and practice of screening for disease. Public Health Paper No. 34, World Health Organization, Geneva, Switzerland

Prevention and Screening of Colorectal Cancer 7

Genetic Predisposition as a Basis for Chemoprevention, Surgical and Other Interventions in Colorectal Cancer

Hansjakob Müller, Martina Plasilova, Anna Marie Russell, Karl Heinimann

Hj. Müller (✉)
Research Group Human Genetics,
Division of Medical Genetics UKBB and of Research,
Department of Clinical-Biological Sciences, University of Basel,
Vesalgasse 1, 4051 Basel, Switzerland

Abstract

Strategies of cancer prevention are generally developed with the population at large in mind. However, special attention is warranted for those persons with rare genetic traits associated with a greatly elevated risk of developing colorectal cancer (CRC) and some other malignancies: Orphan diseases demand Orphan preventive measures! Recent advances in modern genetics have enhanced our understanding of several genes and the specific germ-line mutations responsible for colorectal carcinogenesis. A number of features provide evidence for a genetic predisposition to CRC. These include typical clinical and histological features of a particular syndrome, a familial aggregation of CRC and associated malignancies, young age at onset of CRC, occurrence of multiple neoplasias and/or unusual localisation of the tumour (e.g., right side of the colon). In hereditary colorectal cancer, genetic testing can easily be demonstrated as cost-effective.

Spectrum of Predispositions for Colorectal Cancer and Associated Tumours

Approximately 5%–10% of colon cancers are related to autosomal-dominantly inherited susceptibilities. These can be subdivided into at least two major categories: those displaying hundreds and thousands of colorectal polyps, referred to as polyposis, and those without this preexisting phenomenon (see Table 1). Polyps can either be hamartomatous or adenomatous (neoplastic) in nature. Among the nonpolyposis CRC syndromes, hereditary nonpolyposis colorectal cancer (HNPCC) is a clinically and genetically quite well-characterised entity, whereas familial colorectal cancer (FCR) (Müller et al. 1994) represents a still poorly defined, heterogeneous one.

Table 1. Hereditary colorectal cancer syndromes

Traits	Mutated gene(s)	Histology of polyps	Frequency	Gastro-intestinal cancer risk
Peutz-Jeghers syndrome (PJS)	*LKB1 (STK11)*	Hamartoma	1:120,000	Increased
Juvenile polyposis (JP)	*SMAD4 (MAD4)* *BMPR1A* *PTEN?*	Hamartoma	Rare	~50%
Cowden syndrome (CS) and variants (BRRS)	*PTEN* Others	Hamartoma	Rare	Uncertain
Familial adenomatous polyposis coli (FAP)	*APC* gene	Adenoma	1:5,000/17,000	100%
HNPCC	*hMLH1* *hMLH2* *hMSH6* *hPMS1/2* *Exo1*	Adenoma	1:1,000/10,000	~80%

Hamartoma Polyposis Syndromes (HPS)

Peutz-Jeghers' syndrome (PJS) is characterised by the development of primarily benign polyps with unique histological features which occur throughout the gut, including the small intestine (70%–90% of the patients), the colon (50%), as well as in the stomach, but also by the occurrence of hyperpigmented spots (freckling) of the lips and of the oral mucosa, which become noticeable within the first 5 years of age and often fade during adulthood. Patients with PJS are at a very high risk for gastrointestinal and nongastrointestinal cancers (Giardiello et al. 2000), including breast, ovarian, cervical, colorectal, stomach, and pancreatic cancer. The relative risk of cancer at any site has been estimated to be 18 times that of the general population (Giardiello et al. 1987). The gene mutated in at least some PJS-patients is termed *LKB1* or *STK11* located on chromosome 19p13 (Wang et al. 1999). *LKB1* encodes a serine threonine kinase, the exact cellular function of which still remains to be determined. Interestingly, restoration of normal LKB1 activity in deficient cells results in G1 cell cycle arrest and growth suppression (Tiainen et al. 1999).

For Cowden syndrome (CS) (Eng 2000), the occurrence of hamartomas in various organs is typical as well as the increased risk of neoplasms of the thyroid, breast, uterus and skin (trichilemmonas). Although gastrointestinal hamartomatous polyps can regularly be found in CS patients if systematically searched for (Weber et al. 1998), the polyps are rarely symptomatic, in contrast to the other hamartoma polyposis syndromes. Bannayan-Riley-Ruvalcaca (BRRS) patients suffer from macrocephaly, hamartomatous polyps, lipomatosis, and freckling of the penis. The same mutated gene, called *PTEN* (protein tyrosine phosphatase and tensin homologue), located on chromosome 10q23, causes both syndromes: CS and BRRS. The clinical differences are due to allelic variation (allelic diversity). *PTEN*-mutations can be detected in 80% of the patients with "classic" CS and in 60% of those with BRRS (Marsh et al. 1999).

Juvenile polyposis (JP) is characterised by multiple gastrointestinal hamartomatous polyps of the colon resulting in rectal bleeding late in childhood or early adolescence. In some patients large numbers of polyps can occur throughout the gastrointestinal tract, causing failure to thrive, anaemia, hypoalbuminaemia, and abdominal pain (Stiff et al. 1995). These polyps have the histological characteristics of juvenile polyps with an expanded lamina propria infiltrated with neutrophils, eosinophils, and lymphocytes. The epithelium may show reactive hyperplasia in the presence of inflammation (Desai et al. 1995). A quarter of JP patients have been found to carry a *SMAD4*-germline mutation (Houlston et al. 1998; Friedl et al. 1999). *SMAD4*, localised on chromosome 18q21, encodes a major component in the TGFβ intracellular pathway (Howe et al. 1998). *PTEN* may also be affected in a small number of JP patients (Marsh et al. 1997). Furthermore, mutations of *BMPR1A* on chromosome 10q21-q22, which encodes a bone morphogenic protein receptor serine-threonine kinase, have been observed in JPS-patients without a *SMAD4* (*MADH4*)-defect (Zhou et al. 2001; Howe et al. 2001). Germ-line *BMPR1A* mutations might also occur in a small subset of patients with CS/BRRS and a specific colonic phenotype (Howe et al. 2001).

Familial Adenomatous Polyposis

Familial adenomatous polyposis (FAP) is defined by the presence of adenomatous (neoplastic) polyps in the colon and rectum with the inevitable development of colorectal cancer in some of them. It is estimated to occur between 1 in 8,000 and 1 in 15,000 live births and affects both sexes equally. Genetic variants of FAP include attenuated FAP (AFAP) (Spirio et al. 1993) defined by the presence of less than 100 adenomatous polyps and also the Gardner's syndrome (Gardner 1962) with extracolonic symptoms such as epidermoid skin cysts and benign osteoid tumours of the mandible and long bones. Desmoid tumours are frequent in FAP patients (Jones et al. 1986). Occasional neoplastic manifestations of FAP include hepatoblastoma (Giardiello et al. 1991), papillary carcinoma of the thyroid (Herve et al. 1995), adrenocortical tumours, and cerebellar medulloblastoma. The association with this particular brain tumour is referred to as Turcot syndrome I (Hamilton et al. 1995).

Germ-line mutations of the adenoma polyposis coli (*APC*) gene are found in the majority (approximately 70%) of FAP-patients (Fearnhead et al. 2001). In accordance with Knudson's two-hit hypothesis, somatic mutations or loss of heterozygosity (Müller and Scott, 1992) occur in the neoplastic cells on the other homologous chromosome 5 carrying the wild-type allele. Specific *APC* missense variants have been found in patients without clinical FAP, but with multiple adenomas or a carcinoma developing at young age. The *APC*-gene can be regarded as the gene for colorectal cancer. It encodes a large multidomain protein. Inactivation of APC function seems to underlie both tumour initiation related to an activation of the WNT signal transduction as well as progression through the disruption of intercellular adhesion and stability of the cytoskeleton and through the enhancement of chromosomal instability. Somatic mutations are found in the majority (~ 80%) of sporadic colorectal tumours (Powell et al. 1992).

Hereditary Nonpolyposis Colorectal Cancer

Hereditary nonpolyposis colorectal cancer (HNPCC) represents the most common cancer predisposition syndrome of the colon, and furthermore, is the most common inherited cancer syndrome. It accounts for 3%-5% (range 1%-13%) of all colon cancers (Aaltonen et al. 1998). The HNPCC-phenotype is characterised by a few polyps and early onset of multiple cancers also in the transverse and ascending portions of the colon. Clinical penetrance is high, with an 80%-85% lifetime risk of colorectal cancer and also a 40%-50% risk of endometrial cancer by the age of 80 years. In addition, there is an increased risk of developing a typical spectrum of other extracolonic malignancies, such as cancer of the small bowel, stomach, hepatobiliary tract, renal tract, and the ovaries, as well as tumours of the brain. Stringent criteria have been established for the clinical designation of a family with HNPCC, the so-called Amsterdam criteria I and II (Vasen et al. 1999). Two rare conditions can be included within this entity: The Muir-Torre syndrome, which includes patients with sebaceous gland tumours (Kolodner et al. 1994), and the Turcot syndrome II, which includes family members with glioblastoma multiforme (Hamilton et al. 1995).

HNPCC is caused by germ-line mutations of DNA mismatch repair (MMR)-genes (Jiricny and Nyström-Lahti 2000), of which two major representatives, *hMLH1* and *hMSH2*, account for 50%-70% of HNPCC families (Leach et al. 1993; Heinimann et al. 1999). Several other mismatch repair genes have been assigned to the aetiology of HNPCC, namely *hPMS1*, *hPMS2* (Nicolaides et al. 1994), and *hMSH6* (Palombo et al. 1995). Also, mutations of other genes such as CACR1 (Tomlinson et al. 1999) and TGF-β-type II receptor gene (Lu et al. 1998) may be related to a HNPCC-phenotype. Germ-line mutations of the *EXO1* gene have also been found in patients with HNPCC and atypical HNPCC forms (Wu et al. 2001).

Familial Colorectal Cancer

Their remains a clinically and biologically ill-defined category of familial colorectal cancers (FCRC) where a preexisting polyposis is not apparent and patients do not fulfil the so-called Amsterdam Criteria I or II (Vasen et al. 1999) or the Bethesda Guidelines (Rodriguez-Bigas et al. 1997) in order to be classified to suffer from HNPCC (see below).

Penetrance and Expressivity of Known Cancer Genes

Mutated genes predisposing to hereditary cancer syndromes generally exhibit considerable variation of penetrance and expressivity. This causes serious difficulty when an individual mutation carrier seeks medical help since it is not possible to predict exactly the development of cancer in his/her colon and therefore to suggest the best kind of preventive measures and therapy considering that heroic measures such as colectomy have to be taken into consideration.

The wide variation in phenotypic appearance of FAP in patients with specific APC mutations, even those belonging to the same family, is in relation to polyp number, age of onset, and especially extracolonic manifestations. The modifying factors, genetic or environmental in nature, which may influence the clinical manifestation of a particular so-called monogenetic disposition have yet to be identified. The understanding of the role that different molecular events play in tumour development and their interaction with environmental and dietary components may help to establish preventive strategies more tailored to the particular needs of an individual.

The identification of *Mom1* as a major modifier locus affecting *ApcMin*-induced intestinal neoplasia in the mouse (Dietrich et al. 1993) and the presumption of the secretory phospholipase A2 gene as a candidate for the *Mom1*-locus (MacPhee et al. 1995) prompted us to assess the role of the homologue human gene in 97 FAP patients with variable disease expression. However, since only two silent polymorphisms were found, the *sPLA2*-gene could be excluded as a major modifier in FAP (Dobbie et al. 1996). Linkage analysis in a large Swiss kindred which harbours a 5945delA mutation of the *APC* gene and presents a considerable phenotypic variation indicated the presence of a modifier locus on chromosome 1p35-p36 (Dobbie et al. 1997) which has to be identified and characterised.

We have tried to determine the expression of genes coding for putative anticancer targets including *COX2, iNOS, MMP-7, ODC, PKCβ, PPARγ, RXRα, RXRβ, RXRγ* using TaqMan analysis in normal and adenomatous tissue from FAP patients and healthy individuals (Humar et al. 2001) and observed considerable interindividual variation. However, some of our findings may contribute to the design of future chemoprevention and therapy studies. The data suggests *PKCβ and MMP-7* to be the most suitable cancer targets among the genes studied and that a combination of chemopreventive agents could be more effective than using only one alone.

Since a MMR deficiency does not explain the phenotypic heterogeneity observed among MMR gene mutation carriers, we investigated the influence of various potentially modifying genes on disease expression in HNPCC. Determination of the N-acetyltransferase 2 (*NAT2*) genotype in 26 unaffected and 52 cancer-affected *hMLH1/hMSH2* mutation carriers revealed that slow acetylators were significantly more prevalent in the group of affected mutation carriers, suggesting a protective effect of the NAT2 rapid acetylator phenotype (Heinimann et al. 1999).

Identification of Novel Genetic Pathways and Genes Predisposing to Hereditary and Familial Colorectal Cancer

Most familial cases of colorectal cancer (FCRC) cannot be attributed to these hereditary genetic CRC syndromes and often the underlying predisposition of a clinically suspected syndrome cannot be shown to be caused by the mutation of one of the responsible genes as mentioned in Table 1. This failure is only partly due to the limitations of the conventional mutation detection techniques. This situation causes frustration and uncertainty among the patients, their relatives, and also the responsible physicians. Presymptomatic genetic testing can not be offered as this impedes proper genetic counselling and demands further research to clarify the underlying mechanisms in polyp formation and cancer.

Despite the use of several screening techniques, no pathogenic germ-line mutation in the APC-gene can be found in about 30% of individuals with classical FAP and 90% of those with AAPC/multiple adenomas (Miyoshi et al. 1992; Armstrong et al. 1997; Lamlum et al. 2000; Sieber et al. 2002). Besides the limited sensitivity of the screening methods applied, large genomic deletions/insertions, mutations in regulatory regions, epigenetic gene silencing, as well as an involvement of other predisposition gene(s) may account for the inability to identify APC-germ-line mutations.

Quantitative measures (Yan et al. 2001) showed that at least in some of the affected APC-negative patients the expression of one APC-gene may be impaired by as yet unknown reasons, leading to tumour formation as soon as the normally expressed gene is lost in a colonic cell. Similar decreases in gene expression may be found to cause other hereditary diseases which cannot be detected by conventional mutational analysis.

Similarly, in 15%–55% of HNPCC families fulfilling the Amsterdam criteria, no pathogenic mutation in any MMR-genes can be identified, suggesting involvement of other genes such as EXO1 or TGFβ in the pathogenesis of this syndrome (see above). Thus, the spectrum and sequence of the molecular genetic events involved in tumourigenesis in the yet "mutation-negative" FAP, HNPCC and FCRC patients remain to be determined.

Recommended Options for Prevention

The incidence of neoplasia in PJS patients, most of which occur outside the gastrointestinal tract, is in the range at which surveillance programs have been advocated in other high risk conditions. Also in the other hamartomatous cancer syndromes the improved methods of detection and screening of at-risk individuals represent the progress of present-day medical care. Chemopreventive measures have usually not been considered for HPS patients so far although, e.g., the JP genetic pathway (*SMAD4*) is commonly involved in colorectal carcinogenesis.

The identification of an APC mutation, as confirmation of a clinical diagnosis of FAP following detection of polyps, usually leads to a consideration of prophylactic colectomy as the treatment of choice for adolescents. Because CRC can occur in the rectal segment, most investigators favour proctocolectomy with mucosal proctectomy and ileoanal pullthrough (with pouch formation) or proctocolectomy with Brooke or continent ileostomy (Giardiello et al. 2001). However, colectomy is generally not performed on a polyp-free colon in heterozygotes for APC mutations (Petersen and Brensinger 1996). A careful surveillance of the upper GI tract is indicated in colectomised FAP patients. Annual physical examination of the thyroid along with consideration of ultrasonography is warranted (Giardiello et al. 1993).

A reduction of the number of polyps in FAP-patients has been observed after treatment with the nonsteroidal anti-inflammatory drugs sulindac (Giardiello et al. 1993) and celecoxib (Steinbach et al 2000). However, standard doses of sulindac cannot prevent the development of adenomas in subjects with the FAP-predisposition (Giardiello et al 2002). Therefore, it is not surprising that no authority has advocated the use of these agents for primary treatment of FAP.

Aspirin, which is thought to act as a chemopreventive agent via inhibition of cyclooxygenase-2, is currently assessed for its ability to induce adenoma regression and decrease colorectal cancer mortality in FAP and HNPCC germline mutation carriers [CAPP (Concerted Action Polyp prevention) studies 1 and 2] (Burn et al. 1998). In a recent population based cohort, the reduction in CRC risk appeared to be dose- and duration-dependent. Long-term users of 300 mg or more of aspirin daily exhibit a relative risk of 0.6, whereas no association was found with daily doses of 75 mg and 150 mg aspirin (Rodriguez and Huerta-Alarez 2001). Recently, a novel action mechanism for the antitumourigenic effects of aspirin has been described showing that the drug also activates the NF-kB signalling pathway to induce apoptosis in colon cancer cell lines (Stark et al. 2001). A variety of dietary components, including nonstarch polysaccharide or fibre, vitamins C and E, and calcium, have been observed to prevent or even reverse polyp development (see other chapters of this volume).

Colonoscopic polypectomy is the widely accepted option for the management of patients with germ-line mutations of one of the *MMR*-genes (Giardiello et al. 2001). The improvement in fibre-optics and other technical innovations have greatly improved the efficacy and safety of endoscopy. Based on the very high rate of synchronous and metachronous colon cancer development in HNPCC patients, subtotal colectomy has been recommended at the initial diagnosis of a CRC (Lynch et al. 1997). Others feel that the surgical approach should be offered when a polyp is first detected. The issue of prophylactic colectomy in HNPCC is complex due to the following: penetrance is not 100% in *MMR*-gene mutation carriers; there remains an increased risk of rectal cancer

(Rodrigues-Bias et al. 1997); the flat or plaque like polyps occurring occasionally in HNPCC-patients can more easily be missed by colonoscopy; adenomas in HNPCC patients may grow more rapidly and more aggressively, and finally mortality from the surgical procedure is a risk. Women with an HNPCC predisposition should also be screened for endometrial cancer and cancer of the ovaries. Prophylactic hysterectomy and bilateral salpingo-opherectomy remain viable options to be considered after childbearing (Burke et al. 1997). Endometrial cancer represents the most common clinical manifestation among female hMSH6 mutation carriers (Wijnen et al. 1999), indicating that the prevention of CRC cannot be the only aim in HNPCC.

Chemopreventive or dietary options to be discussed include the beneficial regular use of aspirin (see above), postmenopausal hormone replacement, dietary calcium, and fibre intake (see other chapters of this volume). High intake of red meat and animal fat, obesity, and sedentary lifestyle are considered to be additional risk factors for HNPCC which have to be avoided.

Potential New Areas of Chemoprevention: Prevention or Intensification of Genomic Instability

A potential approach for preventing carcinogenesis in hereditary CRC cancer syndromes is the reintroduction of the wild-type allele into cells suffering from the second hit leading to tumour development by the means of gene therapy or by the introduction of selection barriers which arrest the outgrowth of cancerous cells. A possible alternative preventive measure would be to render malignant cells so genetically unstable that they exceed the threshold of viability so that apoptotic pathways are activated and cell death ensues. Genomic instability could be a promising target for new chemopreventive options, since it is a characteristic of CRC occurring as a consequence of *APC*- or *MMR*-gene germ-line mutations.

Two different types of genomic instability, chromosomal instability (CIN) and microsatellite instability (MIN) can be observed in most cases of CRC. They seem to have in common the ability to increase the rate of progression along the path to clinical cancer.

CIN is related to mutations of the *APC* gene, which are inherited in a heterozygous state in FAP, but also occur in the early stages of sporadic colorectal cancer (Kinzler and Vogelstein 1996). Recent studies have shown that the C-terminus of APC is involved in the maintenance of chromosomal stability during mitosis. APC is localised to the kinetochore of metaphase chromosomes and this localisation is likely to be dependent on the interaction between APC and EB1 (Kaplan et al. 2001). Centrosome abnormalities, the emergence of chromosomal breakage and rearrangements characterise the transit along the path to clinical cancer. This is referred to as chromosomal instability (CIN) (Lengauer 1998). CRC occurring in FAP patients sporadically show mostly complex chromosome aberrations at diagnosis

Another type of genomic instability, which is called microsatellite instability (MIN or MSI), is associated with colon cancer belonging to HNPCC. Inherited mutations of the mismatch-repair (MMR) genes, most frequently *hMSH2* and *hMLH1*, are responsible for this hereditary cancer syndrome, leading to elevated rates (around 1,000-fold) of mutations of specific loci (Bhattacharya et al. 1974), among them the *TGFβR2* gene (Markowitz et al. 1995; Peltomäki 2001). MSI has, therefore, emerged as an important pathway in tumorigenesis and has important implications for diagnosis and treatment of patients with malignancies showing abnormalities in MMR, allowing the prediction of response to conventional therapy (Elsaleh et al. 2000), as well as opening up opportunities for novel forms of CRC treatment (Wantanabe et al. 2001). The presence of a high-frequency MSI (MSI-high) has been shown to be independently predictive of a relatively favourable outcome of sporadic CRC, including reduced likelihood of metastases (Gryfe et al. 2000; Heinimann et al. 2000). Further confirmation in further studies with detailed information on the MMR gene and the MSI status is needed.

Ruschoff et al. (1998) observed that the administration of aspirin resulted in the suppression of microsatellite instability in a subset of MMR-deficient CRC cancer cell lines. The time- and dose-dependent effect on the induction of apoptosis was due to selection for cells that retain stable microsatellites rather than an antiproliferative effect. As yet, however, it is not clear whether the instability phenomenon can be used for the derivation of new strategies for prevention of the initiation of CRC or for the suppression of the clinical onset of CRC.

Conclusions

1. Hereditary colorectal cancers are among the best in vivo models to study colorectal carcinogenesis and the influence of preventive measures. Improved understanding of clinical manifestation, genetics and the biology of cancer predisposition will allow, in time, the delineation and institution of new preventive strategies to reduce the burden of CRC not only in persons with such a trait, but also in the population at large.
2. In hereditary CRC syndromes preventive measures cannot be limited only to the gut since other organs are at an increased cancer risk.
3. A comprehensive understanding of the genetic events prior to, early on, during, or late in colorectal carcinogenesis is a prerequisite for informative DNA screening of stool samples to detect colorectal cancer (Traverso et al. 2002)
4. The benefits of genetic testing and counselling in clinical practice and prevention/intervention strategies of CRC include not only removal of patient uncertainty, greater choice of surgical and other intervention options, and elimination of unnecessary conventional screening, but also provide information for family planning and career decisions.

5. With regard to prevention, consideration must not only be given to medical options, but also to measures the person at risk can take on their own initiative, such as changes in their dietary habits or physical activity.

Acknowledgements. Our research was supported by grants from the Swiss National Foundation (3200-055664.98, 3200-064171.00, 3138-051088.1) and by the Freiwillige Akademische Gesellschaft Basel, by SwissBridge Zürich and by the Krebsforschung Schweiz (932-09-1999).

References

Aaltonen LA (1998) Molecular epidemiology of hereditary non-polyposis colorectal cancer in Finland. Recent Results Cancer Res 154:306–311

Bhattacharya NP, Skandalis A, Ganesh A, Groden J, Meuth M (1994) Mutator phenotype in human colorectal carcinoma cell lines. Proc Natl Acad Sci USA 91:6319–6323

Burke W, Petersen G, Lynch P, Botkin J, Daly M, Garber J, Kahn MJ, McTierman A, Offit K, Thomson E, Varricchio C (1997) Recommendations for follow-up care of individuals with an inherited predisposition to cancer. I. Hereditary nonpolyposis colon cancer. JAMA 277:915–919

Burn J, Chapman PD, Bishop DT, Mathers J (1998) Diet and cancer prevention: the concerted action polyp prevention (CAPP) studies. Proc Nutr Soc 57:183–186

Desai DC, Murday V, Phillips RKS, Neale KF, Milla P, Hodgson S (1998) A survey of phenotypic features in juvenile polyposis. J Med Genet 35:467–481

Dietrich WF, Lander ES, Smith JS, Moser AR, Gould KA, Luongo C, Borenstein N, Dove W (1993) Genetic identification of Mom-1, a major modifier locus affecting Min-induced intestinal neoplasia in the mouse. Cell 75:631–639

Dobbie Z, Heinimann K, Bishop DT, Müller HJ, Scott RJ (1997) Identification of a modifier gene locus on chromosome 1p53-36 in familial adenomatous polyposis. Hum Genet 99:653–657

Dobbie Z, Spycher M, Mary JM, Häner M, Guldenschuh I, Hürlimann R, Amman R, Roth J, Müller Hj, Scott RJ (1996) Correlation between the development of extracolonic manifestations in FAP patients and mutations beyond codon 1403 in the APC gene. J Med Genet 33:274–280

Elsaleh H, Joseph D, Grieu F, Zeps N, Spry N, Iacopetta B (2000) Association of tumor site and sex with survival benefit from adjuvant chemotherapy in colorectal cancer. Lancet 355:1745–1750

Eng C (2000) Will the real Cowden syndrome please stand up: revised diagnostic criteria. J Med Genet 37:828–830

Fearnhead NS, Britton MP, Bodmer WF (2001) The APC of APC. Hum Mol Genet 10:721–733

Friedl W, Kruse R, Uhlhaas S, Stolte M, Schartmann B, Keller KM, et al (1999) Frequent 4-bp deletion in exon 9 of the SMAD4/MADH4 gene in familial juvenile polyposis patients. Genes Chromosomes Cancer 25:403–406

Gardner EJ (1962) Follow-up study of a family group exhibiting dominant inheritance for a syndrome including intestinal polyps, osteomas, firbomas and epidermal cysts. Am J Hum Genet 14:376–390

Giardiello FM, Welsh SB, Hamilton SR, Offenhaus GJ, Gittelsohn AM, Brooker SV, Krush AJ, Yardley JH, Luk GD (1987) Increased risk of cancer in Peutz-Jeghers syndrome. N Engl J Med 316:1511–1414

Giardiello FM, Offerhaus GJ, Krush AJ, Booker SV, Tersmett AC, Mulder JW, Kelley CN, Hamilton SR (1991) Risk of hepatoblastoma in familial adenomatous polyposis. J Pediatr 119:766–768

Giardiello FM, Offerhaus GJA, Lee DH, Krush AJ, Tresmetta AC, Booker SV, Kelley NC, Hamilton SR (1992) Increased risk of thyroid and pancreatic carcinoma in familial adenomatous polyposis. Gut 34:1393–1396

Giardiello FM, Hamilton S, Krush A, Piantadosi S, Hylind L, Celano P, Booker SV, Robinson CR, Offerhaus GJ (1993) Treatment of colonic and rectal adenomas with sulindac in familial adenomatous polyposis. N Engl J Med 328:1313–1316

Giardiello FM, Brensinger JD, Tersmette AC, Goodmann SN, Petersen GM, Brooker SV, Cruz-Correa M, Offerhaus JA (2000) Very high risk of cancer in familial Peutz-Jeghers syndrome. Gastoenterology 119:1447–1453

Giardiello FM, Brensinger JD, Petersen GM (2001) AGA Technical review on hereditary colorectal cancer. Gastroenterology 212:198–213

Giardiello FM, Yang VW, Hylind LM, Krush AJ, Petersen GM, Trimbath JD, Piantadosi S, Garrett E, Geiman DE, Hubbard W, Offerhausen JA, Hamilton SR (2002) Primary chemoprevention in familial adenomatous polyposis with sulindac. N Engl J Med 346:1054–1059

Gryfe R, Kim H, Hsieh ET, Aronson MD, Holowaty EJ, Bull SB, Redston M, Gallinger S (2000) Tumor microsatellite instability and clinical outcome in young patients with colorectal cancer. N Engl J Med 342:69–77

Hamilton SR, Liu B, Parsons RE, Papadopoulos N, Jen J, Powell SM, Krush AJ, Berk T, Cohen Z, Tetu B, et al (1995) The molecular basis of Turcot's syndrome. New Engl J Med 332:839–847

Heinimann K, Scott RJ, Buerstedde JM, Weber W, Siebold K, Attenhofer M, Müller Hj, Dobbie Z (1999) Influence of selection criteria on mutation detection in patients with hereditary nonpolyposis colorectal cancer. Cancer 85:2512–2518

Heinimann K, Scott RJ, Chappuis P, Weber W, Müller HJ, Dobbie Z, Hutter P (1999) N-actyltransferase 2 influences cancer prevalence in hMLH1/hMSH2 mutation carriers. Cancer Res 59:3038–3040

Heinimann K, Müller Hj, Dobbie Z (2000) Microsatellite instability in colorectal cancer. N Engl J Med 342:1607–1608

Herve R, Farret O, Mayaudon H, Helie C, Denee JM, Bauduceau B, Molinie C (1995) Association of Gardner syndrome and thyroid carcinoma. Presse Med 24:415

Houlston RS, Tomlinson IP (1998) Modifier genes in humans: strategies for identification. Eur J Hum Genet 6:80–88

Howe JR, Bair JL, Sayed MG, Anderson ME, Mitros FA, Petersen GM, Velulescu VE, Traverso G, Vogelstein B (2001) Germline mutations of the gene encoding bone morphogenetic protein receptor 1A in juvenile polyposis. Nat Genet 28:184–187

Howe JR, Roth S, Ringold JC, Summers RW, Järvinen HJ, Sistonen P, Tomlinson IPM, Houlston RS, Bevan S, Mitros FA, Stone EM, Aaltonen LA (1998) Mutations in the SMAD4/DPC4 gene in juvenile polyposis. Science 280:1086–88

Humar B, D'Orazio D, Albrecht C, Bauerfeind P, Müller Hj, Dobbie Z, Bendik I (2001) Expression of putative anticancer targets in familial adenomatous polyposis and its association with the APC mutation status. Int J Oncol 19:1179–1186

Jiricny J, Nyström-Lahti M (2000) Mismatch repair defects in cancer. Curr Opin Genet Dev 10:157–161

Jones IT, Jagelman DG, Fazio VW, Lavery IC, Weakley FL, McGannon E (1986) Desmoid tumors in familial polyposis coli. Ann Surg 204:94–97

Kaplan KB, Burds AA, Swedlow JR, Bekir SS, Sorger PK, Näthke IS (2001) A role for the Adenomatous Polyposis Coli protein in chromosome segregation. Nat Cell Biol 3:429–432

Kinzler KW, Vogelstein B (1996) Lessons from hereditary colorectal cancer. Cell 87:159–170

Kolodner RD, Hall NR, Lipford J, Kane MF, Rao MR, Morrison P, Wirth L, Finan PJ, Burn J, Chapman P (1994) Structure of the human MSH2 locus and analysis of two Muir-Torre kindreds for msh2 mutations. Genomics 24:516–526

Lamlum H, Tassan AI, Jaeger E, Frayling I, Sieber O, Reza FB, Eckert M, Rowan A, Barclay Y, Atkin W, Williams C, Gilbert J, Cheadle J, Bell J, Houlston R, Bodmer W, Sampson J, Tomlinson I (2000) Germline APC variants in patients with multiple colorectal adenomas, with evidence for the particular importance of E1317Q. Hum Mol Genet 9:2215–2221

Leach FS, Nicholaides NC, Papadopoulos N, Liu B, Jen J, Paarson R, Peltomaki P, Sistonen P, Aaltonen LA, Nystrom-Lahti M, et al (1993) Mutations of the Mut S homolog in hereditary non-polyposis colorectal cancer. Cell 75:1215–1225

Lengauer C, Kinzler KW, Vogelstein B (1998) Genetic instability in human cancers. Nature 396:643–649

Lu SL, Kawabata M, Imamura T, Akiyama Y, Nomizu T, Miyazono K, Yuasa Y (1998) HNPCC associated with germline mutation in the TGF-beta type II receptor gene. Nat Genet 19:17–18

Lynch HT, Smyrk T, Lynch J (1997) An update of HNPCC (Lynch syndrome) Cancer Genet Cytogenet 93:84–99

MacPhee M, Chepenik KP, Liddell RA, Nelson KK, Siracusa LD, Buchberg AM (1995) The secretory phospholipase A2 gene is a candidate for the Mom1 locus, a major modifier of ApcMin-induced intestinal neoplasia. Cell 81:957–966

Markowitz S, Wang J, Myeroff L, Parsons R, Sun L, Lutterbaugh J, Fan RS, Zborowska E, Kinzler KW, Vogelstein B, et al (1995) Inactivation of the type II TGF-α receptor in colon cancer cells with microsatellite instability. Science 268:1336–1338

Marsh DJ, Dahia PLM, Zheng Z, Liaw D, Parsons R, Gorlin RJ, Eng C (1997) Germline mutations in PTEN are present in Bannayan-Zonana syndrome. Nat Genet 16:333–334

Marsh DJ, Kum JB, Lunetta KL, Bennett MJ, Gorlin RJ, Ahmed SF, Bodurtha J, Crowe C, Curtis MA, Dasouki M, Dunn T, Feit H, Geraghty MT, Graham JM Jr, Hodgson SV, Hunter A, Korf BR, Manchester D, Miesfeldt S, Murday VA, Nathanson KL, Parisi M, Pober B, Romano C, Eng C, et al (1999) PTEN mutation and genotype-phenotype correlations in Bannayan-Ruvalcaba syndrome suggest a single entity with Cowden syndrome. Hum Mol Genet 8:1461–1472

Miyoshi Y, Ando H, Nagase H, Nishisho I, Horii A, Miki Y, Mori T, Utsunomiya J, Baba S, Petersen G, et al (1992) Germ-line mutations of the APC gene in 53 familial adenomatous polyposis patients. Proc Natl Acad Sci USA 89:4452–4456

Müller Hj, Heinimann K, Dobbie Z (2000) Genetics of hereditary colon cancer – a basis for prevention? Eur J Cancer 36:1215–1223

Müller Hj, Scott R (1992) Hereditary conditions in which loss of heterozygosity may be important. Mutat Res 284:15–24

Müller Hj, Scott R, Weber W, Meier R (1994) Colorectal cancer: lessons for genetic counseling and care for families. Clin Genet 46:106–114

Nicolaides NC, Papadopoulos N, Liu B, Wei YF, Carter KC, Ruben SM, Rosen CA, Haseltine WA, Fleischmann RD, Fraser CM, et al (1994) Mutations of two PMS homologues in hereditary nonpolyposis colon cancer. Nature 37:75–80

Palombo F, Gallinari P, Iaccarino I, Lettieri T, Hughes M, D'Arrigo A, Truong O, Hsuan JJ, Jiricny J (1995) GTBP, a 160-kilodalton protein essential for mismatch-binding activity in human cells. Science 268:1912–1914

Peltomäki P (2001) Deficient DNA mismatch repair: a common etiologic factors in colon cancer. Hum Mol Genet 10:735–740

Petersen GM, Brensinger JD (1996) Genetic testing and counseling in familial adenomatous polyposis. Oncology 10:89–94

Powell SM, Zilz N, Beazer-Barclay Y, Bryan TM, Hamilton SR, Tribodeau SN, Vogelstein B, Kinzler KW (1992) APC mutations occur early during colorectal tumorigenesis. Nature 359:235–237

Rodriguez LAG, Huerta-Alvarez C (2001) Reduced risk of colorectal cancer among long-term users of aspirin and nonaspirin nonsteroidal antiinflammatory drugs. Epidemiology 12:88–93

Rodriguez-Bigas MA, Boland CR, Hamilton SR, Henson JR, Jass JR, Khan PM, Lynch H, Perucho M, Smyrk T, Sobin L, Srivasta S (1997) A National Cancer Institute workshop on hereditary nonpolyposis colorectal cancer syndrome: meeting highlights and Bethesda guidelines J Natl Cancer Inst 89:1758–1762

Ruschoff J, Wallinger S, Dietmaier W, Bocker T, Brockhoff G, Hofstadter F, Fishel R (1998) Aspirin suppresses the mutator phenotype associated with hereditary nonpolyposis colorectal cancer by genetic selection. Proc Natl Acad Sci USA 95:11301–11306

Sieber OM, Lamlum H, Crabtree MD, Rowan AJ, Barclay E, Lipton L, Hodgson S, Thomas HJ, Neale K, Phillips RK, Farrington SM, Dunlop MG, Mueller Hj, Bisgaard ML, Bulow S, Fidalgo P, Albuquerque C, Scarano MI, Bodmer W, Tomlinson IP, Heinimann K (2002) Whole-gene APC deletions cause classical familial adenomatous polyposis, but not attenuated polyposis or "multiple" colorectal adenomas. Proc Natl Acad Sci USA 99:2954-2958

Spirio L, Olschwang S, Groden J, Robertson M, Samowitz W, Joslyn G, Gelbert L, Thliveris A, Carlson M, Otterud B, et al (1993) Alleles of the APC gene: an attenuated form of familial polyposis. Cell 75:951-957

Stark LA, Din FVN, Zwacka RM, Dunlop MG (2001) Aspirin-induced activation of the NF-kB signalling pathway: a novel mechanism for aspirin-mediated apoptosis in colon cancer cells. FASEB J 15:1273-1275

Steinbach G, Lynch PM, Phillips RK, Wallace MH, Hawk F, Gordon GB, et al (2000) The effect of celecoxib, a cyclooxygenase-2 inhibitor, in familial adenomatous polyposis. N Eng J Med 342:1946-1952

Stiff GJ, Alwafi A, Jenkins H, Lari J (1995) Management of infantile polyposis syndrome. Arch Dis Child 73:253-254

Tiainen N, Ylikorkala Y, Makela TP (1999) Growth suppression by Lkb1 is mediated by a G1 cell cycle arrest. Proc Natl Acad Sci USA 96:9248-9251

Tomlinson I, Rahman N, Frayling I, Mangion J, Barfoot R, Hamoudi R, et al (1999) Inherited susceptibility to colorectal adenomas and carcinomas: Evidence for a new predisposition gene on 15q14-q22. Gastroenterology 116:789-795

Traverso G, Shuber A, Levin B, Johnson C, Olsson L, Schoetz DJ Jr, Hamilton SR, Boynton K, Kinzler KW, Vogelstein B (2002) Detection of APC mutations in fecal DNA from patients with colorectal tumors. N Engl J Med 346:311-320

Vasen HFA, Watson P, Mecklin JP; Lynch HAT and the ICG-HNPCC (1999) New clinical criteria for hereditary nonpolyposis colorectal cancer (HNPCC, Lynch syndrome) proposed by the International Collaborative Group on HNPCC. Gastroenterology 116:1453-1456

Wang ZJ, Chrchman M, Avizienyte E, McKoewn C, Davies S, Evans DG, Ferguson A, Ellis I, Xu WH, Yan ZY, Aaltonen LA, Tomlinson IP (1999) Germline mutations of the LKB1 (STK11)gene in Peutz-Jeghers patients. J Med Genet 36:365-368

Watanabe T, Wu TT, Catalano PJ, Ueki T, Satriano R, Haller DG, Benson AB 3rd, Hamilton SR (2001) Molecular predictors of survival after adjuvant chemotherapy for colon cancer. N Engl J Med 344:1196-1206

Weber HC, Marsh D, Lubensky I, Lin A, Ent C (1998) Germline PTEN/MMAC1/TEP1 mutations and association with gastrointestinal manifestations in Cowden disease. Gastroenterology Suppl 114S:G2902

Wijnen J, de Leeuw W, Vasen H, van der Klift H, Moller P, Storkmorken A, Meijers-Heijboer H, Lindhout D, Menko F, Vossen S, Moslein G, Tops C, Brocker-Vriends A, Wu Y, Hofstra R, Sijmons R, Cornelisse C, Morreau H, Fodde R (1999) Familial endometrial cancer in female carriers of MSH6 germline mutations. Nat Genet 23:142-144

Wu Y, Berends MJW, Post JG, Mensink RG, Verlind E, Van der Sluis T, Kempinga C, Sijmons H, Van der Zee AGJ, Holleman H, Kleibeuker JH, Buys HCM, Hofstra RMW (2001) Germline mutations of EXO1 gene in patients with hereditary nonpolyposis colorectal cancer (HNPCC) and atypical HNPCC forms. Gastroenterology 120:1580-1587

Yan H, Dobbie Z, Gruber SB, Markowitz S, Romans K, Giardiello FM, Kinzler KW, Vogelstein B (2002) Small changes in expression affect predisposition to tumorigenesis. Nat Genet 30:25-26

Fecal Occult Blood Screening – Trial Evidence, Practice and Beyond

Gad Rennert

G. Rennert (✉)
Department of Community Medicine and Epidemiology,
Carmel Medical Center and Technion Faculty of Medicine,
and Clalit Health Services (CHS) National Cancer Control Center,
7 Michal St., Haifa 34362, Israel

Abstract

Colorectal cancer is a leading cause of morbidity and mortality in Western countries. Primary prevention and early detection of this malignancy has been shown in multiple research set-ups, and using different modalities, to be effective in reducing the incidence and mortality rates of this disease. Three randomized controlled trials have been conducted over the last 30 years to evaluate the efficacy of periodic screening with fecal occult blood tests (FOBT). These studies have consistently demonstrated mortality reduction with biennial as well as annual testing after 8–18 years of follow-up. A significant primary prevention effect through reduction of colorectal cancer incidence was also reported. The results of the Israeli population-based screening program using Hemocclut Sensa show that it is possible to achieve a high detection rate in a well-organized community set-up and, in addition, also a shift in tumor stage towards smaller tumors, a low positivity rate, and an acceptable false positivity rate. FOBT is cheap and performs very well in cost effectiveness analyses evaluating the cost of detecting one cancer. This is quite a rare situation where mortality reduction can be achieved with a simple rather than a sophisticated technology. Research to further enhance the cancer detection capabilities of FOBT through the incorporation of molecular testing of the stool for tumor genes is underway. Multiple policymakers are already recommending this procedure for routine screening of average risk population. Taking their recommendations into action is of major importance.

Trial Evidence

Three randomized controlled trials have been conducted over the last 30 years to evaluate the contribution of periodic screening with fecal occult blood tests (FOBT) to the reduction in mortality of colorectal cancer in the studied population. The studies were conducted in the United States, England, and Denmark by three independent research teams.

United States: Minnesota Colon Cancer Control Study

During 1976–1977, this study [1] recruited 46,551 participants, 50–80 years of age, to one of three arms: annual FOBT, biennial FOBT, and no FOBT. The FOBT used was Hemoccult II. The test was analyzed after rehydration, a procedure shown to increase sensitivity but decreases specificity [2]. The test sensitivity for cancer detection was estimated at about 90% [3]. After 13 years, a significantly lower cumulative mortality per 1,000 from colorectal cancer was found among the annually screened group (5.88 vs. 8.83) [1]. After 18 years, the biennial group had also shown a significant 21% decrease in colorectal cancer mortality rate compared to the control group [4]. It was estimated that 75%–84% of the mortality reduction effect was due to the FOBT screening and not due to chance [5]. In addition, FOBT, either annual or biennial, was found to significantly reduce incidence of cancer by about 20% [6].

UK: Nottingham Study

Between 1981 and 1991 this study [7] recruited 152,850 people, aged 45–74 years, to one of two arms: biennial screening or no screening. Hemoccult II tests were not rehydrated in this study. About 60% of the screening group actually performed the test at least once, while 38.2% completed all offered test rounds. After a median follow-up period of 7.8 years, a significant mortality reduction of 15% (CI=0.74–0.98) was registered [7].

Denmark: Funen Study

In 1985, this study [8] recruited 62,000 people, aged 45–75 years, who were randomized to biennial Hemoccult II (nonrehydrated) or no screening. Five screening rounds were performed over a 10-year period. In total, 67% of the screening group performed at least one test. After 10 years, colorectal cancer mortality was significantly reduced by 18% (CI=1%–32%) [8]. After 14 years and seven screening rounds, colorectal cancer mortality was further reduced by 30% compared to the controls [9].

These highly consistent data from the three trials show strong evidence of a significant reduction in mortality with biennial as well as annual testing after 8–18 years of follow-up. The effect of biennial tests took more follow-up time and more screening rounds to be expressed. A significant primary prevention effect through reduction of colorectal cancer incidence was also reported.

Practice

While studies are usually conducted in an expert environment and under strict quality standards, moving a technology from the research field into routine practice can influence its performance.

When FOBT tests were first shown to have a potentially positive effect on colon cancer detection, the largest HMO-type organization in Israel (Clalit Health Services, CHS) decided to initiate an early detection pilot activity. This was done to study the field performance and yield of this technology in the general asymptomatic population. Crucial to the success of a population-based screening program are high-quality detection and good population compliance levels. Hemoccult Sensa (SKD Inc.) was offered to all CHS insurees, aged 50–74, through their primary care clinics. Hemoccult Sensa is a newer FOBT product developed to increase sensitivity of the test, avoiding the need for rehydration employed in one of the RCTs. In a comparative study of a variety of FOBT kits, Hemoccult Sensa was found to have a better sensitivity than the regular Hemoccult I or II tests, either rehydrated or not [10]. The test kits were provided to participants with written instructions. Two technicians read all cards. Positive tests were reported back to the primary care physicians and were followed up by the National Cancer Control Center for appropriate clinical evaluation.

A total of 45,166 tests were performed in the National Cancer Control Center of CHS. Of these, 22,193 tests were first tests and 23,088 were repeated screens. Seventy-eight cancers, 60 adenomas, and 163 polyps were diagnosed in the studied population [11].

This screening program has managed to maintain a low positivity rate, with 4.7% of the first round tests positive in one or more of the six test windows. This is compared with similar positivity rates in the RCTs using nonrehydrated Hemoccult II tests and is better than the reported rate of the rehydrated Hemoccult II. Low positivity rate is of utmost importance for population screening activities, as it is an indicator of the extent of the burden on the medical system that results from unnecessary tests and the burden of false positive results on the patient.

The detection rate for colorectal cancer in the first round was 2.61/1,000. The sensitivity and specificity of the test in the prevalence round were 85.3% and 95.5%, leading to a positive predictive value of 5.5% for cancer and 26.6% for all tumors (Table 1). The highest sensitivity was in the left colon (87.9%), also in line with findings of the RCTS (Table 2).

In the prevalence round more than 60% of the screen-detected tumors were in situ or Dukes stages A and B. Stage distribution was far improved in the repeated (incidence) rounds of the screening with only 40% of the tumors detected at stages Dukes B or higher (Table 3). Detection of a high proportion of potentially curable tumors marks a potential positive effect on mortality reduction in the future.

Table 1. Detection utilities (and 95% CI) of fecal occult blood test in a screening set-up

Round	Specificity	Sensitivity[a]	PPV cancer	PPV tumor[b]
Prevalence (n=22,193)	95.5 (90.6–100.0)	85.3 (76.9–93.7)	5.5 (0.0–11.0)	26.6 (20.2–32.9)
Incidence (n=10,780)	96.6 (86.7–100)	69.2 (62.3–94.3)	2.4 (0.0–10.7)	19.0 (7.5–30.4)

PPV, positive predictive value.
[a] Sensitivity based on a median follow-up period of 35 months for round 1, 25 months for round 2.
[b] Cancer, adenoma, polyp.

Table 2. Location in colon of prevalence round colorectal cancers

Location	Screen-detected	Screen-missed	Sensitivity
Right and transverse colon	11 (21.6%)	3 (30%)	78.6%
Left and sigmoid colon	29 (56.9%)	4 (40%)	87.9%
Rectum	11 (21.6%)	3 (30%)	78.6%

Table 3. Stage distribution of screen-detected colorectal cancers in prevalence and incidence rounds

Stage at diagnosis	Prevalence round	Incidence rounds
In situ	7 (13.0%)	2 (11.8%)
A	17 (31.5%)	8 (47.1%)
B	10 (18.5%)	4 (23.5%)
C	15 (27.8%)	2 (11.8%)
D	5 (9.3%)	1 (5.9%)
Unknown	4	0

The results of this program show that it is possible to achieve a high detection rate in a well-organized community set-up. The detection rate of 2.6/1,000 in the prevalence round was, as expected, about 1.5 times higher than the incidence rate reported by the Israel Cancer Registry for this age group [11].

Our population-based screening program managed to achieve, in addition to a high detection rate, a shift in tumor stage towards smaller tumors, a low positivity rate, and an acceptable false positivity rate.

Discussion

Public health theory calls for screening tests to be employed only if they comply with certain requirements. Tests need to have good detection qualities, i.e., be relatively sensitive and specific, need to be shown in randomized controlled trials to be effective in reducing mortality from the disease, need to be acceptable to the population and need to be feasible and affordable to the health system. Fecal occult blood tests of the newer generations are exhibiting sensitivity rates of 80%–90% for cancer and specificity rates of 95% or more.

Sensitivity and specificity figures of the same magnitude are the current practice with mammography screening for breast cancer, for example. FOB tests have been shown in three independent randomized controlled trials to achieve a significant and meaningful mortality reduction of colorectal cancer. While requiring the handling of feces, these noninvasive tests are decently acceptable as shown in the high adherence rates achieved in the trials. The achieved adherence rate of 70% is the same level currently achieved with mammography screening in most countries. FOBT is cheap and performs very well in cost effectiveness analyses evaluating the cost of detecting one cancer [12, 13]. Manpower requirements for the performance of these tests on a national level are quite small, including the need for endoscopic evaluation of only a small fraction (<5%) of positive cases, which makes the test reasonably feasible. This is quite a rare situation, where mortality reduction can be achieved with a simple rather than a sophisticated technology. Additional effort is needed to achieve the means of further enhancing the cancer detection capabilities of FOBT. This can possibly be achieved by incorporating molecular testing of the stool for tumor genes. Such efforts are currently underway [14–17]. These molecular tests will probably enable a better detection of premalignant lesions, which are currently detected less often by FOBT than by endoscopy. The detection of premalignant lesions, currently achieved by endoscopy or virtual endoscopy, has the merit of contributing to primary prevention of colorectal cancer and presents a relative advantage over the mere early detection of tumors. These technologies, however, are invasive and many times unpleasant. They are also very expensive to be employed for average risk population screening while achieving high compliance rates. Current evidence clearly supports the incorporation of FOBT in national cancer control policies of Western countries for routine screening of the population at ages 45–80, for which evidence exists. It is, at the same time, important to evaluate the possible contribution of additional technologies to the further reduction of colorectal cancer mortality. Policies in support of FOBT screening have recently been issued by the U.S. Centers for Disease Control [18], the European Group for Colorectal Cancer Screening [19], U.S. Preventive Services Task Force [20], the Canadian Task Force [21] and the United Kingdom National Health Service [22].

References

1. Mandel JS, Bond JH, Church TR, Snover DC, Bradley GM, Schuman LM, Ederer F (1993) Reducing mortality from colorectal cancer by screening for faecal occult blood. N Engl J Med 328: 1365–1371
2. Mandel JS, Bond JH, Bradley M, Snover DC, Church TR, Williams S, Watt G, Schuman M, Ederer F, Gilbertsen V (1989) Sensitivity, specificity, and positive predictivity of the Hemoccult test in screening for colorectal cancers. The University of Minnesota's Colon Cancer Control Study. Gastroenterology 97:597–600
3. Church TR, Ederer F, Mandel JS (1997) Fecal occult blood screening in the Minnesota study: sensitivity of the screening test. J Natl Cancer Inst 89:1440–1448

4. Mandel JS, Church TR, Ederer F, Bond JH (1999) Colorectal cancer mortality: effectiveness of biennial screening for fecal occult blood. J Natl Cancer Inst 91:434–437
5. Ederer F, Church TR, Mandel JS (1997) Fecal occult blood screening in the Minnesota study: role of chance detection of lesions. J Natl Cancer Inst 89:1423–1428
6. Mandel JS, Church TR, Bond JH, Ederer F, Geisser MS, Mongin SJ, Snover DC, Schuman LM (2000) The effect of fecal occult-blood screening on the incidence of colorectal cancer. N Engl J Med 343:1603–1607
7. Hardcastle JD, Chamberlain JO, Robinson MHE, Moss SM, Amar SS, Balfour TW, James PD, Mangham CM (1996) Randomised controlled trial of faecal occult blood screening for colorectal cancer. Lancet 348:1472–1477
8. Kronborg O, Fenger C, Olsen J, Jorgensen OD, Sondergaard O (1996) Randomised study of screening for colorectal cancer with faecal occult blood test. Lancet 348:1467–1471
9. Jorgensen OD, Kronborg O, Fenger C (2002) A randomized study of screening for colorectal cancer using faecal occult blood testing: results after 13 years and seven biennial screening rounds. Gut 50:29–32
10. St John DJ, Young GP, Alexeyeff MA, Deacon MC, Cuthbertson AM, Macrae FA, Penfold JC (1993) Evaluation of new occult blood tests for detection of colorectal neoplasia. Gastroenterology 104:1661–1668
11. Rennert G, Rennert HS, Miron E, Peterburg Y (2001) Population colorectal cancer screening with fecal occult blood test. Cancer Epidemiol Biomarkers Prev 10:1165–1168
12. Cost effectiveness of colorectal cancer screening (1999) In: Conseil d'evaluation des technologies de la sante du Quebec. CETS, Montreal
13. Whynes DK, Neilson AR, Walker AR, Hardcastle JD (1998) Faecal occult blood screening for colorectal cancer: is it cost effective? Health Econ 7:21–29
14. Traverso G, Shuber A, Olsson L, Levn B, Johnson C, Hamilton SR, Boynton K, Kinzler KW, Vogelstein B (2002) Detection of proximal colorectal cancers through analysis of faecal DNA. Lancet 359:403–404
15. Lev Z, Kislitsin D, Rennert G, Lerner A (2000) Utilization of K-ras mutations identified in stool DNA for the early detection of colorectal cancer. J Cell Biochem Suppl 34:35–39
16. Traverso G, Shuber A, Levin B, Johnson C, Olsson L, Schoetz DJ Jr, Hamilton SR, Boynton K, Kinzler KW, Vogelstein B (2002) Detection of *APC* mutations in fecal DNA from patients with colorectal tumors. N Engl J Med 346:311–320
17. Ahlquist DA, Skoletsky JE, Boynton KA, Harrington JJ, Mahoney DW, Pierceall WE, Thibodeau SN, Shuber AP (2000) Colorectal cancer screening by detection of altered human DNA in stool: feasibility of a multitarget assay panel. Gastroenterology 119:1219–1227
18. CDC (1999) Screening for colorectal cancer – United States, 1997. MMWR Morb Mortal Wkly Rep 48:116–121
19. The European Group for Colorectal Cancer Screening (1999) Recommendation to include colorectal cancer screening in public health policy. J Med Screen 6:80–81
20. Guide to clinical preventive services (1996) Report of the U.S. Preventive Services Task Force, 2nd edn. Williams & Wilkins, Baltimore, pp 89–103
21. The Canadian Task Force on the Periodic Health Examination Preventive Health Care, 2001 Update: Colorectal cancer screening (2001) CMAJ 65:206–207
22. UK National Health Service. UK National Screening Committee. Second Report

Is FOB Screening Really the Answer for Lowering Mortality in Colorectal Cancer?

Philippe Autier, Peter Boyle, Marc Buyse, Harry Bleiberg

P. Autier (✉)
Centre for Research in Epidemiology (CRESIS),
Luxembourg Health Institute, Luxembourg, Luxembourg

Abstract

In the three trials that tested screening with biennial fecal occult blood test (FOBT), follow-up of control patients for colorectal cancer (CRC) differed: in the Minnesota (United States) trial, the follow-up was equivalent to patients in the intervention groups, while in the Nottingham (United Kingdom) and Funen (Denmark) trials, control patients just received usual care. In the two latter trials, mortality from colorectal cancer was lower in subjects with interval colorectal cancer than in control subjects, while in the Minnesota trial, survival was equivalent in patients with interval CRC and in control patients. We examined whether better disease awareness of subjects allocated to the intervention group contributed to changes in colorectal cancer mortality observed in the FOBT trials. In the Nottingham and Funen trials, we evaluated the amount of colorectal cancer mortality reduction attributable to better survival of subjects in whom an interval colorectal cancer developed. In the Minnesota trial, we examined whether earlier detection of colorectal cancer in control subjects could explain the small (6%) reduction in colorectal cancer mortality observed with biennial FOBT. In the Nottingham and Funen trials, about one-quarter of the reduction in colorectal cancer mortality could be attributed to better awareness of patients with interval colorectal cancer. After correction for the effects of disease awareness, the absolute reduction in colorectal cancer mortality due to FOBT itself was 12% instead of 16%, and was no longer statistically significant ($P>0.05$). The results from biennial FOBT in the Minnesota trial published in 1993 would probably have been similar to those obtained in the Nottingham and Funen trials if disease awareness had not influenced the stage at diagnosis of colorectal cancers found in the control group. Better awareness of colorectal cancer contributes to the reduction of colorectal cancer mortality and should be encouraged. Because of a study design effect, the decrease in colorectal cancer mortality attributable to the FOBT itself is about 25% lower than that reported in the Nottingham and Funen trials. Therefore,

Recent Results in Cancer Research, Vol. 163
© Springer-Verlag Berlin Heidelberg 2003

recommending general population screening with biennial FOBT is still an open question.

Introduction

In most industrialized countries, colorectal cancer (CRC) is the third commonest malignancy in men and women. When surgical resection of CRC is possible, survival is largely dependent on disease stage: 5-year survival rate is 82% in patients with Dukes' A tumors, and 64%, 37%, and 4% in patients with Dukes' B, C, and D tumors, respectively (Kune et al. 1990). Given these sharp differences in prognosis according to stage at diagnosis, early detection of cancerous, or detection of precancerous lesions of the large bowel, are appealing methods for reducing CRC mortality.

Because of their ability to detect occult blood in the stools, guaiac-impregnated paper slides or immunochemical tests (i.e., the fecal occult blood tests, hereafter abbreviated "FOBT") have been proposed as methods for detecting CRC at an earlier stage. Because the test is relatively inexpensive and easy to use, in the early 1980s randomized clinical trials were mounted to test whether FOBT was capable of reducing CRC mortality.

The Minnesota trial was the first randomized trial on screening with FOBT (Mandel et al. 1993). In total, 46,551 volunteers were randomly allocated to a biennial rehydrated FOBT, an annual rehydrated FOBT, and a control group, and followed up during 13 years. The annual FOBT resulted in a 33% ($P<0.05$) decrease in CRC mortality and the biennial FOBT resulted in a nonsignificant 6% ($P>0.05$) decrease in CRC mortality.

Population screening with biennial nonrehydrated FOBT was tested in the Nottingham and Funen trials (Hardcastle et al. 1996; Kronborg et al. 1996). The Nottingham trial randomized 151,637 subjects aged 45–74 years to either FOBT screening or to the control group. The Funen trial performed a similar randomization of 61,933 subjects of the same age. Reductions in mortality from CRC achieved by these trials were statistically significant ($P<0.05$), but modest, on the order of 16%.

Should FOBT become a routine screening tool, implemented through either large-scale organized screening programs or through better reimbursement modalities? Before debating that question, it is crucial to establish whether FOBT actually succeeded in significantly reducing mortality from CRC or whether there are alternative explanations worthy of consideration, such as the biases produced by disease awareness.

Colorectal Cancer Awareness in the Nottingham and Funen Trials

In the Nottingham and Funen trials, the modest impact of FOBT on CRC mortality was mainly attributable to the poor sensitivity of the biennial FOBT. In both trials, in subjects who accepted at least one FOBT, that test detected 48%

of all CRCs while interval CRCs represented the remaining 52%. Given their numerical importance, interval CRCs could have influenced the mortality from CRC in the intervention groups, if the prognosis of subjects with interval CRC was different from that of subjects with screen-detected CRC. In earlier works on cancer screening, it was thought that for a variety of reasons, interval cancers would have a poorer prognosis than cancers diagnosed in unscreened subjects (Eddy 1980; DeGroote et al. 1983). First, these cancers could be fast growing tumors with greater malignant potential than average. Second, a negative screening test could give a false sense of security, possibly leading to the dismissal of early signs of presence of the cancer, an attitude that could delay the diagnosis. The breast cancer screening trials and the breast cancer screening programs implemented outside the context of randomized trials showed that the survival of women with interval breast cancer was about the same as that of control women (Shapiro et al. 1982; Holmberg et al. 1986) or of women not participating in mammographic screening (Brekelmans et al. 1995; Burrell et al, 1996; Yoshida et al. 1990; Peeters et al. 1989).

In the Nottingham trial, subjects with interval CRC had CRC-specific survival as good as the entire intervention group (Fig. 2 of the published report – Hardcastle et al. 1996), and in the Funen trial, subjects with interval CRC had CRC-specific survival intermediate between the control group and the entire intervention group (Fig. 3 of the published report – Kronborg et al. 1996). Why such a discrepancy between the CRC-specific survival observed in these two trials and earlier works on cancer screening or the observations done in breast cancer screening? Of all potential explanations, it seems worthwhile to consider that a fraction of the lower mortality among subjects with interval CRC could be due to an increased level of awareness of CRC. Physicians and perhaps many screened subjects knew they were part of a study. This was not the case for control subjects who were not told about the study and continued to use health care facilities as usual. Furthermore, most physicians involved in the study were aware of the likelihood of interval cancers with a test known for its low sensitivity. Therefore, it is probable that among screened subjects, more attention was paid to early symptoms of the eventual presence of interval CRC, prompting more precocious diagnosis of malignant lesions. Data from the two trials support this hypothesis (Table 1); the stage distribution of interval CRCs was intermediary between screen-detected CRCs and CRCs diagnosed in nonresponders. The most salient feature was that Dukes' A tumors were more frequent in subjects with interval CRCs than among nonresponders or controls who developed the disease. Given that 52% of CRCs in subjects who had at least one FOBT were interval cancers, it could well be that part of the reduction in mortality from CRC observed in the intervention group was not directly attributable to the efficacy of the FOBT itself, but to a difference in CRC awareness of both screened subjects and physicians, as compared to control subjects.

Table 1. Dukes' A colorectal cancers (CRCs) in the Nottingham and Funen trials

	Origins of colorectal cancers in screening group				Controls
	Subjects with ≥1 screening test			Nonresponders[a]	
	Total	Screen detected	Interval		
Nottingham trial (Hardcastle et al. 1996)					
Number of subjects	75,253	44,838		30,415	74,998
All CRCs	885	236	249	400	836
Number (%) Dukes' A	178 (20)	97 (41)	39 (16)	42 (11)	95 (11)
Dukes' B	286 (32)	71 (30)	76 (31)	139 (35)	285 (33)
Dukes' C	211 (24)	51 (22)	71 (29)	89 (22)	264 (31)
Dukes' D	191 (22)	13 (6)	61 (22)	117 (29)	179 (21)
Not known	19 (2)	4 (2)	2 (1)	13 (3)	33 (4)
P value*	<0.0001	<0.0001	0.07	0.65	—
P value**	0.0001	<0.0001	0.81	0.15	—
Funen trial (Kronborg et al. 1996)					
Number of subjects	30,967	20,672		10,295	30,966
All CRCs	481	138	148	195	483
Number (%) Dukes' A	105 (22)	53 (38)	31 (21)	21 (11)	54 (11)
Dukes' B	164 (34)	52 (38)	46 (31)	66 (34)	177 (37)
Dukes' C	90 (19)	20 (14)	35 (24)	35 (18)	111 (23)
Dukes' D	98 (20)	11 (8)	27 (18)	60 (31)	114 (24)
Not known	24 (5)	2 (1)	9 (6)	13 (7)	27 (6)
P value*	<0.0001	<0.0001	0.002	0.88	—
P value**	0.001	<0.0001	0.03	0.21	—

[a] Subjects allocated to the screening group but who were never screened with the fecal occult blood test.
* χ^2 Test for percentage of Dukes' A CRCs compared with controls.
** χ^2 Test for trend comparing Dukes' distribution with controls.

Correcting for the Colorectal Cancer Awareness Bias

In order to assess the true impact of FOBT on mortality from CRC, results of these trials must be corrected by removing the bias introduced by the CRC awareness. The most direct strategy would consist of applying to the interval CRCs the case-fatality rate observed in controls who developed a CRC, i.e., 49% [100 (420/856)] in the Nottingham trial and 52% [100 (249/483)] in the Funen trial (Table 2). The resultant would have allowed estimating the CRC mortality in subjects with interval CRC if disease awareness had not been present. Unfortunately, the published articles did not report the number of deaths due to CRC that occurred in subjects with screen-detected or interval CRC, or in subjects who refused screening.

However, the CRC-specific survival rates at study end reflect the CRC death rates during the study. Using the published CRC-specific survival curves, it was possible to estimate the CRC-specific survival rate at study end of subjects with screen-detected or interval CRCs, or in subjects who refused screening (Table 2). In the absence of screening, the expected CRC-specific survival rate would have been the one observed in the control groups, and thus, the gain in survival rate can be calculated as the difference between survival rates in the intervention and the control group. For estimating what proportion of the gain in survival observed in the intervention groups was attributable to the better survival of interval CRCs, the gain in survival rate in the interval CRCs was divided by the gain in survival in both the screen-detected and the interval CRCs (fourth column of Table 2). The formula used in the fourth column of the Table 2 assumes that the number of screen-detected equals the number of interval CRCs. Hence, the ratio (interval/screen-detected CRCs) was necessary to adjust for the differences in the numbers of screen-detected and of interval CRCs. Finally, the number of CRC deaths that did not occur in the intervention groups because the interval CRCs tended to be detected earlier than the CRCs in the control groups could be calculated as the difference in CRC deaths between the intervention and the control groups times the proportion of the gain in CRC-specific survival rate attributable to the interval CRCs, adjusted for the differences in the number of screen-detected and interval CRCs.

Correcting for the observation bias yielded corrected mortality ratios of 0.89 in the Nottingham trial, and 0.86 in the Funen trial, which were no longer statistically significant (i.e., $P>0.05$). Also, the absolute reduction in CRC mortality to be expected from the FOBT itself became smaller than that reported in the published articles, around 12% instead of around 16%.

Colorectal Cancer Awareness in the Minnesota Study

In the biennial screening group of the Minnesota trial, 61% of CRCs were not detected by the FOBT (Fig. 4 of Mandel et al. 1993). Since 90% of volunteers completed at least one screening, most of these CRCs were interval cancers. In

Table 2. Reported efficacy of Nottingham and Funen trials with fecal occult blood test and correction for disease awareness bias

	Number of CRCs	Deaths from CRC	% CRC-specific survival probability at study end[a]	% of gain in CRC-specific survival from interval cancers	Ratio interval/ screen-detected CRCs	Avoided deaths due to better disease awareness	Corrected number of deaths from CRC
Nottingham trial (Hardcastle et al. 1996)							
Intervention group (n=75,253)							
Total	885	360	48%	100*(48−38)	(249/236)=1.06	(420−360)* 0.23*1.06≡ 15	375
Screen-detected	236	na	71%				
Interval	249	na	48%	(48−38) + (71−38)=23%			
Nonresponders	400	na	32%				
Control group (n=74,998)	856	420	38%				420
Relative risk (95% CI)		0.85 (0.74−0.98)[b]					0.89 (0.77−1.02)[c]
Funen trial (Kronborg et al. 1996)							
Intervention group (n=30 967)							
Total	481	205	46%	100*(40−32)	(148/138)=1.07	(249−205)* 0.17*1.07≡ 8	213
Screen-detected	138	na	70%				
Interval	148	na	40%	(40−32)+(70−32)=17%			
Nonresponders	195	na	28%				
Control group (n=30,966)	483	249	32%				249
Relative risk (95% CI)		0.82 (0.68−0.99)[b]					0.86 (0.72−1.03)[c]

CRC, colorectal cancer; na, data not reported in publication.
[a]Estimated from published CRC-specific survival figures; study end is 14 years in the Nottingham trial and 10 years in the Funen trial.
[b]P<0.05; [c]P=0.10.

Table 3. Survival of control subjects with colorectal cancer in the fecal occult blood test trials

| | Study duration (years) | Age at entry | % Survival probability of[a] | | | % Dukes' A |
			Screen-detected CRCs	Interval CRCs	Controls with CRC	CRCs in controls
Minnesota trial[b]	13	50–80	71%	58%	59%	22%
Nottingham trial[c]	14	45–75	71%	48%	38%	11%
Funen trial[d]	10	45–75	70%	40%	32%	11%

[a] Survival probability for the entire study duration.
[b] Data from Figs. 4 (biennial screening) and 5 of Mandel et al. 1993.
[c] Data from Table 4 and Fig. 2 of Hardcastle et al. 1996.
[d] Data from Table 4 and Fig. 3 of Kronborg et al. 1996.

contrast to the Nottingham and Funen trials, in the Minnesota study, survival was similar for interval CRCs and for CRCs diagnosed among control subjects (Table 3). Although patients were somewhat older in the Minnesota study, mortality among control subjects with CRC was lower: Dukes' A CRCs were twice more frequent in the Minnesota control group than in the Nottingham and Funen control groups. Interestingly, there was virtually no difference in survival among screen-detected cancers between the three trials.

These contrasts may find an explanation in differences in the way control subjects were managed: in the Minnesota trial, similarly to subjects allocated to the two intervention arms, control subjects were contacted annually about their vital status or about eventual diagnosis of CRC or colonic adenoma. In the Nottingham and Funen trials, control subjects were not told they had participated in a human experiment and continued to use health care services as usual. Thus, in the Minnesota trial, it is not impossible that better attention to gastrointestinal symptoms given to all subjects, regardless of the randomization arm, led to earlier detection of most CRCs, which resulted in lower mortality from CRC. As a consequence, control subjects with CRC finally resembled subjects of the intervention arm who developed an interval CRC. It is tempting to hypothesize that in the Minnesota study, if the control group had been managed as a "usual care group" without any particular follow-up after randomization, results in the biennial screening arm could have been similar to those obtained by the Nottingham and Funen trials, and could have been more impressive in the annual screening arm.

Discussion

Our reassessment of the FOBT trials suggests that in the Nottingham and Funen trials, about three-quarters of the reduction in CRC mortality was attributable to the FOBT itself, and the remaining quarter was attributable to better CRC awareness. Hence, the reduction in colorectal cancer mortality attributable to the FOBT itself is lower than that reported in the published reports. Therefore, there is a need to critically review all available data before proposing the biennial nonrehydrated FOBT for general population screening.

In the Minnesota trial, CRC awareness has probably concealed a part of the impact of rehydrated FOBT itself on CRC mortality. In that respect, results from that trial were probably better than initially reported by Mandel and coworkers (1993). However, the question remains as to whether the results obtained with the annual screening with rehydrated FOBT are applicable to general population surveillance, since the acceptability of the numerous complete bowel examinations induced by the high proportion of falsely positive tests is not guaranteed (Hardcastle et al. 1996; Simon 1998).

A general decline in CRC mortality is noticeable since the 1950s and 60s in the United Kingdom, Germany, France, the United States and Canada (CCS 1997; Chu et al. 1994; Coleman et al. 1993). The etiology of the decline is multifactorial, with contributions from changes in dietary patterns, occasional removal of polyps, earlier diagnosis, and improved management of CRC. It is difficult to know which of these factors accounts for what proportion of the observed decline in mortality, but increasing awareness of colorectal cancer among lay public and health professionals has probably contributed to the reinforcement of each of these aspects. Changes in CRC awareness are witnessed by reports consistently showing a time-trend towards higher proportions of Dukes' A CRCs at diagnosis (Robinson et al. 1993; Clarke et al. 1992; Cappel and Goldberg 1992; Ohman 1982; Lea et al. 1982). Our reassessment of the FOBT trials further supports the view that better CRC awareness may contribute to reduce CRC mortality. CRC awareness should thus be encouraged in the medical community and in the general population.

In the context of clinical trials, however, better disease awareness may distort the true relationship between a screening method and the disease-specific mortality it is supposed to reduce. It should therefore be considered an "observation bias." A key question is to know whether there is a need to dissect out the respective influence of the screening method itself and of better disease awareness on the study results, and not just consider the bias introduced by better disease awareness as being an inherent part of the screening process.

The evaluation of the efficacy of a screening test in a randomized trial should not be influenced by factors depending on the trial design, such as the modalities of follow-up of subjects according to their allocation in the intervention or in the control group: the differences in the way control subjects were followed up resulted in an increase in the apparent impact of FOBT screening in the Nottingham and Funen trials, as compared to a reduction in the apparent impact of FOBT screening in the Minnesota trial. Also, better disease awareness is likely to vary according to the cultural and medical background of settings where studies on screening efficiency are implemented. Such difference in trial design may render difficult the comparison of results between studies testing the same screening method.

Secondly, it is not sure whether the degree of CRC awareness observed in the FOBT trials will be retrieved in the routine medical practice. Thirdly, the disease awareness bias may be present even when a screening tool without efficacy is used, possibly leading to the wrong conclusion that the tool is somewhat efficient.

Disease awareness bias is expected to occur in any situation where physicians know which of their patients are part of a randomized clinical trial and to which randomization arm they were allocated to. Patients may also know they are part of a randomized trial. As a consequence, physicians and patients may have a different attitude towards the health problem under study. In clinical trials testing new drugs, to overcome observation biases, it is common practice to keep both patients and study endpoint assessors ignorant of the study arm to which a patient has been allocated to (i.e., the "double blind" randomized trial). If endpoint assessors are not blinded for the randomization status, they may provide different levels of attention to patients receiving or not receiving the tested drug. Failure to implement blinding procedures may contribute to invalidating the conclusions of a trial. Unfortunately, in most trials testing screening methods, it is impossible to implement the blinding procedures used in trials testing new drugs. Therefore, evaluating how disease awareness may have influenced results may improve the critical analysis of studies testing screening methods.

Acknowledgements. This study was conducted within the framework of support from the Associazione Italiana per la Ricerca sul Cancro.

References

Brekelmans CT, Peeters PH, Deurenberg JJ, Collette HJ (1995) Survival in interval breast cancer in the DOM screening programme. Eur J Cancer 31A:1830–1835

Burrell HC, Sibbering DM, Wilson AR, et al (1996) Screening interval breast cancers: mammographic features and prognosis factors. Radiology 199:811–817

Cappel MS, Goldberg ES (1992) The relationship between the clinical presentation and spread of colon cancer in 315 consecutive patients. A significant trend of earlier cancer detection from 1982 through 1988 at a university hospital. J Clin Gastroenterol 14:227–235

CCC Canadian Cancer Society (1997) Canadian cancer statistiques, 1997. Toronto

Chu KC, Tarone RE, Chow W, Hankey BF, Reis LAG (1994) Temporal patterns in colorectal cancer incidence, survival and mortality from 1950 through 1990. J Nat Cancer Inst 86:997–1006

Clarke PJ, Dehn TC, Kettlewell MG. Changing patterns of colorectal cancer in a regional teaching hospital (1992) Ann R Coll Surg Engl 74:291–293

Coleman MP, Esteve J, Dameicki P, Arslan A, Renard H (1993) Trends in cancer incidence and mortality. International Agency for Research on Cancer. IARC Scientific Publications No 121, Lyon

DeGroote R, Rush BF Jr, Milazzo J, Warden MJ, Rocko JM (1983) Interval breast cancer: a more aggressive subset of breast neoplasia. Surgery 94:543–547

Eddy DM (1980) Screening for cancer: theory, analysis and design. Prentice-Hall, Englewood Cliffs, New Jersey

Hardcastle JD, Chamberlain JO, Robinson MHE, et al (1996) Randomised controlled trial of faecal-occult-blood screening for colorectal cancer. Lancet 348:1472–1477

Holmberg LH, Tabar L, Adami O, Bergström R (1986) Survival in breast cancer diagnosed between mammographic screening examinations. Lancet 2:27–30

Kronborg O, Fenger K, Olsen J, Jorgensen OD, Sondergaard O (1996) Randomised study of screening for colorectal cancer with faecal-occult-blood test. Lancet 348:1467–1471

Kune GA, Kune S, Fields B, White R, Brough W, Schellemberg R, Watson LF (1990) Survival in patients with large-bowel cancer. Dis Colon Rectum 33:938–946

Lea JW 4th, Covington K, McSwain B, Scott HW Jr (1982) Surgical experience with carcinoma of the colon and rectum. Ann Surg 195:600–607

Mandel JS, Bond JH, Church TR, et al (1993) Reducing mortality from colorectal cancer by screening for fecal occult blood. New Eng J Med 328:365–371

Ohman U (1982) Colorectal carcinoma: trends and results over a 30-year period. Dis Colon Rectum 25:431–440

Peeters PH, Verbeek AL, Hendriks JH, Holland R, Mravunac M, Vooijs GP (1989) The occurrence of interval cancers in the Nijmegen screening programme. Br J Cancer 59:929–932

Robinson MH, Thomas WM, Hardcastle JD, Chamberlain J, Mangham CM (1993) Change towards earlier stage at presentation of colorectal cancer. Br J Surg 80:1610–1612

Shapiro S, Venet W, Strax P, Venet L, Roeser R (1982) Ten to fourteen year effect of screening on breast cancer mortality. J Nat Cancer Inst 69:349–355

Simon JB. Should all people over the age of 50 have regular fecal occult-blood tests? (1998) New Eng J Med 338:1151–1152

Yoshida K, Abe R, Taguchi, et al (1990) Comparisons of interval cancers with other breast cancers detected through mass screening and in outpatients clinics in Japan. Japan J Clin Oncol 20:374–379

Summary and Conclusions

Rudolf Morant

R. Morant (✉)
Center for Tumor Detection and Prevention, Rorschacherstr. 150,
9006 St. Gallen, Switzerland

Tumor prevention is gathering momentum, and conferences such as this one help to provide new insights, crossfertilize laboratory and clinical research projects, and acquaint participants with the people leading the field. This 3-day conference, the second in St. Gallen, attracted 270 participants from 30 countries. The conference was cosponsored by the International Society of Cancer Chemoprevention (President: F. Meysken, Irvine, United States), the European School of Oncology (Director: A. Costa, Pavia, Italy) and by the local host, St. Gallen Oncology Conferences, represented by H.J. Senn and R. Morant (St. Gallen, Switzerland).

The participants represented various backgrounds ranging from basic scientists and geneticists to clinical urologists, gynecologists, medical oncologists, surgeons, and epidemiologists, offering an opportunity for interesting interactions and discussions necessary to advance this field and to broaden clinical applications.

The topics covered the search for and the assessment of new cancer susceptibility genes and preclinical models of cancer chemoprevention. A more detailed discussion involved clinical chemoprevention and screening efforts of skin tumors, breast cancer, prostate cancer, and colorectal carcinomas.

Breast Cancer

D.L. Wickerham (NSABP, Pittsburgh, United States) discussed the current large STAR trial. This randomized study compares tamoxifen to raloxifene in the prevention of breast cancer in high-risk women and has already randomized more than 12,000 women (target: 22,000). He noticed that the findings of the NSABP-P1 study, which showed a significant reduction of breast cancer incidence by nearly 50% with tamoxifen prevention [1], were not yet widely incorporated into clinical practice. Many practitioners are apparently reluctant to prescribe a drug with potential serious side effects, such as thromboembolic events and endometrial carcinoma, for prevention, especially as

Recent Results in Cancer Research, Vol. 163
© Springer-Verlag Berlin Heidelberg 2003

other trials with similar designs in Europe have been negative so far. T. Powles (Royal Marsden Hospital, London, United Kingdom) warned that there were no data yet to prove the efficacy of tamoxifen in the subgroup of women with high-penetrance breast cancer predisposing gene mutations. J. Cuzick (Imperial Cancer Research Fund, London, United Kingdom) discussed the planned IBIS-2 trial, which will study the very promising drug anastrozole. This aromatase inhibitor has been recently proven superior to tamoxifen in the adjuvant setting (ATAC trial) [2].

A very lively discussion, moderated by M. Osborne (Strang Cancer Prevention Center, New York, United States) and J. Cuzick, about the value of mammography screening highlighted controversial views by the epidemiologist A. Miller (Deutsches Krebsforschungszentrum Heidelberg, Germany) and the radiologist S. Feig (Mount Sinai Medical Center, New York, United States).A public controversy had been initiated by two similar *Lancet* papers (2000, 2001) by Gotzsche and Olsen [3, 4]. The discussion centered around whether it was justified to disregard the positive results of some older studies because of minor methodological flaws. The vast majority of active researchers in the field, however, continue to support mammography screening. This view is also supported by many professional organizations and Cancer Leagues. This scientific controversy, propagated by many media releases to the general public, however, has delayed the introduction of state screening programs in some countries, such as Switzerland, and has discredited one of the few screening methods with a proven survival benefit to a significant minority of the lay public.

G. Rennert (National Breast Cancer Screening Program, Haifa, Israel) discussed the political dimensions and influences on screening programs, e.g., the fact that the United States Congress forced the National Cancer Institute to recommend mammography screening starting at the age of 40 years (instead of 50 years as in most other countries), contradictory to the conclusions of its scientific committee.

Prostate Cancer

E. Klein (Cleveland Clinic, United States), chairman of the current SELECT trial, discussed the chemoprevention of prostate cancer with selenium and/or vitamin E. Results of this large randomized United States trial, initiated by the SWOG (South West Oncology Group), are not to be expected before the year 2013. G. Bartsch (Innsbruck, Austria) reported a significant drop in mortality from prostate cancer following the introduction of PSA mass screening at no cost in 1993 in the federal state of Tyrol and gave an update of the screening results among men aged 45–75 years. H.P. Schmid (Kantonsspital St. Gallen, Switzerland), advised against introducing mass screening of PSA until the data from the large randomized trials in Europe (European Randomized Study of Screening for Prostate Cancer, ERSPC) and America (Prostate, Lung, Colon and Ovary Cancer Screening Project, PLCO) are available.

Colorectal Carcinomas

The session involved a very insightful presentation of its epidemiology (P. Boyle, Istituto Europeo di Oncologia, Milano, Italy), followed by a review of genetics (HJ Müller, Basle University, Switzerland) and possible approaches to chemoprevention based on laboratory findings (M. Lipkin, Strang Cancer Prevention Center, New York, United States). The influence of diet, especially the Mediterranean diet, was discussed with respect to epidemiological data. Potential preventive methods using selective Cox-2 inhibitors, supplementation of calcium and folic acid were reviewed. G. Rennert (National Cancer Control Center, Haifa, Israel) reported the encouraging results of a well-organized screening program testing for fecal occult blood (FOB) in Israel. Stool samples were sent by mail to over 2,000 participating primary care physicians. He stressed that centralized testing for traces of hemoglobin in stool samples by experienced technicians and standardized conditions were essential for the success of this screening method. This low-technology, cost-effective method has been shown to lower mortality rates from colorectal cancer in several randomized trials by 15%–30% [6]. An alternative method of screening was presented by J. Cuzick with the current mass screening trial using flexible sigmoidoscopy.

Prevention is getting stronger and becoming mainstream – the future of primary cancer prevention and screening is bright and we are already looking forward to new insights that will be presented and discussed at the next conference: The Third International Conference on Tumor Prevention and Genetics is already scheduled to be held on 12–14 February 2004, again at the University of St. Gallen, Switzerland.